# The Golden Guide to Oncologic Pharmacy

Carolina Witchmichen Penteado Schmidt • Kaléu Mormino Otoni
Editors

# The Golden Guide to Oncologic Pharmacy

Springer

*Editors*
Carolina Witchmichen Penteado Schmidt
Pediatric Oncology Pharmacist & Writer, Curitiba, Paraná, Brazil

Kaléu Mormino Otoni
Jesus Maria José Maternity Hospital, Quixadá, Ceará, Brazil

Postgraduate Program in Integrated and Multidisciplinary Care for Women's and Children's Health, Federal University of Ceará, University Campus – Rectory, PICI, Fortaleza, CE, Brazil

ISBN 978-3-030-98595-0 ISBN 978-3-030-98596-7 (eBook)
https://doi.org/10.1007/978-3-030-98596-7



This Springer imprint is published by the registered company Springer Nature Switzerland AG
The registered company address is: Gewerbestrasse 11, 6330 Cham, Switzerland

# Preface

Oncology is an area of high complexity, where more and more specific knowledge is required. The time is short, the area is embracing and deep, and the books for pharmacists are few. *The Golden Guide to Oncologic Pharmacy*, edited by Carolina Witchmichen Penteado Schmidt and Kaléu Mormino Otoni, is a book by oncology pharmacists for oncology pharmacists. We, editors, have years of experience in the daily practice and teaching of oncology in postgraduate courses and publishing scientific knowledge to help professionals have the information we would like to have had when we started, and also years later, for quick search. So, we gathered a team of experienced pharmacists and other healthcare professionals who work in this area of high complexity. This book fills a gap, and it's the first one aimed at oncology pharmacists' daily practice. If you also work with pediatric patients, please check *Pediatric Oncology Pharmacy: A Complete Guide to Practice* as well.

This essential guide will support oncologic pharmacists, clinical pharmacists, and hospital pharmacists in their daily practice with every area that involves chemotherapy, such as oncology, hematology, rheumatology, stem cell transplantation, ICU, and surgery center, as well as approaches without chemotherapy for cancer, such as CAR-T cells. The essential knowledge has been gathered in this volume, being essential also for postgraduate students, residents, and even undergraduate students.

Curitiba, Brazil Carolina Witchmichen Penteado Schmidt
Quixadá, Ceará, Brazil Kaléu Mormino Otoni

# Contents

# Editors and Contributors

## About the Editors

**Carolina Witchmichen Penteado Schmidt** Author of several Springer books in pediatric oncology. Editor of the book Chemotherapy and Pharmacology for Leukemia in Pregnancy: Guidelines and Strategies for Best Practices. Pediatric Oncology Pharmacist with extensive experience in chemotherapy for children. Oncological Hospital Pharmacy specialist with experience in chemotherapy for adults. MBA in Planning and Business Management. Substantial experience at hospitals and clinics, with pharmacy, drug interactions, pediatrics, oncology, hematology, stem cell transplantation, neonatology, intensive health care and infectology. Academic experience in pharmacy, pediatrics, oncology and hematology; teaching for specialists including pharmacists, physicians and nurses. Author of numerous children's books about cancer, under the pen name Carola Schmidt, such as Chubby's Tale: The true story of a teddy bear who beat cancer, which was defined as "one of the best leukemia books of all time" by Book Authority, and Bald is Beautiful: A letter for a fabulous girl, which was featured by Crayola Education. Check out more about her work at kidscancerbooks.com

**Kaléu Mormino Otoni** Oncology pharmacist with experience at major centers of excellence for cancer treatment, e.g., AC Camargo Cancer Center and Nove de Julho Hospital. Regional representative of the Brazilian Society of Pharmacists in Oncology

(SOBRAFO) for the State of São Paulo (2018-2019). Specialist in oncology hospital pharmacy at AC Camargo Cancer Center and MBA in Health Management from the University of São Paulo (USP) and Master's student in Women's and Children's Health at the Federal University of Ceará/Brazil Experience in chemotherapy manipulation, clinical oncology pharmacy, pediatric oncology and hematology, adult oncohematology, and intensive care unit oncology. He is currently the general director of Hospital Maternity Jesus Maria José and a professor of postgraduate courses in oncology pharmacy, and he offers training for health professionals.

## Contributors

**Marcus Rafael Lobo Bezerra** Postgraduate Program in Biotechnology and Natural Resources, Federal University of Ceará, Fortaleza, Brazil

Fiocruz Ceará, Precabura, Eusébio, Brazil

**Marlize Brandão Ribeiro Cardoso** Salvador, Bahia, Brazil

**MérciaPatrícia Ferreira Conceição** Translational Research Center in Oncology, ICESP – Instituto do Câncer do Estado de São Paulo, São Paulo, Brazil

FMUSP – Faculdade de Medicina da Universidade de São Paulo, São Paulo, Brazil

**Ellen Mayara Corrêa** São Caetano do Sul, SP, Brazil

**Priscila Pinto Costa** Salvador, Bahia, Brazil

**Douglas Coutinho Ribeiro da Costa** Hospital Samaritano, João Pessoa, PB, Brazil

**Guilherme Aparecido Monteiro Duque da Fonseca** Periodontology Department, School of Dentistry, Universidade Guarulhos, São Paulo, Brazil

**Pedro Mikael da Silva Costa** Postgraduation Program in Biotecnology – RENORBIO, Laboratório de Oncologia Experimental, Núcleo de Pesquisa e Desenvolvimento de Medicamentos (NPDM), Fortaleza, CE, Brazil

**Gabriela Sandoval da Silva** Pharmacy, Hospital Israelita Albert Einstein, São Paulo, SP, Brazil

Department of Oncology Pharmacy, Albert Einstein Hospital, São Paulo, Brazil

**Samanta Oliveira da Silva** Guarulhos, SP, Brazil

**Cristiane Souza de Agostinho** Salvador, Bahia, Brazil

**Daniel Rodrigues de Bastos** Translational Research Center in Oncology, ICESP – Instituto do Câncer do Estado de São Paulo, São Paulo, Brazil

FMUSP – Faculdade de Medicina da Universidade de São Paulo, São Paulo, Brazil

**José de Brito Vieira Neto** Postgraduate Program in Pharmacology, Department of Physiology and Pharmacology, Faculty of Medicine, Federal University of Ceará, Laboratory of Experimental Oncology, Center for Research and Development of Medicines (NPDM), Fortaleza, CE, Brazil

**Celina de Jesus Guimarães** Postgraduate Program in Pharmacology, Department of Physiology and Pharmacology, Faculty of Medicine, Federal University of Ceará, Laboratory of Experimental Oncology, Center for Research and Development of Medicines (NPDM), Fortaleza, CE, Brazil

Hospital Pharmacy, Fundação Centro de Controle de Oncologia do Estado do Amazonas (FCECON-AM), Manaus, AM, Brazil

**Thais de Leles Balisa** Graduate Program in Pharmaceutical Sciences, Faculdade Unida de Campinas, Goiânia, Golas, Brazil

**Danilo de Oliveira Cerqueira** Department of Clinical Pharmacy and Oncology, HSC – Hospital São Camilo, São Paulo, Brazil

Department of Education in Pharmacy Oncology, IPESSP – Instituto de Pesquisa e Ensino em Saúde de São Paulo, São Paulo, Brazil

**Nataly Any Barros Garrido de Paula** Department of Clinical Pharmacy and Oncology, ICESP – Instituto do Câncer do Estado de São Paulo, São Paulo, Brazil

**Bruna de Sousa Lima** Fiocruz Ceará, Precabura, Eusébio, Brazil

Undergraduate Program in Pharmacy, Federal University of Ceará, Fortaleza, Brazil

**Felipe de Souza Alves** Graduate Program in Pharmaceutical Sciences, Universidade Paulista, São Paulo, Brazil

**Renan Gomes do Nascimento** Department of Clinical Pharmacy and Oncology, HSC – Hospital São Camilo, São Paulo, Brazil

Department of Education in Pharmacy Oncology, SENAC – Serviço Nacional de AprendizagemComercial, São Paulo, Brazil

Department of Education in Pharmacy Oncology, IPESSP – Instituto de Pesquisa e Ensino em Saúde de São Paulo, São Paulo, Brazil

**Amanda Nascimento dos Reis** Brazilian Society of Pharmacists in Oncology, ONCOMINAS - Instituto Sul Mineiro de Oncologia, São Paulo, Brazil

**Flávio dos Santos Silvério** Brazilian Society of Pharmacists in Oncology, Samaritano Hospital, São Paulo, Brazil

**Fred Soares dos Santos** Graduate Program in Pharmaceutical Sciences, Federal University of Golas, Goiânia, Brazil

**Sandna Larissa Freitas dos Santos** Graduate Program in Pharmaceutical Sciences, Federal University of Ceará, Fortaleza, CE, Brazil

**Giovani Marino Favero** General Biology Department, Universidade Estadual de Ponta Grossa, Parana, Brazil

**Lygia Leão Fernandes** Pharmacy, Hospital Salvalus (Grupo NotreDame Intermédica), São Paulo, SP, Brazil

**Lucio Frigo** Associação Paulista de Cirurgiões Dentistas School of Dentistry (FAOA), São Paulo, Brazil

**Gilvan Pessoa Furtado** Fiocruz Ceará, Precabura, Eusébio, Brazil

**Maria Inês Rodrigues Gato** Brazilian Society of Oncology Pharmacists (Sobrafo), São Paulo, Brazil

**Breno Magalhães Gomes** Fortaleza, Ceara, Brazil

**Anderson Cavalcante Guimarães** Chemistry Department, Exact Science Instituit, Universidade Federal do Amazonas, Manaus, AM, Brazil

**Fumiko Takahashi Ito** Brazilian Society of Pharmacists in Oncology, São Paulo, Brazil

**Flávia Mendes Leite** Salvador, Bahia, Brazil

**Kathia Ferraro Lopes** Brazilian Society of Pharmacists in Oncology, Institute Racine, São Paulo, Brazil

**Maria Liliane Luciano** Graduate Program in Pharmaceutical Sciences, Federal University of Ceará, Fortaleza, CE, Brazil

**Durvanei Augusto Maria** Molecular Biology Laboratory, Instituto Butantan, São Paulo, Brazil

**Laura Alegria Martins** Hospital de Clínicas de Porto Alegre – HCPA, Porto Alegre, Brazil

SOBRAFO (Sociedade Brasileira de Farmacêuticos em Oncologia), São Paulo, Brazil

College of Pharmacy – Universidade Federal do Rio Grande do Sul – UFRGS, Porto Alegre, Brazil

Oncology Pharmacy – Institute of Education and Research Hospital Moinhos de Vento - IEP/HMV, Porto Alegre, Brazil

Institute of Education and Research Hospital Moinhos de Vento, Porto Alegre, Brazil

**Alessandro Menegon** Clinical Pharmacist of Pharmaceutical Assistance Department, July 9th Hospital, São Paulo, São Paulo, Brazil

**Cintia Vecchies Morassi** Department of Oncology Pharmacy, Albert Einstein Hospital, São Paulo, Brazil

**Karla Bruna Nogueira Torres Mormino** Catholic University Center of Quixadá, Unicatólica, Quixadá, Ceará, Brazil

**Mariana Perez Esteves Silva Motta** Department of Oncology Pharmacy, Albert Einstein Hospital, São Paulo, Brazil

**Wanessa Ferraz Neres** Graduate Program in Pharmaceutical Sciences, Universidade Paulista de Brasilia, UNIP, Brasília, Brazil

**Sandro Luis Ribeiro Ness** Hospital de Clínicas de Porto Alegre – HCPA, Porto Alegre, Brazil

College of Medicine – Universidade Federal do Rio Grande do Sul – UFRGS, Porto Alegre, Brazil

Hospital Pharmacy and Clinical Oncology – IBRAS, Ponta Grossa, PR, Brazil

Oncology Pharmacy – Centro Universitário São Camilo, São Paulo, Brazil

SOBRAFO (Sociedade Brasileira de Farmacêuticos em Oncologia), São Paulo, Brazil

Clinical Pharmacy by SBRAFH (Sociedade Brasileira de Farmácia Hospitalar e Serviços de Saúde), São Paulo, Brazil

**Kaléu Mormino Otoni** Jesus Maria José Maternity Hospital, Quixadá, Ceará, Brazil

Postgraduate Program in Integrated and Multidisciplinary Care for Women's and Children's Health, Federal University of Ceará, University Campus – Rectory, PICI, Fortaleza, CE, Brazil

**Rafael Duarte Paes** Oncoclínicas, Sao Paulo, Brazil

**Taynna Tatiane Pereira** Pharmacy, Hospital Israelita Albert Einstein, São Paulo, SP, Brazil

**Larissa Queiroz Pontes** Postgraduate Program in Biotechnology and Natural Resources, Federal University of Ceará, Fortaleza, Brazil

Fiocruz Ceará, Precabura, Eusébio, Brazil

**Larissa Zuppardi Lacerda Sabino** Oncology and Hematology Center, Albert Einstein Hospital, São Paulo, Brazil

**Carolina Witchmichen Penteado Schmidt** Pediatric Oncology Pharmacist & Writer, Curitiba, Paraná, Brazil

**Igor Cabral Studart** Postgraduate Program in Biotechnology and Natural Resources, Federal University of Ceará, Fortaleza, Brazil

Fiocruz Ceará, Precabura, Eusébio, Brazil

**Joyce Ferreira Viana** Clínica São Germano Oncologia, São Paulo, SP, Brazil

**Hebe Mizuno Watanabe** Hospital Beneficência Portuguesa de São Paulo, São Paulo, SP, Brazil

# The Pharmacist in Oncology and Hematology

# 1

Carolina Witchmichen Penteado Schmidt

## 1.1 The Oncology Pharmacist

The history of the oncology pharmacy is relatively new, and we are still building our place and roles in this area. There are different roles the pharmacists play throughout the world and in (adult and pediatric) oncology, hematology, and chemotherapy for other specialized areas, like rheumatology. As cancer knowledge becomes more complex, there are more areas in which specialists are needed. Pharmacists are needed in diverse stages of cancer treatment, from the research, production of chemotherapeutic drugs in the industry, logistics, hospital management, clinical pharmacy with oncologic patients, chemotherapy handling, follow-up and management of side effects, and support drugs even when the patient is at home. Another relatively new area where the pharmacist is essential is stem cell transplantation. Furthermore, for those cases in which all the possibilities of treatment ended, the pharmacist has much work in palliative care, especially the clinical pharmacist. Many countries and many oncology centers only allow pharmacists specialized in oncology to be responsible for chemotherapy handling, since the professional doing this work needs to know drug interaction, han-

C. W. P. Schmidt (✉)
Pediatric Oncology Pharmacist & Writer, Curitiba, Paraná, Brazil
e-mail: carola@kidscancerbooks.com



C. W. P. Schmidt, K. M. Otoni (eds.), *The Golden Guide to Oncologic Pharmacy*, https://doi.org/10.1007/978-3-030-98596-7_1

dling, chemistry, microbiology, and, among other areas, especially a deep knowledge in pharmacology that only pharmacists have. The specialization and graduation courses have been modernized to include the new high complexity needs. As well as we cannot imagine another professional administrating chemotherapy but an oncology/hematology nurse, and it is unimaginable another professional defining the protocol and prescribing the chemotherapy but an oncology/hematology physician, it is impossible to imagine nowadays another professional handling chemotherapy but the oncology/hematology pharmacist. Unfortunately, some countries have so many health issues and social problems that barely have cancer treatment, even more pharmacists handling chemotherapy. In the past, when cancer was treated with less complexity than today, nurses were the healthcare professionals who used to handle chemotherapy. In 1979, it was published the first convincing evidence, in a small but controlled study, that mutagenic activity was found in the urine of patients who received chemotherapy as well as in the nurses who administered it. Since then, there was evidence of significant risk by occupational exposure published all around, and the safety of professionals involved in the chemotherapy treatment and also of the patients was improved. The main routes of cytotoxic drug exposure occur through skin contact and absorption, inhalation, ingestion, and sharp injuries. In the 1980s, the USA Occupational Safety and Health Administration (OSHA) was concerned about chemotherapy preparation practices, and the analysis of the procedures showed facilities failing in protecting the pharmacists. A safe handling program was implemented, described in the American Journal of Hospital Pharmacy, and it became the basis for the first American Society of Hospital Pharmacists (ASHP) Technical Assistance Bulletin on Handling Cytotoxic Drugs [1].

## 1.2 The Roles of an Oncology Pharmacist

The Oncology Pharmacy Team consists of specialty-trained pharmacists and their team of pharmacy technicians, and it is an integral component of the multidisciplinary healthcare team. Involved with all aspects of cancer patient care, this team works to guarantee quality in patient care, safety, and local regulatory compliance. The International Society of Oncology Pharmacy Practitioners (ISOPP) developed a statement to guide five key areas: oncology pharmacy practice as a pharmacy specialty, contributions to patient care, oncology pharmacy practice management, education and training, and contributions to oncology research and quality initiatives to involve this team. Their position statement advocates that the oncology pharmacy team be fully incorporated into the multidisciplinary team to optimize patient care, educational and healthcare institutions develop programs to educate the members of this team continually, and regulatory authorities develop certification programs to recognize the unique contributions of the oncology pharmacy team in cancer patient care [2].

An oncology pharmacist is responsible for evaluating the prescriptions and protocols and if they are appropriate for the patient, evaluating the doses, drug interactions, chemical compatibility, volume, and, if it is not adequate, contact the physician who prescribed it to suggest changes and politely discuss the reasons and mechanisms and work as a team for the well-being of the patient. Before calling the physician, the pharmacist should be sure about what he has to discuss and be open to hear the feedback and analyze the protocol as a team working for the patient. The pharmacist is co-responsible for every drug the patient will receive, so if the therapy is harmful and the physician is not able to identify an error, it is the role of the pharmacist to talk as much as it is necessary with them or contact a preceptor or the rest of the team to discuss the therapy. At the same time that a pharmacist evaluates the appropriateness of the therapy, including pre-chemotherapy and support drugs, the pharmacist should evaluate if he can contribute to this therapy to make it better for that patient. Maybe the patient has a volume restriction, and the protocol can be handled in a more concentrated way. Maybe the patient will benefit from another combination of support drugs due to a reduced drug interaction. Maybe another formula can be better for that patient. If there are ways to improve the therapy, the pharmacist should call the physician who prescribed to suggest that. The pharmacist should have in mind an optimization of the patient's adherence to anticancer therapy and the different formulas and support drugs that can help this. A clinical pharmacist can monitor drug therapy's adverse effects and pharmacovigilance-related activities. Verifying, reviewing, and recommending strategies for food and drug interactions before and throughout therapy is also essential. Implement patient-specific management of treatment-related adverse effects, and ensure supportive care is planned and implemented is important. Promoting patient and caregiver advocacy is also a pharmacist's role, together with the whole team [2].

It is also the role of an oncology pharmacist to define practices and standards for safe practice and train the team. The oncology pharmacist should develop strategies to mitigate, manage, and prevent medication errors, drug-related problems, and drug-related morbidity. Standard operating procedures (SOP) are necessary and should be written and studied by all the team. It is important to reread the SOPs and do new training to guarantee a safe practice from time to time. The oncology pharmacist needs to guarantee the quality of the drugs, promoting appropriate storage and handling and dispensing of medication. The drugs and the environment should be controlled regarding temperature, microorganisms, and the drugs handled should be sterile. The pharmacist needs to have critical thinking, certify the procedures and the references used, and modernize it according to the advance of science. A good oncology pharmacist is ahead; they do not just follow the legislation and only the minimum standard. A good oncology pharmacist is creative and can adapt and make the best possible with the minimum resources. Education and training are necessary for the pharmacist, and it is also essential that they promote knowledge for their team inside the pharmacy, the multidisciplinary team, and the patients. Good pharmacists learn and teach; they share knowledge always. Moreover, they are humble enough to understand that what they do is always for the patient's health and the community, the collective health. However, they are also strong enough not to be tricked by false knowledge or accept situations that can harm their own health or the patients. The safety of them and their teams is the most critical priority. To take care of the others, you need to take care of yourself first. That story of the oxygen masks in the airplanes, to put your mask before helping your kid or another person, is the perfect metaphor for the oncology pharmacists. Nobody should accept to work in harmful conditions. The work of an oncology pharmacist can be extended for research. They can conduct and facilitate oncology-related research activities [2].

## 1.3 Becoming an Oncology Pharmacist

The first thing to have in mind when becoming an oncology pharmacist is to check the local law and what it demands. Then, what the institutions ask. In general, a pharmacist can become an oncology pharmacist completing a post-graduation, residency program, or a structured traineeship in the area. The kind of certification the countries ask in law may vary. Official organizations recognize and certificate pharmacists after a test or validating their own certifications achieved by courses. To become a pediatric oncology pharmacist, knowledge in pediatrics and neonatal is also needed, as well as the knowledge specifically in pediatric oncology, which differs a lot from adult oncology. The most common of childhood cancer types are hematological. Children receive, in general, higher doses of chemotherapy than adults since their cellular renewal is faster. Pediatric oncology is more complex than adult oncology and has much more details. Pediatric oncology books, courses, training, experience, and internship help a lot. Formal training in pediatric oncology is still not standard everywhere, and many pharmacists search for education in oncology in post-graduation courses that include pediatric oncology and focus all their work in pediatric oncology, studying books, making research or their monography or another kind of final course assignment in this area, as well as an internship. Residence programs for pharmacists in pediatric oncology are not standard everywhere, but some countries have it available more commonly. Independent from the method available and chosen, the important is to be qualified to offer high-quality therapy for the patients and be allowed by law to work in this area.

## 1.4 Resources

It is important that oncology pharmacists surround themselves with trustworthy resources that help them find the correct information quickly, such as books, articles, journals, and protocols. An investment must be made in good resources to guarantee that the oncology pharmacist will have support when they need it. Springer Nature (https://link.springer.com/) has packages for hospitals and universities to sign up for their clinical medicine database and access trustworthy books and journals; it is a great resource that can be available at the pharmacist's workplace, and it can be found out talking to the librarian. National Cancer Institute (https://www.cancer.gov/) has a lot of good material available for free. The International Society of Oncology Pharmacy Practitioners (ISOPP) (https://www.isopp.org/) has many resources available for memberships. American Society of Clinical Oncology (ASCO) (https://beta.asco.org/) has resources to keep informed. There are wonderful books that help pharmacists a lot; one of them, which helps to check doses and concentrations quickly, is the Lexicomp Drug Information Handbook for Oncology. Since the oncology area is all based on protocols, the pharmacist must be present in congresses and events that present the most recent research and be a part of research groups if possible.

## 1.5 Oncology Pharmacist: A Valuable Resource in the Workforce

The pharmacist is a valuable resource for many different subareas in oncology and hematology, making a difference in the treatment of patients in the most diverse ways.

A study evaluated the incorporation of a clinical oncology pharmacist into an ambulatory care pharmacy in pediatric hematology-oncology and transplant clinic. It published the results of the professional playing an integral role in minimizing the adverse effect and reduction in readmission into the hospital, which was especially important because this study was performed in Pakistan, which is defined by the authors of the study as an underdeveloped country. This is a relatively new expansion of the pharmacist's role in 2019 and was published in 2020. During the five months analyzed, 1820 visitations were performed for pediatric patients. The clinical oncology pharmacist documented 1665 pharmacist interventions in the 980 direct patient interviews performed. Most of the documented clinical oncology pharmacist interventions were reviews of medication histories (24%) and dose adjustments of deferiprone (24%). Genomic profiling interventions were also among the commonly reported activities by the professional. For beta-thalassemia patients undergoing hydroxyurea therapy, genomic profiling was performed to assess whether the hydroxyurea treatment was clinically effective or not (23%) [3].

A study performed in Japan aimed to demonstrate the differences in clinical pharmacy services provided by oncology and non-oncology pharmacists for patients and physicians. The study also defined the potential impact of these services on medical costs. It concluded that although both oncology pharmacists and non-oncology pharmacists provided a service that contributed greatly to cancer therapy and reduction in medical costs, the service provided by oncology pharmacists was of higher quality. The impact of the service provided by both oncology pharmacists and non-oncology pharmacists may exceed the medical fees currently being charged for their services. Clinical pharmacy service for outpatients who undergo chemotherapy may not only provide better clinical management for patients but also reduce medical costs [4].

A pharmacist-led program open to adult outpatients with refractory chemotherapy-induced nausea and vomiting was implemented at the University of Wisconsin. Pharmacists conducted baseline and follow-up assessments, provided patient education, and started, discontinued, and/or adjusted antiemetic drugs according to the clinical necessary for all enrolled patients. A retrospective chart review described the proportion of patients whose chemotherapy-induced nausea and vomiting improved through the intervention. The effect of the program on antiemetic adherence was analyzed as well and the duration of patient enrollment. Forty-six patients were enrolled in this program. 89.1% had an overall reduction in their nausea and vomiting. 23.9% met the criteria for non-adherence to prescribed antiemetic drugs at baseline, and all patients were adherent in the end. One hundred eleven interventions were made. The most common intervention was the addition of a breakthrough antiemetic drug. The least common intervention was dose escalation of a previously prescribed antiemetic drug. The average number of interventions made per patient was 2.5. On average, patients were enrolled in the program for 16.6 days and met with a pharmacist three times. The implementation of this program standardized and streamlined pharmacist involvement with refractory chemotherapy-induced nausea and vomiting, resulting in a measurable reduction in nausea and/or vomiting for those patients [5].

## References

1. da Conceição AV, Bernardo D, Lopes LV, et al. Oncology pharmacy units: a safety policy for handling hazardous drugs and related waste in low- and middle-income African countries-Angolan experience. Ecancer Med Sci. 2015;9:575. 10.3332/ecancer.2015.575. PMID: 26557873; PMCID: PMC4631569.
2. Holle LM, Bilse T, Alabelewe RM, Kintzel PE, Kandemir EA, Tan CJ, Weru I, et al. International Society of Oncology Pharmacy Practitioners (ISOPP) position statement: Role of the oncology pharmacy team in cancer care. J Oncol Pharm Pract. 2021:785–801. https://doi.org/10.1177/10781552211017199.
3. Ali K, Al-Quteimat O, Naseem R, Malhi SM, Mehwishwajdi NJ, Ansari SH, Shamsi TS. Incorporating a clinical oncology pharmacist into an ambulatory care pharmacy in pediatric hematology–oncology and transplant clinic: assessment and significance. J Oncol Pharm Pract. 2021;27:815–20. https://doi.org/10.1177/1078155220934167.
4. Kaya M, Nakamura K, Nagamine M, et al. A retrospective study comparing interventions by oncology and non-oncology pharmacists in outpatient chemotherapy. Cancer Rep. 2021;4(4):e1371. https://doi.org/10.1002/cnr2.1371.
5. Quinn, Caroline S, Jason J Bergsbaken, Emily J Blessinger, and Jennifer K Piccolo. Implementation of a clinical pharmacist-led service to optimize management of refractory chemotherapy-induced nausea and vomiting in Adult Hematology/Oncology Clinic. J Oncol Pharm Pract. 2021. https://doi.org/10.1177/10781552211029702.

# Oncological Diseases 2

Maria Inês Rodrigues Gato,
Amanda Nascimento dos Reis,
Flávio dos Santos Silvério,
Fumiko Takahashi Ito,
and Kathia Ferraro Lopes

## 2.1 Breast

### 2.1.1 Introduction and Epidemiology

This is a malignant tumor that develops due to genetic changes in the breast cells, which undergo an abnormal growth. Most breast cancers begin in the lobules (milk glands) or in the ducts that connect the lobules to the nipple [2]. If diagnosed early and treated in

M. I. R. Gato (✉)
Brazilian Society of Oncology Pharmacists (Sobrafo), São Paulo, Brazil

A. N. dos Reis
Brazilian Society of Pharmacists in Oncology, ONCOMINAS - Instituto Sul Mineiro de Oncologia, São Paulo, Brazil

F. dos Santos Silvério
Brazilian Society of Pharmacists in Oncology, Samaritano Hospital, São Paulo, Brazil

F. T. Ito
Brazilian Society of Pharmacists in Oncology, São Paulo, Brazil

K. F. Lopes
Brazilian Society of Pharmacists in Oncology, Institute Racine, São Paulo, Brazil



C. W. P. Schmidt, K. M. Otoni (eds.), *The Golden Guide to Oncologic Pharmacy*, https://doi.org/10.1007/978-3-030-98596-7_2

a timely manner, the prognosis is positive, and the cure rate is high. Despite being diagnosed in a few cases, men should also be alert to possible symptoms of the disease.

According to the IARC publication, 2,261,419 new cases of breast cancer were estimated in 2020, equivalent to 12.5% of all estimated cancers and 684,996 deaths corresponding to 6.9% of the deaths of all cancers [3].

### 2.1.2 Risk Factors

There is not only one risk factor for breast cancer; however, the age above 50 years is considered the most important. Other factors that contribute to the increased risk of developing the disease are:

- Genetic factors (*BRCA1* and *BRC2* gene mutations) and hereditary factors
- Late menopause
- Obesity
- Sedentary lifestyle
- Frequent exposure to ionizing radiation [4]

### 2.1.3 Signs and Symptoms

Breast cancer typically has no symptoms when the tumor is small and most easily treated, and that is why screening is important for early detection [2, 5].

- Changes in the skin that covers the breast (such as redness or retractions).
- On the nipple, an aspect similar to orange peel.
- Spontaneous release of abnormal fluid through the nipples.
- Palpable nodes with or without pain in the breast or armpit.
- Presence of a fixed and generally painless node is the main manifestation of the disease, which is present in about 90% of cases when cancer is noticed by the woman herself.

- Abnormal calcifications and/or structural distortion in routine mammography.

### 2.1.4 Detection

Breast cancer diagnosis is based on clinical examination combined with imaging studies and confirmed by histopathological evaluation. Anamnesis (with special attention to the menopausal condition and family history of breast and ovarian cancer) and physical examination should be performed, which should include bimanual palpation of the breasts and regional lymph nodes. At the same time, a search should be made for signs and symptoms that may indicate potential sites of metastatic disease.

A minimal blood evaluation (complete blood count, liver and kidney function tests, alkaline phosphatase, and calcium level tests) is recommended prior to surgery and also a definition of the systemic (neo) adjuvant treatment. A bilateral mammography should be performed and, if necessary, complement it with a breast ultrasound scan. Breast magnetic resonance imaging (MRI) is not routinely indicated and can be considered in special situations [6].

### 2.1.5 Staging

The staging system used for breast cancer is the TNM system of the *American Joint Committee on Cancer* (AJCC) that considers the clinical and pathological staging. In 2018, the staging system was updated to include details about the tumor such as estrogen and progesterone receptor status, HER2 status [7].

- The *pathological stage*, also called surgical stage, is determined by the analysis of the tissue sample removed during surgery.
- If surgery is not possible, the tumor receives the *clinical staging*, which is based on the physical examination, biopsy, and

imaging results. The clinical stage is used in the treatment planning. However, when the disease is disseminated, the clinical stage does not have the same accuracy as the pathological stage to predict prognosis.

In both staging systems, the following prognostic factors were adopted:

- *T:* Indicates the primary tumor size and if it is spread to other areas.
- *N*: Describes if there is disease dissemination to regional lymph nodes.
- *M*: Indicates if metastasis is present in other organs, such as lungs or liver.
- *ER*: The tumor is an estrogen receptor.
- *PR*: The tumor is a progesterone receptor.
- *HER2*: The tumor has HER2 protein.
- *G*: The grade indicates how much cancer cells look like normal cells.

Due to the high complexity of the new staging for breast cancer prognosis, we present the Anatomical Staging (AS) solely based on the anatomical extension as defined by TNM and according to data from clinical history, physical examination, and imaging studies (when indicated) [6].

**Definition of the Primary Tumor (T): Clinical and Pathological** [6]

- *TX:* Primary tumor cannot be assessed.
- *T0*: No evidence of primary tumor.
- *Tis (DCIS)*: Ductal carcinoma in situ (lobular carcinoma in situ was excluded from the new TNM, and it is characterized as a benign disease).
- *T1*: $T \leq 20$ mm in the greatest dimension.
- *T1mi* (microinvasion): $T \leq 1$ mm.
- *T1*: $> 1$ and $\leq 20$ mm.
- *T2*: $> 20$ and $\leq 50$ mm.
- *T3*: $> 50$ mm.

- *T4*: Any size, with direct extension to the thoracic wall and/or skin or inflammatory cancer. Dermis invasion alone does not qualify it as T4.

**Clinical Definition of Regional Lymph Nodes (cN)** [6]
- *cNX*: Regional lymph nodes (LNs) cannot be assessed.
- *cN0*: No regional metastasis (by physical or imaging examination).
- *cN1*: Metastasis to movable ipsilateral axillary LNs levels I and II.
- *cN2*: Metastasis to ipsilateral LNs levels I and II that are clinically fixed or coalescent or metastasis to internal breast LNs in the absence of axillary metastases.
- *cN3*: Metastasis to LNs of the ipsilateral infraclavicular chain (level III), with or without involvement of the axillary chain (level I or II) or clinically apparent metastasis in the ipsilateral internal breast chain, in the presence of clinically positive metastasis in the axillary region or metastasis in the ipsilateral supraclavicular chain, with or without involvement of the axillary or internal breast chain.

**Definition of Distant Metastasis (M)** [6]
- *M0*: No metastasis by clinical or radiological criterion of distant metastasis.
- *cM1(i+)*: No metastasis by clinical or radiological criteria in the presence of tumor cells or tumor deposits not greater than 0.2 mm detected microscopically or by molecular techniques in the blood, bone marrow, or other non-regional lymph node tissue in a patient with or without symptoms or signs of metastasis.
- *M1*: Distant metastasis detected by clinical or radiological criterion (cM) and/or histological criterion with deposit greater than 0.2 mm (pM).

**Stage Grouping** [8, 9]

*Stage zero (0):* Describes disease that is only in the breast tissue ducts and has not spread to the surrounding tissue of the breast. It is also called non-invasive or in situ cancer (Tis, N0, M0).

Invasive breast cancer is classified in the following stages, according to the disease extent:

- *IA:* (T1, N0, M0).
- *IB:*(T0 or T1, N1mi, M0).
- *IIA:* (T0, N1, M0);(T1, N1, M0) or (T2, N0, M0).
- *IIB:*(T2, N1, M0) or (T3, N0, M0).
- *IIIA:*(T0, T1, T2, or T3; N2; M0) or (T3, N1, M0).
- *IIIB:*(T4; N0, N1, or N2; M0).
- *IIIC:* (any T, N3, M0).

Stages *IA*, *IB,* and *IIA* are generally considered early-stage breast cancer and stages *IIIA*, *IIIB,* and *IIIC*, a locally advanced disease. Stage IIB can be classified as initial stage if the tumor is >20 mm, but ≤50 mm, and if it is disseminated to 1–3 axillary lymph nodes (T2 N1 M0), or as a locally advanced disease if the tumor has >50 mm without axillary lymph node involvement (T3 N0 M0) [5].

In general, the new staging system classifies triple-negative breast cancer (estrogen-receptor-negative, progesterone-receptor-negative, and HER2-negative) at a higher stage and classifies most hormone-receptor-positive breast cancer at a lower stage.

Although breast cancer most commonly spreads to nearby lymph nodes, it can also spread further through the body to areas such as the bones, lungs, liver, and brain. This is called metastatic or stage IV breast cancer and is the most advanced type of breast cancer (any T, any N, M1). If breast cancer comes back after initial treatment, it can recur locally, mainly in the same breast and/or regional lymph nodes. It can also recur elsewhere in the body, called a distant recurrence or metastatic recurrence [8].

### 2.1.6 Histopathological and Molecular Classification [10]

#### 2.1.6.1 Non-invasive Breast Conditions

Also called carcinoma in situ. These are precancerous conditions, where the cells look like cancer cells, but have not invaded nearby tissues.

- *Ductal carcinoma in situ* (DCIS): abnormal cells in the breast ducts may develop into invasive breast cancer.
- *Lobular carcinoma in situ* (LCIS): abnormal cells in the breast lobules increase the risk of developing cancer in either breast.

#### 2.1.6.2 Invasive Breast Cancer

There are two main types of invasive breast cancer. They are named after the area of the breast they start in:

- *Invasive ductal carcinoma* (IDC): starts in the ducts/accounts for about 80% of breast cancers.
- *Invasive lobular carcinoma* (ILC): starts in the lobules/makes up about 10% of breast cancers.

There are other less common types of breast cancer. These include inflammatory breast cancer, Paget's disease of the nipple, medullary carcinoma, mucinous carcinoma, and papillary carcinoma.

#### 2.1.6.3 Molecular Classification

Breast cancer molecular classification can be performed in the histopathological material by genetic analysis and, more commonly, by immunohistochemistry. Different molecular subtypes of breast cancer are described, which differ in their clinical evolution and prognosis. The five molecular subtypes are luminal A, luminal B, luminal HER, receptor of human epidermal growth factor 2 (HER-2), and triple negative; however, in clinical practice, for defining the breast cancer treatment, in addition to the clinical-pathological criteria, the estrogen (ER) and progesterone (PR) hormone receptors status and the HER-2 status evaluation are mainly used.

## 2.2 Cervix Uteri

### 2.2.1 Introduction and Epidemiology

Uterine cancer is considered the most common invasive gynecological cancer among American women. Endometrial cancer accounts for approximately 90% of all uterine cancers.

Recent advances indicate that the disease etiology is heterogeneous and consists of at least two major subgroups. This heterogeneity extends to important racial differences in both incidence and survival, probably associated with genetic factors [11].

The incidence of uterine cancer is higher in North America and Europe, intermediate in Southern Europe and South America, lower in South and East Asia and higher in part of Africa. This probably reflects differences in the prevalence of risk factors, including obesity and reproductive patterns. In the USA it is the fourth most diagnosed type of cancer, which had an estimate of 63,230 cases in 2018 (life-threatening to 1 in 40 women). The disease is considered rare before the age of 45, but the risk increases sharply among women of all races aged 40–60 years. In 2012 uterine cancer was ranked as the sixth most common in the world [11]. GLOBOCAN estimated 604,127 new cases of Uterine Cancer (3.1%) and 341,831 new deaths (3.4%) related to the disease in 2020 [12].

### 2.2.2 Risk Factors

Some of the factors below may increase a woman risk of developing uterine cancer:

- Age
- Obesity
- Race
- Genetics
- Diabetes
- Other cancers
- Use of tamoxifen
- Radiotherapy
- Diet and nutrition
- Progesterone
- Estrogens

### 2.2.3 Signs and Symptoms [13, 14, 15]

- Difficulty and pain to urinate
- Vaginal bleeding
- Pain during sexual intercourse
- Pelvic pain (usually a symptom in the more advanced stages of the disease)
- Unexplained weight loss (usually a symptom of the more advanced stages of the disease)

### 2.2.4 Detection

*Ultrasound*: Often it is one of the first tests used to visualize the uterus, ovaries, and fallopian tubes in women with possible gynecological problems. Vaginal ultrasound offers a better view of the uterus, to see if the organ contains any mass (tumor) or if the endometrium is thinner than normal, and which may indicate an endometrium cancer [16].

*Endometrial biopsy*: this is the most used test for endometrium cancer and very accurate in postmenopausal women and can be performed in the doctor's office [16].

*Hysteroscopy*: the surgeon can have a privileged view and can biopsy something abnormal.

*Dilation and curettage*: if endometrial biopsy does not provide sufficient tissue or suggest cancer, but the results are not conclusive, dilation and curettage should be performed [16, 17].

### 2.2.5 Staging [16]

Two systems are used for endometrial cancer staging, FIGO (*International Federation of Gynecology and Obstetrics*) and AJCC, and their staging is practically the same.

The endometrial cancer stage system considers the clinical and pathological staging.

- *TX:* The main tumor cannot be assessed due to lack of information.
- *T0:* No evidence of primary tumor.
- *NX:* Regional lymph node cannot be assessed due to lack of information.

- *Stage I:* cancer grows inside the uterus, and can also grow within the cervix glands, but not inside the connective tissues supporting the cervix (T1), and it has not spread to nearby lymph nodes (N0) or to distant tissues (M0).
- *Stage IA:* cancer remains in the endometrium (inner lining of the uterus) and may have a growth less than half of the underlying muscle layer of the uterus [(myometrium), T1a], N0 and M0.
- *Stage IB:* cancer grew from the endometrium to the myometrium and more than half of the myometrium but did not spread beyond the body of the uterus (T1b), to the nearby lymph nodes (N0) and not to distant tissues (M0).
- *Stage II:* cancer has spread from the body of the uterus and grows in the connective tissue supporting the cervix but has not spread out of the uterus (T2), to nearby lymph nodes (N0) and not to distant tissues (M0).
- *Stage III:* cancer has spread out of the uterus, but not to the inner lining of the rectum or urinary bladder (T3), to nearby lymph nodes (N0) and not to distant tissues (M0).
- *Stage IIIA:* cancer has spread to the outer surface of the uterus (serosa) and/or to the fallopian tubes or ovaries (T3a), has not spread to nearby lymph nodes (N0) or distant tissues (M0).
- *Stage IIIB:* cancer has spread through the vagina or tissues around the uterus (parametrium: T3b), has not spread to nearby lymph nodes (N0) or distant tissues (M0).
- *Stage IIIC1:* cancer grows in the body of the uterus. May have spread to some nearby tissues, but it is not growing inside the bladder or rectum (T1 to T3). It has also spread to the pelvic

lymph nodes (N1, N1mi or N1a), but not to the lymph nodes around the aorta or distant sites (M0).

- *Stage IIIC2:* cancer is growing in the body of the uterus. May have spread to some nearby tissues, but it is not growing inside the bladder or rectum (T1 to T3). It has also spread to the lymph nodes around the aorta (N2, N2mi or N2a), but not to distant sites (M0).
- *Stage IVA:* cancer has spread to the inner lining of the rectum or urinary bladder (mucous membrane), (T4). It may or may not have spread to the nearby lymph nodes (any N), but it has not spread to distant sites (M0).
- *Stage IVB:* cancer has spread to the inguinal lymph nodes (groin), upper abdomen, omentum or organs distant from the uterus, such as lungs, liver, or bones (M1). Cancer can be of any size (T) and may or may not have spread to other lymph nodes (any N).

### 2.2.6 Histopathological and Molecular Classification

Endometrial tissue samples are removed by biopsy or by dilation and curettage and are observed under a microscope. If cancer is found, the pathology laboratory will report the stage and type, and grade of endometrial cancer that is classified on a scale of 1–3 according to the normal state of the endometrium [16].

#### 2.2.6.1 Types of Endometrial Cancer [18, 19]

*Endometrioid:* It can be called endometrial cancer type 1, accounting for 75–80% of cases, and its genetic changes include microsatellite instability, mutations of PTEN gene, Kras, and beta catenin.

*Serous papillary:* Accounting for 1–5% of cases, it is known as endometrial cancer type 2; the p53 gene mutation is an early event and characterizes aggressive tumors. Papillary cell architecture with the presence of psammoma bodies in 30% of cases.

*Clear cells:* 5 to 10% of cases, this is a type 2 endometrial cancer; the p53 gene mutation is an early event, and cells have tubulocystic cell architecture, papillary or large solid areas.

*Mixed tumors:* Those whose serous component corresponds to more than 10% and less than 50%, with a controversial prognosis and rare histology.

*Histological subtypes:* Endometrioid adenocarcinoma, clear cell carcinoma, serous adenocarcinoma, mixed adenocarcinoma, squamous carcinoma, mucinous adenocarcinoma, transitional cell carcinoma, small cell adenocarcinoma, and undifferentiated carcinoma.

## 2.3 Colorectum

### 2.3.1 Introduction and Epidemiology

Colorectal cancer usually begins with polyps that can develop on the inner wall of the colon and rectum, which make up the large intestine, and can be called precancerous polyps. Colorectal cancer can be prevented by removing adenomatous polyps or precancerous adenomas, lesions that are usually and easily found in screening colonoscopy in the form of lumps in the colon. About 10% of polyps are flat and difficult to detect by colonoscopy and can progress to a malignant tumor.

Most colon and rectal cancers are called adenocarcinoma, which is the tumor of the cells lining the internal tissue of the colon and rectum [20].

Colorectal cancer is the third most common incident of all cancers, according to IARC. The change in social lifestyle of the world population and the income increase are clear indicators of the colorectal cancer incidence. An estimated growth of 60% of cases is expected, reaching 2.2 million new cases and 1.1 million deaths by 2030 [21].

Colorectal cancer mainly affects older adults, but there is an increasing incidence among younger adults. While rates decreased 3.6% each year in adults aged 55 and over, there was a 2% increase each year in those under 55 [1]. When early diagnosed, colorectal cancer has a 54% cure expectation, which may increase in the face of higher screening rates and new treatments [20].

### 2.3.2 Risk Factors

The cause of colorectal cancer is not well known. Most colorectal tumors (about 95%) are considered sporadic, which means that genetic changes develop by chance and there is no risk of transmitting them to descendants. Lifestyle and health care contribute to reducing the risk of developing the disease. However, the following factors may increase an individual risk of developing colorectal cancer [20, 22].

- Age between 45 and 85 years
- Male gender
- Family history of colorectal cancer
- Inflammatory intestinal diseases
- Familiar adenomatous polyps
- White or black (African American) or Latin/Hispanic race
- Sedentary lifestyle and obesity
- High-fat diet processed foods and red meats, low-fiber diet
- Smoking

### 2.3.3 Signs and Symptoms

Many people do not show symptoms until the disease is advanced, and the initial signs and symptoms are like numerous diseases of the gastrointestinal tract, making early diagnosis difficult. A regular screening is recommended. The most common signs and symptoms of colorectal cancer are [20]:

- Change of intestinal habit
- Diarrhea, constipation, or feeling of non-emptying of the intestine at evacuation
- Presence of blood in the stool or darkened staining
- Change in the feces type

- Abdominal discomfort, presence of gauze, flatulence, and abdominal swelling
- Unexplained weight loss
- Weakness, fatigue, and anemia

### 2.3.4 Detection

The most effective and safe method of diagnosing colorectal cancer is through biopsy, which can be preceded by colonoscopy with or without biopsy at the same time, in addition to including molecular tests of the collected sample. In the blood test, a sign of anemia hemorrhage and the increased level of carcinoembryonic antigen (CEA) can be identified, and although this is not a specific and exclusive marker of colorectal cancer, high levels of this protein are identified in 60% of patients with the disease. CT scan and MRI can help visualize the tumor size, as well as its location [20].

Somatic and germinal mutations that lead to microsatellite repair deficiency incompatibility or instability and RAS pathway mutations have a personalized approach for diagnosing and treating colorectal cancer and have an emphasis for the treatment definition [23].

### 2.3.5 Staging

The staging system used for colorectal cancer is the AJCC TNM system [20].

The T classification describes the primary tumor growth depth in the intestine lining [24]:

- *TX:* Primary tumor cannot be assessed.
- *T0:* No evidence of primary tumor.
- *Tis:* Carcinoma in situ, intramucosal carcinoma (involvement of lamina propria with no extension through muscularis mucosae).

- *T1:* Tumor invades submucosa (through the muscularis mucosa but not into the muscularis propria).
- *T2:* Tumor invades muscularis propria.
- *T3:* Tumor invades through the muscularis propria into the pericolorectal tissues.
- *T4a:* Tumor invades through the visceral peritoneum.
- *T4b:* Tumor directly invades or adheres to other adjacent organs or structures.

Classification N describes the involvement of lymph nodes near the colon and rectum and regional lymph nodes [24]:

- *NX:* Regional lymph nodes cannot be assessed.
- *N0*: No regional lymph node metastasis.
- *N1a*: Metastasis in 1 regional lymph node.
- *N1b*: Metastasis in 2–3 regional lymph nodes.
- *N1c*: No regional lymph nodes are positive, but there are tumor deposits in the subserosa, mesentery, or non-peritonealized pericolic or perirectal/mesorectal tissues.
- *N2a*: Metastasis in 4–6 regional lymph nodes.
- *N2b*: Metastasis in 7 or more regional lymph nodes.

Classification M describes the presence of distant metastasis [24]:

- *M0*: No distant metastasis by imaging; no evidence of tumor in other sites or organs.
- *M1a*: Metastasis confined to 1 organ or site without peritoneal metastasis.
- *M1b*: Metastasis to 2 or more sites or organs is identified, without peritoneal metastasis.
- *M1c*: Metastasis to the peritoneal surface is identified alone or with other site or organ metastases.

**Stage Grouping** [24]

- *Stage 0*: (Tis, N0, M0).
- *I*: (T1–T2, N0, M0).

- *IIA*: (T3, N0, M0).
- *IIB*: (T4a, N0, M0).
- *IIC*: (T4b, N0, M0).
- *IIIA*: (T1–T2, N1/N1c, M0); (T1, N2a, M0).
- *IIIB*: (T3–T4a, N1/N1c, M0); (T2–T3, N2a, M0); (T1–T2, N2b, M0).
- *IIIC*: (T4a, N2a, M0); (T3–T4a, N2b, M0); (T4b, N1–N2, M0).
- *IVA*: (Any T, Any N, M1a).
- *IVB*: (Any T, Any N, M1b).
- *IVC*: (Any T, Any N, M1c).

### 2.3.6 Histopathological and Molecular Classification

Most colorectal tumors are carcinomas, and more than 90% are adenocarcinoma; and a relative minority are hamartoma, endocrine, mesenchymal, or lymphoma [25].

#### 2.3.6.1 Histological Classification (OMS, 2010) [26]

- Adenocarcinoma
- Mucinous/colloid carcinoma
- Signet-ring cell carcinoma
- High-grade neuroendocrine carcinoma (small or large cells)
- Squamous carcinoma
- Adenosquamous carcinoma
- Medullary carcinoma
- Undifferentiated carcinoma

The histological grade of differentiation considers the distribution of diffusely immunostained CEA granules in the cellular cytoplasm and with the few polarized, those showing cellular distribution with the impossibility of differentiating from conventional histology. The *College of American Pathologists* (CAP) and the American Joint Committee on Cancer (AJCC)/Union for International Cancer Control (UICC) establish the use of a four-level grading system [25]:

- *Grade 1:* Well-differentiated (> 95% of granules formation)
- *Grade 2*: Moderately differentiated (50–95% of granules formation)
- *Grade 3*: Poorly differentiated (<50% of granules formation)
- *Grade 4:* Undifferentiated (no granules formation; with no squamous or neuroendocrine differentiation)

#### 2.3.6.2 Molecular Classification

Molecular analysis is not part of the pathological staging of colorectal cancer; it provides complementary information with predictive usefulness of therapeutic response and prognostic evaluation. The only factors that are used for clinical decision-making today are the status of DNA incompatibility repair proteins (MMR) and BRAF and RAS mutations that are prognostic and predictive factors of chemotherapy efficacy [25].

## 2.4 Kidney

### 2.4.1 Introduction and Epidemiology

Renal cell carcinoma (RCC), also known as renal cell cancer or renal cell adenocarcinoma, is a renal malignancy that arises in the renal parenchyma/cortex, accounting for about 85% of renal cancers [27].

Approximately 54% of diagnosed kidney tumors are confined to the kidney, 20% are locally advanced (affecting regional ganglia near the kidney), and 25% already have metastasis, mainly to the lungs, liver, and bones.

The American Cancer Society's most recent estimates for kidney cancer in the United States for 2021 are [28]:

- About 76,080 new cases of kidney cancer (48,780 in men and 27,300 in women) will be diagnosed.
- About 13,780 people (8790 men and 4990 women) will die from this disease.

These numbers include all types of kidney and renal pelvis cancers.

Most people with kidney cancer are older. The average age of people when they are diagnosed is 64 with most people being diagnosed between ages 65 and 74. Kidney cancer is about twice as common in men than in women, and it is more common in African Americans and American Indian/Alaska Natives [28].

### 2.4.2 Risk Factors [27, 29, 30, 31]

Smoking is the most well-established risk factor for RCC. Other factors are known, among them:

- Exposure to toxic chemicals (cadmium, asbestos, lead, and aromatic hydrocarbons).
- Renal transplantation and end-stage kidney disease with dialysis.
- Obesity.
- Hypertension.
- Family history of RCC.
- Von Hippel-Lindau syndrome is a genetic and rare disease characterized by the formation of tumors with a lot of vascularization in several different parts of the body.
- Pelvic radiation (low risk).
- Obstetric history/exposure to estrogen.
- Gender.
- Race: African Americans have a slightly higher rate of RCC than do whites.
- Gene changes (mutations).
- Tuberous sclerosis: Tuberous sclerosis is a disease that causes seizures and mental retardation, as well as the formation of tumors in many different organs.

### 2.4.3 Signs and Symptoms [32, 33, 34]

Kidney cancer usually does not have signs or symptoms in its early stages. In time, signs and symptoms may develop, including:

- Blood in urine
- Pain in the area between the ribs and the hip (on the flank)
- Loss of appetite
- Unexplained weight loss
- Tiredness
- Fever
- Polycythemia due to high levels of erythropoietin
- Hypercalcemia
- A lump in the lower back or side of the waist

### 2.4.4 Detection

Most renal tumors are diagnosed by imaging tests such as ultrasound, computerized tomography, and magnetic resonance imaging of the abdomen/pelvis. Preoperative renal biopsy is usually not performed and is only necessary in exceptional situations in order to differentiate malignant from benign lesions, which would not require treatment [29].

A urine sample is tested to see if it contains blood. Blood tests are done to count the number of each different kind of blood cells, and also look at different electrolytes [5].

### 2.4.5 Staging [35]

Kidney cancer is typically given a *clinical stage* based on the results of a physical exam, biopsy, and imaging tests. If surgery is done, the *pathologic stage* is determined by examining tissue removed during the operation.

- *T1*
- *T1a:* Tumor found only in the kidney and is ≤ 4 cm.
- *T1b:* Tumor found only in the kidney and is > 4 e ≤ 7.

- *T2*
- *T2a:* Tumor only in the kidney and is > 7 and ≤ 10 cm.
- *T2b:* Tumor only in the kidney and is >10 cm.

- *T3*
- *T3a:* Tumor extends into the renal vein, or its segments, either invades the pyelocaliceal system, or invades perirenal fat or renal sinus fat, but does not exceed the Gerota fascia.
- *T3b:* Tumor extends to inferior vena cava below diaphragm.
- *T3c:* Tumor extends into the vena cava above the diaphragm or invades the vena cava wall.

- *T4:* Tumor surpasses the Gerota fascia including ipsilateral adrenal gland.
- *NX:* Regional lymph nodes cannot be assessed.
- *N0:* No metastasis in regional lymph nodes.
- *N1:* Regional lymph node involvement.
- *M0:* No distant metastasis.
- *M1:* Distant metastasis.

**Stage Grouping**
- *Stage I:* (T1, N0, M0).
- *Stage II:* (T2, N0, M0).
- *Stage III:* (T1 or T2, N1, M0) or (T3, any N, M0).
- *Stage IV:* (T4, any N, M0) or (any T, any N, M1).

**Recurrent** Recurrent cancer is cancer that has come back after treatment. It may be found in the kidney area or in another part of the body. If the cancer does return, there will be another round of tests to learn about the recurrence extent. These tests and scans are often similar to those done at the time of the original diagnosis.

### 2.4.6 Histopathological and Molecular Classification

#### 2.4.6.1 Histopathological Classification
There are over a dozen subtypes of renal cell carcinoma. The most common types are [36]:

- *Clear cell renal cell carcinoma*: About 70% of kidney cancers are made up of clear cells. Clear cells range from slow growing (grade 1) to fast growing (grade 4).

- *Papillary*: Papillary kidney cancer is found in 10–15% of patients. It is divided into 2 different subtypes, called type 1 and type 2.
- *Chromophobe*: Chromophobe is another uncommon cancer that may form indolent tumors that are unlikely to spread but are aggressive if they do.
- *Clear cell papillary*: Approximately 2–4% of all cases. A new subtype with features of both papillary and clear subtypes. These are often less aggressive.
- *Collecting duct RCC*: Approximately 1% of all cases. Aggressive type arising from the collecting system that forms irregular tubules.
- *Medullary carcinoma*: Approximately 1% of cases. An extremely aggressive type often occurring in young African Americans with sickle trait.
- *Unclassified*: Approximately 2–3% of tumors that do not fit into any other category.

#### 2.4.6.2 Other Types of Kidney Cancers [37]

*Urothelial carcinoma*: This is also called transitional cell carcinoma. It accounts for 5–10% of kidney cancers diagnosed in adults. Urothelial carcinoma begins in the area of the kidney where urine collects before moving to the bladder, called the renal pelvis.

*Sarcoma*: Sarcoma of the kidney is rare. This type of cancer develops in the soft tissue of the kidney; the thin layer of connective tissue surrounding the kidney, called the capsule; or surrounding fat.

*Wilms tumor (nephroblastoma)*: Wilms tumor is most common in children and is treated differently from kidney cancer in adults. Wilms tumors make up about 1% of kidney cancers.

*Lymphoma*: Lymphoma can enlarge both kidneys and is associated with enlarged lymph nodes, called lymphadenopathy, in other parts of the body, including the neck, chest, and abdominal cavity. In rare cases, kidney lymphoma can appear as a lone tumor mass in the kidney and may include enlarged regional lymph nodes.

#### 2.4.6.3 Molecular Classification [38]

The initial genetic event in most clear cell renal carcinomas is inactivation of the VHL tumor suppressor gene. Subsequent cooperating genetic events include gain of chromosome 5q, loss of chromosome 14q, and intragenic mutations affecting various chromatin modifiers, such as PBRM1 and BAP1, and genes linked to the mTOR pathway.

## 2.5 Liver

### 2.5.1 Introduction and Epidemiology

The liver is the largest human internal organ, responsible for several essential functions to the body such as processing, converting, and storing nutrients absorbed in the intestine; bile production; toxins removal from the body; maintaining adequate blood glucose levels, among others. Primary liver cancer refers to the tumor with origin in this organ, although the most common is that primary tumors of other organs, such as pancreas, colon, stomach, and breast, spread to the liver (metastasis) [39].

Hepatocarcinoma is the most frequent and aggressive type, representing the fourth leading cause of cancer-related deaths in the world [40, 41]. Cholangiocarcinoma develops from bile duct cells, and represents about 10–20% of primary liver cancers in adults; and angiosarcoma, less frequent, grows rapidly from blood vessels in the liver [39].

According to the IARC publication, 905,677 new cases of liver cancer were estimated worldwide for 2020, equivalent to 5.0% of all cancers and 830,180 deaths corresponding to 8.4% of deaths of all cancers [42]. In the United States, liver cancer is the fifth leading cause of cancer-related deaths in men and the seventh among women, with a 5-year disease-free survival rate of 18% [39]. The incidence, however, varies according to geographic region with about 5% of cases in Latin America, 5% in North America, 8% in Africa, 10% in Europe, and 72% in Asia [43].

In this chapter we will address primary liver tumors with emphasis on hepatocellular carcinoma (HCC), the most common type.

### 2.5.2 Risk Factors

Several factors can increase the risk of liver cancer, such as [39, 41]:

- Chronic viral hepatitis
- Cirrhosis
- Non-alcoholic fatty liver disease
- Exposure to aflatoxins (dietary toxins)
- Primary biliary cirrhosis
- Gender
- Race/ethnicity
- Tobacco use
- Obesity
- Type 2 diabetes
- Certain rare diseases (such as tyrosinemia, alpha1-antitrypsin deficiency, porphyria cutanea tarda, glycogen storage diseases, Wilson disease)

The risk of developing hepatocarcinoma increases as one or more risk factors are associated; these factors are cumulative [39].

### 2.5.3 Signs and Symptoms

Signs and symptoms include but are not limited to [39, 41]:

- Abdominal pain
- Unexplained weight loss
- Loss of appetite
- Nausea or vomiting

- Feeling very full after a small meal
- Liver and spleen enlarged
- Swelling or fluid build-up in the abdomen
- Jaundice (yellowing of the skin and eyes)

Some of these symptoms may be caused by cirrhosis and not necessarily by the tumor. Among them we can mention the fluid accumulation and swelling of the abdomen (requiring the use of diuretics), hepatic encephalopathy, and bleeding from the esophagus or stomach [39].

### 2.5.4 Detection

In the early stages, HCC often shows no symptoms, which hinders early detection and results in diagnosis already in more advanced stages of the disease. For individuals at high risk of developing liver cancer, for example, those with cirrhosis and severe liver dysfunction, consider monitoring every 6 months with surveillance tests, but above all the appropriate selection of which individuals should be monitored to avoid overdiagnosis of HCC [41, 44].

Currently, the HCC diagnosis can be established by imaging and/or pathological tests. In symptomatic patients the physical examination of the abdomen allows the doctor to check for swelling or changes in the liver, spleen, and other nearby organs, accumulation of fluid in the abdomen, and signs of jaundice, such as yellowish skin and eyes. Blood tests are added to the physical examination to assess liver function, which include alpha-fetoprotein (AFP), blood count, liver function test, and hepatitis B and C serologies. And imaging, CT scans with contrast or magnetic resonance imaging adapted to assess liver injury [39, 41, 44].

A biopsy of the lesion may not be necessary when it demonstrates specific characteristics, through imaging, CT, or MRI, and by AFP examination strongly indicating HCC. In these cases, most surgeons opt for biopsy as part of surgery if the liver or a piece is removed, and not as an isolated procedure [41]. For nodules with an inconclusive pattern through imaging or those present in patients without cirrhosis, the diagnosis should be based on biopsy [44].

In patients with cirrhosis and who have lesions smaller than 1 cm, active watch and wait surveillance is recommended, with ultrasound imaging every 3 or 4 months. If the lesion remains stable for 12 months, conventional surveillance may be resumed every 6 months [44].

### 2.5.5 Staging

There are some proposed systems for the staging of liver cancer, but all have limitations. Ideally, staging systems should quantify tumor load, extent of liver dysfunction, and performance status to adequately estimate survival. It is essential to distinguish patients with well-preserved liver function from those with more advanced liver disease [44]. Among the systems adopted for HCC staging are the TNM *system* (AJCC), *The Barcelona Clinic Liver Cancer* (BCLC) *System*, *The Cancer of the Liver Italian Program* (CLIP) *System*, *The Okuda System*, *The Hong Kong Liver Cancer (HKLC) Staging System*, the MELD (*Model for End-Stage Liver Disease*) score, and the *Model to Estimate Survival in Ambulatory HCC Patients* (MESIAH) score [41, 44, 45, 46].

Currently the BCLC system is the most widely used, and despite its limitations, it shows robust prospective validation, classifies the disease in five stages, and estimates the median survival and the type of treatment for each stage. It comprises the *Child-Pugh* and TNM classifications with the performance status. Therefore, we detail below the BCLC and TNM systems, the only one validated in independent cohorts of patients undergoing liver resection or transplantation [41, 44].

**BCLC** *System* **(Adapted from Augusto Villanueva, Hepatocellular Carcinoma)** [44]

- *Stage 0* (very early stage): Single tumor of less than 2 cm.

- *Stage A* (early stage): Single tumor or 2 to 3 nodules ≤3 cm.
- *Stage B* (intermediate stage): Multinodular, no metastasis.
- *Stage C* (advanced stage): Portal invasion or metastasis.
- *Stage D* (terminal stage): Non-transplantable HCC.

**TNM System AJCC 8th edition (2018)** [45]
- *StageIA:* T1a, N0 and M0.
- *Stage IB:* T1b, N0 and M0.
- *Stage II:* T2, N0 and M0.
- *Stage IIIA:* T3, N0 and M0.
- *Stage IIIB:* T4, N0 and M0.
- *Stage IVA:* any T, N1 and M0.
- *Stage IVB:* any T, any N and M1.

**Primary Tumor Classification (T)**
- *TX*: Primary tumor cannot be assessed.
- *T0*: No evidence of primary tumor.
- *T1a:* Solitary tumor ≤2 cm.
- *T1b*: Solitary tumor >2 cm without vascular invasion.
- *T2*: Solitary tumor >2 cm with vascular invasion, or multiple tumors, none >5 cm.
- *T3*: Multiple tumors, at least one of which is >5 cm.
- *T4*: Single tumor or multiple tumors of any size involving a major branch of the portal vein or hepatic vein or tumor(s) with direct invasion of adjacent organs other than the gallbladder or with perforation of visceral peritoneum.

**Regional Lymph Nodes (N)**
- *NX*: Regional lymph nodes cannot be assessed.
- *N0*: No regional lymph node metastasis.
- *N1*: Regional lymph node metastasis.

**Distant Metastasis (M)**
- *M0:* No distant metastasis.
- *M1:* Distant metastasis.

### 2.5.6 Histopathological and Molecular Classification

The HCC development process is complex and arises from multiple genetic and epigenetic changes that culminate in the formation of dysplastic nodules, which are genuine preneoplastic lesions. These changes may be favored by sustained liver inflammation, fibrosis, and aberrant regeneration of hepatocytes, which are common conditions in patients with chronic liver diseases. Primary liver tumors can be classified, from the type of cell from which they develop, into four main types: hepatocellular carcinoma, cholangiocarcinoma, angiosarcoma, and hepatoblastoma (it is a rare type, more common in early-life children) [39, 44, 47].

#### 2.5.6.1 Molecular Classification

From resected specimens of patients in the early stages of the disease, different molecular subtypes of HCC related to clinical characteristics have been identified. However, molecular pathogenesis is not well understood, although much is known about the changes of the etiological agents responsible for most cases (such as excessive alcohol consumption and viral infections by hepatitis B and C) and the cellular changes that lead to HCC. Their use in clinical practice is limited because they have not been completely tested as predictive factors of response to systemic therapy [44, 47].

These molecular subtypes can be divided into two main classes: the proliferation class, common in patients with HBV infection, and the nonproliferation class, tumors with more mutations in *CTNNB1* (beta-catenin) and gene expression patterns similar to normal hepatocytes. The proliferation class has a more aggressive behavior, with clinical and histological characteristics that include HBV infection, high serum levels of alpha-fetoprotein, poor cell differentiation, chromosomal instability, TP53 mutations, activation of oncogenic pathways, and worse clinical outcome. And the non-proliferation class, on the other hand, shows as clinical and histological characteristics better clinical outcome, low tumor grade, lower frequency of vascular invasion, commonly associated with hepatitis C and alcohol abuse [44].

## 2.6 Lung

### 2.6.1 Introduction and Epidemiology

Lung cancer is the third most common cancer in the world and has the highest mortality among all types of cancer (25% of cancer deaths). The mean age at diagnosis is 70 years with good prognosis for cases diagnosed at an early stage [48].

The disease may start in the bronchi, bronchioles, or alveolus and spread to another pulmonary lobe, lymph nodes, other lung, and other parts of the body such as liver, bones, and central nervous system [49].

It is classified according to its cell type in small cell and non-small cell lung cancer; the latter corresponds to about 85% of lung cancer cases and is usually diagnosed in more advanced stages of the disease and survival is low [49].

### 2.6.2 Risk Factors [50, 51]

- Smoking is the most important risk factor; this is impacting even if the individual has abandoned the habit. It depends on the exposure intensity and includes individuals who are passively exposed in the risk group.
- Chemical agents and occupational exposure: asbestos, arsenic, chromium, beryllium, nickel, soot, coal, radiation, and pollution. The individual who has combined the exposure to one of these risk factors and smoking has a higher risk of developing lung cancer.
- Age.
- Family history of the disease.

### 2.6.3 Signs and Symptoms

Less than 5% of patients are symptomatic at diagnosis:

- Dyspnea

- Persistent and/or bloody cough
- Repeated pneumonias
- Chest pain
- Hoarseness
- Fatigue
- Unexplained loss of appetite and weight

If cancer has spread, symptoms vary from bone pain, changes in the central nervous system, jaundice to swelling of the lymph nodes [52]. Some lung cancers may cause a group of specific symptoms described as syndromes [53]:

- *Horner syndrome* (or Pancoast tumors): Fall of an eyelid, constriction of the pupil and decreased sweating of the affected side of the face, severe pain in the shoulder.
- *Superior vena cava syndrome*: Can cause swelling in the face, neck, arms, and upper chest, as well as headache, dizziness, and altered consciousness if it affects the brain. This is a condition that develops slowly, but in some cases can be life-threatening.
- *Paraneoplastic syndromes*: Characterized by inappropriate antidiuretic hormone secretion syndrome, Cushing's syndrome, changes in the nervous system (Lambert-Eaton syndrome), paraneoplastic cerebellar degeneration, hypercalcemia, and blood clots.

### 2.6.4 Detection

Combines medical history and physical examination, and if there is a suspicion, it will be necessary to follow with imaging tests and/or lung biopsy [53, 54]:

- *Imaging tests to look for lung cancer:* Chest x-ray, computerized tomography (CT) scan, magnetic resonance imaging (MRI) scan, positron emission tomography (PET) scan, bone scan

- *Tests to diagnose lung cancer:* Sputum cytology, thoracentesis, needle biopsy (fine needle aspiration (FNA) biopsy, core biopsy, transthoracic needle biopsy), and bronchoscopy
- *Tests to find lung cancer spread in the chest:* Endobronchial ultrasound, endoscopic esophageal ultrasound, mediastinoscopy and mediastinotomy, thoracoscopy
- *Lab tests of biopsy and other samples*: Molecular tests for gene changes (EGFR, ALK, ROS1, RET, BRAF, MET) and PD-L1 protein
- *Tests to determine a person's overall health to have a surgery:* Lung function tests, blood tests (complete blood count); blood chemistry tests (liver and kidneys function, calcium and alkaline phosphatase)

### 2.6.5 Staging

*Small cell cancer*: The staging currently used is based on the 8th Edition of AJCC 2017 that classifies it through the limited versus extensive dissemination stage. The stage through the TNM system is not important for this type of cancer [53].

*Limited stage:* The tumor is present in only one lung and may also be present in supraclavicular lymph nodes that are on the same side of the affected lung.

*Extensive stage*: The tumor spread in the same lung or lymph nodes, to another lung or to other organs including bone marrow.

*Non-small cells cancer*: Clinical stage based on TNM classification regarding the results of a physical exam, biopsy, imaging tests, and pathologic stage if surgery has been done [53].

TNM system consists of informing the size and extent of the main tumor (T); propagation to nearby lymph nodes (N); metastasis to distant sites (M): brain, bones, adrenal glands, liver, or another lung.

Classification follows the guidelines of the AJCC (January 2018):

- *TX N0 M0:* Occult cancer
- *Stage 0*: Tis N0 M0.

- *Stage IA1:* T1mi N0 M0; T1a N0 M0.
- *Stage IA2:* T1b N0 M0.
- *Stage IA3:* T1c N0 M0.
- *Stage IB:* T2a N0 M0.
- *StageIIA:* T2b N0 M0.
- *Stage IIB:* T1a / T1b /T1c N1 M0; T2a / T2b N1 M0; T3 N0 M0.
- *Stage IIIA:* T1a / T1b /T1c N2 M0; T2a / T2b N2 M0; T3 N1 M0; T4 N0 or N1 M0.
- *Stage III B:* T1a/T1b/T1c N3 M0; T2a/T2b N3 M0; T3 N2 M0; T4 N2 M0.
- *Stage IIIC:* T3 N3 M0; T4 N3 M0.
- *Stage IVA:* AnyT, AnyN, M1a; AnyT, AnyN, M1b.
- *Stage IVB:* AnyT, AnyN, M1c.

**Classification T**

- *T1mi*: T ≤ 3 cm across, invaded ≤ 0,5 cm (minimally invasive adenocarcinoma).
- T1a: T ≤ 1 cm; *T1b*: T > 1 cm and 2 cm; *T1c*: T > 2 cm and ≤ 3 cm. It has not reached the membranes that surround the lungs, and it does not affect the main branches of the bronchi.
- *T2a:* T > 3 cm and ≤ 4 cm; *T2b:* T > 4 cm and ≤ 5 cm, and/or it has grown into a main bronchus or the visceral pleura, and/or is partially clogging the airways.
- *T3:* T > 5 cm and ≤ 7 cm, and/or it has grown into the chest wall, parietal pleura, the phrenic nerve, or parietal pericardium, and/or there are 2 or more separate tumor nodules in the same lobe of a lung.
- *T4*: T > 7 cm, and/or it has grown into the mediastinum, heart, aorta, trachea, esophagus, diaphragm, backbone, or the carina; and/or there are 2 or more separate tumor nodules in different lobes of the same lung.

**Classification N**

- *N0*: Cancer is not spread to nearby lymph nodes.
- *N1*: It has spread to lymph nodes within the lung and/or the hilar lymph nodes; these are on the same side as the cancer.

- *N2*: It has spread to lymph nodes around the carina, or in the mediastinum, and these are on the same side as the main lung tumor.
- *N3*: It has spread to lymph nodes near the collarbone on either side of the body, and/or has spread to hilar or mediastinal lymph nodes on the other side of the body from the main tumor.

**Classification M**

- *M0*: It has not spread to distant parts of the body.
- *M1a*: It has spread to the other lung or malignant pleural effusion, or malignant pericardial effusion is present.
- *M1b*: It has spread as a single tumor outside of the chest, such as to a distant lymph node or an organ such as the liver, bones, or brain.
- *M1c*: It has spread as more than one tumor outside the chest, such as to distant lymph nodes and/or to other organs such as the liver, bones, or brain.

**Note:**

- T0: There is no evidence of a primary tumor.
- NX: Nearby lymph nodes cannot be assessed due to lack of information.

### 2.6.6 Histopathological and Molecular Classification

#### 2.6.6.1 Histopathological Classification

*Non-small cells carcinoma*: There are three types of non-small cell lung cancer: adenocarcinomas, squamous cell carcinoma, and large-cell carcinomas [7].

Adenocarcinoma develops on the outside of the lung, has slow growth, and prognosis is better when diagnosed in situ. Squamous cell carcinoma tends to grow in the central part of the lung near the bronchi. And large-cell carcinoma (undifferentiated) grows faster, and one of its subtypes, neuroendocrine, is similar to that of small cells [53].

*Oat cell cancer*: It has a rapid growth profile, is considered aggressive and often associated with paraneoplastic syndromes. If cancer is limited, there is a greater potential for cure. Metastasis can occur to the lymph nodes of the mediastinum, liver, bones, adrenals, and brain. Approximately 60–70% of patients have disseminated disease at diagnosis [53].

#### 2.6.6.2 Molecular Classification

Numerous genetic changes are found in lung cancer that impact the treatment choice, such as target therapies. Therefore, a predictive immunohistochemical analysis is necessary, which differs from the analysis used to identify the tumor type and cell line [53].

Useful analyses for lung cancer are the mutations found in the following genes: EGFR, ALK, ROS 1, BRAF, KRAS, MET, RET, and PD-L1 protein. Liquid biopsy is an alternative method in collecting material to avoid the risks of conventional needle biopsy [54, 55].

## 2.7 Melanoma

### 2.7.1 Introduction and Epidemiology

Melanoma is one of the most severe types of skin cancer. The skin is the largest organ in our body and consists of three main layers: epidermis, dermis, and hypodermis. In the deepest layer of the dermis are melanocytes, which produce the pigment that maintains the color of the skin. Melanoma begins when healthy melanocytes undergo transformation and multiply disorderly forming a malignant tumor. The disease can develop from a normal stain, from the change in shape, size, color, and with undefined edges [56].

The incidence of melanoma has increased considerably in the last 30 years [57]. The rate of new cases was 22.8 per 100,000 inhabitants per year, and the mortality rate was 2.3 per 100,000 inhabitants per year; these rates have been adjusted for age and are based on the incidence of cases and deaths from 2014 to 2018 [58]. Melanoma is the fifth most common cancer in men and the sixth in women; 20 times more common in whites than in blacks. In the United States, in 2020, more than 100,000 cases of melanoma were estimated [56].

The mean age of melanoma diagnosis is for individuals over 50 years of age. The 5-year survival rate is 92% after detection, which depends on the primary melanoma depth, possible lymph node involvement, and the spread of melanoma to distant sites [56].

### 2.7.2 Risk Factors

Risk factors for melanoma may be extrinsic and intrinsic [56, 57, 58]:

**Extrinsic**
- Sun exposure
- Artificial tanning
- Immunosuppression
- Various environmental exposures

**Intrinsic**
- Pigmentary characteristics (spots)
- Family history
- Fair skin, blond or red hair, blue eyes, and freckles
- Race or ethnic origins
- Age

### 2.7.3 Signs and Symptoms

Although melanoma can occur in any part of the body, in women, it occurs most commonly in the extremities and, in men, in the torso or head and neck [59]. The first sign of melanoma is a change in the size, shape, or color of an existing stain, and also the presence of itching, bleeding, or ulcerations [56, 58]. The stain can become irregular and hard and is usually painless [56].

### 2.7.4 Detection

Melanoma diagnosis occurs basically through the lesion biopsy for pathological examination, histological examination, and microstaging according to the five levels described by Clark and by tumor thickening in millimeters, according to Breslow's classification. The lesion should never be scraped or cauterized [59]. Based on the results of the physical evaluation, family history, and pathological report, additional tests such as ultrasound, computerized tomography, magnetic resonance imaging, or positron emission tomography may also be included, according to the patient clinical status and the severity of the disease [56].

When the lesion is larger than 1 mm thick or ulcerated, it is recommended to research lymph node [56].

### 2.7.5 Staging

Clinical staging of neoplasms is based on the tumor spreading to regional lymph nodes or distant sites. For the disease that is clinically at the primary site, the chance of lymph node involvement or the presence of systemic metastases increases as the thickness and depth of local invasion increase, with a worse prognosis. The microstage of malignant melanoma is determined on histological examination by the vertical thickness of the lesion in millimeters (Breslow) and/or by the anatomical level of local invasion (Clark) [56].

Melanoma staging is based on clinical and pathological criteria, closely corresponding to the classification by the traditional TNM system, developed by the AJCC.

**Classification T** [60]

- *TX:* Primary tumor cannot be assessed (e.g., curettage or severely regressed melanoma).
- *T0*: No evidence of primary tumor.
- *Tis*: Melanoma in situ.
- *T1a*: Thickness ≤ 1.0 mm, Breslow <0.8 mm without ulceration.
- *T1b:* Thickness ≤ 1.0 mm, Breslow 0.8–1.0 mm with or without ulceration or ≤ 0.8 mm with ulceration.
- *T2a*: Thickness > 1.0–2.0 mm, without ulceration.
- *T2b*: Thickness > 1.0–2.0 mm, with ulceration.
- *T3a*: Thickness > 2.0–4.0 mm, without ulceration.
- *T3b*: Thickness > 2.0–4.0 mm, with ulceration.
- *T4a*: Thickness > 4.0 mm, without ulceration.
- *T4b*: Thickness > 4.0 mm, with ulceration.

**Classification N** [60]

- *NX*: Patients in whom the regional nodes cannot be assessed (e.g., previously removed for another reason).
- *N0*: No regional metastases detected.
- *N1a*: 0–1 node, clinically occult, no MSI (any satellite, locally recurrent, or in transit lesions).
- *N1b*: 0–1 node, clinically detected, no MSI.
- *N1c*: 0–1 node, 0 nodes, MSI present.
- *N2a*: 1–3 nodes, 2–3 nodes clinically occult, no MSI.
- *N2b*: 1–3 nodes, 2–3 nodes clinically detected, no MSI.
- *N2c*: 1–3 nodes, 1 node clinical or occult, MSI present.
- *N3a*: >1 node, >3 nodes, all clinically occult, no MSI.
- *N3b*: >1 node, >3 nodes, ≥1 clinically detected or matted, no MSI.
- *N3c*: >1 node, >1 node clinical or occult, MSI present.

**Classification M** [60]

- *MO*: No evidence of distant metastasis.
- *M1a:* Distant metastasis to skin, soft tissue including muscles, and/or nonregional lymph node.
- *M1b*: Distant metastasis to lung with or without M1a sites of disease.

- *M1c*: Distant metastasis to non-CNS visceral sites with or without M1a or M1b sites of disease.
- *M1d*: Distant metastasis to CNS with or without M1a, M1b, or M1c sites of disease.

**Clinical Staging** [60]
- *Stage 0*: (Tis, N0, M0).
- *IA*: (T1a, No, M0).
- *IB*: (T1b, No, M0); (T2a, N0, M0).
- *IIA*: (T2b, N0, M0); (T3a, N0, M0).
- *IIB*: (T3b, N0, M0); (T4a, N0, M0).
- *IIC*: (T4b, N0, M0).
- *III*: (Any T, N $\geq$ 1, M0).
- *IV*: (Any T, Any N, M1).

**Pathologic Staging** [60]
- *Stage 0*: (Tis, N0, M0).
- *IA*: (T1a, N0, M0); (T1b, N0, M0).
- *IB*: (T2a, N0, M0).
- *IIA*: (T2b, N0, M0); (T3a, N0, M0).
- *IIB*: (T3b, N0, M0); (T4a, N0, M0).
- *IIC*: (T4b, N0, M0).
- *IIIA*: (T1-T2a, N1a, M0); (T1-T2a, N2a, M0).
- *IIIB*: (T0, N1b-N1c, M0); (T1-T2a, N1b-N1c, M0); (T1-T2a, N2b, M0); (T2b-T3a, N1a-N2b, M0).
- *IIIC*: (T0, N2b-N2c, M0); (T0, N3b-N3c, M0); (T1a-T3a, N2c-N3c, M0); (T3b-T4a, Any N, M0); (T4b, N1a-N2c, M0).
- *IIID*: (T4b, N31-N3c, M0).
- *IV*: (Any T, Any N, M1).

### 2.7.6 Histopathological and Molecular Classification

Melanoma cells are generally classified according to histological types, and approximately, 70% of confirmed melanomas are of superficial dissemination subtype, which is the most common type, and corresponds to stage 0 melanoma [61].

#### 2.7.6.1 Melanoma Subtypes [60]

*Superficial spreading*: Arises from existing nevus.

*Nodular*: Absence of a radial growth phase, variable presentation, and robust vertical invasion.

*Lentigo maligna*: Typically demonstrates slow progression, and frequently appears in sun-exposed areas (i.e., face, head, etc.).

*Acral lentiginous*: Has higher incidence in patients with darker skin pigmentation and frequently occurs on the palms, soles, and subungual spaces.

*Amelanotic*: Characteristic absence of pigmentation and are considered rare.

*Desmoplastic*: Rare melanoma seen in older adults that is characterized by scant spindle cells and minimal cellular atypia.

#### 2.7.6.2 Molecular Subtypes [56]

Melanoma can also be classified into molecular subtypes that are classified based on different genetic changes or mutations of melanoma cells. These genetic changes include [60]:

- *BRAF mutations*: About 50% of cutaneous melanomas.
- *NRAS mutations*: Around 20% of people with melanoma.
- *NF-1 mutations*: Around 10–15% of people with melanoma.
- *KIT mutations*: Occurs more commonly in melanomas that develop from mucus membranes, melanomas on the hands or feet, or melanomas that occur in chronically sun-damaged skin, such as lentigo maligna melanoma.

## 2.8 Prostate Cancer

### 2.8.1 Introduction and Epidemiology

Prostate is a small gland, whose main function is the production of semen, a liquid that assists in the protection and transport of spermatozoa. This is located below the bladder, in front of the rectum, and behind the penis base, and urethra passes between it. According to age, prostate size changes and has approximately the size of a walnut in the younger ones and an increased size in the older ones. Prostate enlargement in older men may be associated with a condition known as *benign prostatic hypertrophy* (BPH), which can cause urethra blockage; however this condition does not increase the risk of developing prostate cancer [62, 63].

Prostate tumor may be benign or malignant. The vast majority of prostate cancers are adenocarcinoma type, which develops from the glandular cells of the prostate, and there are the rarest types like small cell carcinomas, neuroendocrine tumors (other than small cell carcinomas), transitional cell carcinomas, and sarcomas [63].

Globally, prostate cancer represents the second most common type of cancer among men. According to the IARC publication, 1,414,259 new cases of prostate cancer were estimated worldwide for 2020, equivalent to 7.8% of all estimated cancers, and 375,304 deaths corresponding to 3.8% of deaths from all cancers [64]. For 2021, the number of new cases estimated by the *American Cancer Society* in the USA is approximately 248,530 and a total of 34,130 deaths [65]. About 60% of cases are diagnosed in men aged 65 years and over [62].

### 2.8.2 Risk Factors

Several factors may affect a man's risk of getting prostate cancer, such as [ 62, 63, 66]:

- Age: Rare in men younger than 40, more common in men older than 65.
- Endogenous hormone balance.
- Race/ethnicity: More often in African American men and in Caribbean men of African ancestry than in men of other races.
- Geography: North America, northwestern Europe, Australia, and on Caribbean islands the prostate cancer is most common.
- Family history: Prostate cancer develops because of a combination of shared genes and shared environmental or lifestyle factors. Having a father or brother with prostate cancer more than doubles a man's risk of developing this disease.
- Gene change.

And some factors with less clear effects on prostate cancer risk, such as [63]:

- Eating habits/diet
- Obesity
- Smoking
- Chemical exposures
- Inflammation of the prostate

### 2.8.3 Signs and Symptoms

Signs and symptoms include but are not limited to [62, 63]:

- Urine: Trouble urinating, frequent urination, weak or interrupted urine flow, the urge to urinate frequently at night
- Blood in the urine
- Weakness or numbness in the legs or feet, or even loss of bladder or bowel control from cancer pressing on the spinal cord
- Erectile dysfunction
- Discomfort or pain when sitting, caused by an enlarged prostate

Some of these symptoms are not only caused by prostate cancer, but they may also, for example, be related to other conditions such as urinary tract infections and benign prostatic hyperplasia [62, 63].

### 2.8.4 Detection

Often, a tumor in the prostate grows slowly, does not spread rapidly through other parts of the body, and does not cause symptoms for years. For this reason, men with prostate cancer can live with good quality of life for a long time [63]. In patients with suspected prostate cancer, initial tests include total prostate-specific antigen (serum PSA) level (a protein released by prostate tissues), rectal examination (DRE), and biomarkers. Most healthy men have blood PSA levels below 4 ng/L of blood; however this does not guarantee that a man does not have prostate cancer. Blood PSA levels between 4 and 10 ng/L (borderline range) increase the risk by 25%, and if the PSA is above 10 ng/L, the chance of having prostate cancer is greater than 50%. There are controversies for screening prostate cancer through PSA dosage in patients without signs and symptoms of the disease. This screening can detect tumors in early stages, very slow growth and without risk of life, but results in unnecessary treatments that can cause side effects and affect the patient's quality of life. Therefore, the *American Cancer Society* (ASCO) and the *American Urological Association* recommend that individuals, before starting a screening with the PSA test, should evaluate with the physician the risks and benefits [62, 63].

Another test option includes the free PSA dosage, found in the bloodstream, and not bound to proteins, which measures the free PSA rate compared to total PSA [62, 63].

Rectal examination is not exactly accurate, but allows evaluating possible changes in gland size, since prostate cancer usually begins at the back of the gland and can be felt during a rectal examination [62, 63].

Other laboratory tests include complete blood count, renal function (urea, creatinine), liver function (bilirubin, coagulogram, albumin, AST, and ALT), renal function, alkaline phosphatase, and testosterone [67].

Biomarker tests for prostate cancer include the *Prostate Health Index* (PHI) and the 4 K score. In general, these two tests combine results from different types of PSA to get an overall score of a man's chance of having prostate cancer [62, 63]. For abnormal results of PSA and DRE tests, imaging scans such as prostate magnetic resonance imaging (MRI) scan and transrectal ultrasound (TRUS) are generally requested, and, according to the results, a biopsy is made for a definitive diagnosis [62]. For individuals with advanced prostate cancer, ASCO recommends performing one or more imaging tests between full-body bone tomography, CT scan, *magnetic resonance imaging* (MRI), and positron emission tomography (PET) or PET-CT scan [62].

### 2.8.5 Staging

The TNM system developed by AJCC (2018) evaluates the clinical and pathological prognostic stage from histological examination of the surgical resection sample [62]. The TNM System classifies prostate cancer into 4 stages (I, II, III, and IV) that combine TNM grouping at PSA levels and risk groups (according to Gleason Score) [68]. Gleason Score is based on the characteristics of the cells found in the biopsy, how much they look healthy or not when analyzed under a microscope, and is closely related to their clinical behavior [62].

Clinical staging (cT) is done from physical examinations, such as rectal examination (DRE); laboratory tests, such as PSA serum dosage and Gleason Score. From these results it is possible to identify whether imaging tests, such as x-rays, bone scans, CT scans, or MRI, may be required. And the pathological staging (pT) is done from the pathological analysis of prostate tissue, removed during surgery, and some lymph nodes usually included in the surgery [62, 63, 68].

#### 2.8.5.1 TNM Classification [62, 63, 68]

**Primary Tumor Classification (T): Clinical T (cT)**

- *TX*: Primary tumor cannot be assessed.
- *T0*: No evidence of primary tumor.
- *T1:* Clinically inapparent tumor that is not palpable; *T1a:* Tumor incidental histologic finding in 5% or less of tissue resected; *T1b:* Tumor incidental histologic finding in more than 5% of tissue resected; *T1c:* Tumor identified by needle biopsy found in one or both sides, but not palpable.
- *T2:* Tumor is palpable and confined within the prostate; *T2a:* Tumor involves one-half of one side or less; *T2b:* Tumor involves more than one-half of one side but not both sides; *T2c:* Tumor involves both sides.
- *T3:* Extra prostatic tumor that is not fixed or does not invade adjacent structures; *T3a:* Extra prostatic extension (unilateral or bilateral); *T3b:* Tumor invades seminal vesicle(s).

- *T4*: Tumor is fixed or invades adjacent structures other than seminal vesicles such as external sphincter, rectum, bladder, levator muscles, and/or pelvic wall.

**Primary Tumor Classification (T): Pathological T (pT)**

- *T2*: Organ confined.
- *T3*: Extra prostatic extension; *T3a*: Extra prostatic extension (unilateral or bilateral) or microscopic invasion of bladder neck; *T3b*: Tumor invades seminal vesicle(s).
- *T4*: Tumor is fixed or invades adjacent structures other than seminal vesicles such as external sphincter, rectum, bladder, levator muscles, and/or pelvic wall.

**Regional Lymph Nodes (N)**

- *NX*: Regional nodes were not assessed.
- *N0*: No positive regional nodes.
- *N1*: Metastases in regional node (s).

**Distant Metastasis (M)**

- *M0*: No distant metastasis.
- *M1*: Distant metastasis; *M1a*: Non-regional lymph node(s); *M1b*: Bone(s); *M1c*: Other site(s) with or without bone disease.

#### 2.8.5.2 TNM Stages of Prostate Cancer [63]

*Stage I:* cT1a-c, cT2a; N0; M0; PSA $<$ 10; Grade Group 1 *or* pT2; N0; M0; PSA $<$ 10; Grade Group 1. Early stage and PSA levels are low.

*Stage IIA:* cT1a-c, cT2a, pT2; N0; M0; $10 \leq$ PSA $<$ 20; Grade Group 1 *or* cT2b-c, pT2; N0; M0; PSA $<$ 20; Grade Group 1. Cancer cells are well differentiated, and PSA levels are medium.

*Stage IIB:* T1–2; N0; M0; PSA $<$ 20; Grade Group 2. Cancer cells are moderately differentiated, and PSA levels are medium.

*Stage IIC:* T1–2; N0; M0; PSA $<$ 20; Grade Group 3 *or* T1–2; N0; M0; PSA $<$ 20; Grade Group 4. Cancer cells are moderately or poorly differentiated and PSA levels are medium.

*Stage IIIA:* T1–2; N0; M0; PSA ≥ 20; Grade Group 1–4. A locally advanced cancer, and PSA level is high.

*Stage IIIB:* T3–4; N0; M0; any PSA; Grade Group 1–4. A locally advanced cancer, it is grown outside of the prostate gland and may have invaded nearby structures, such as the bladder or rectum.

*Stage IIIC:* any T; N0; M0; any PSA; Grade Group 5. Tumor cells are poorly differentiated, and they look very different the healthy cells.

*Stage IVA:* any T; N1; M0; any PSA; any Grade Group. Cancer has spread to the regional lymph nodes.

*Stage IVB:* any T; any N; M1; any PSA; any Grade Group. Cancer has spread to distant lymph nodes, other parts of the body, or to the bones.

#### 2.8.5.3 Gleason Score [69]

Gleason Score assesses the histological grade of prostate cancer, and its stratification correlates the pathological stage and prognosis. The score ranges from 3 to 5, based on tissue analysis from two different locations, and the scores are summed up to get an overall score ranging from 6 to 10. Then 5 distinct grades (Grade Group) are determined, where group 5 indicates a more aggressive tumor and therefore worse prognosis, and group 1 a less aggressive tumor, with a higher grade of differentiation and better prognosis [62, 63, 69].

- *Gleason 6*: Cells are well differentiated. Cancer is likely to grow very slowly, if at all.
- *Gleason 7*: Cells are moderately differentiated. Cancer is likely to grow at a moderate rate.
- *Gleason 8:* Some cells look abnormal. Cancer might grow quickly or at a moderate rate.
- *Gleason 9 or 10:* Cells are poorly differentiated or undifferentiated.

#### 2.8.5.4 Grade Groups [69, 70]

- *Grade group 1:* Gleason 6 (3 + 3 = 6).
- *Grade group 2:* Gleason 7 (3 + 4 = 7).
- *Grade group 3:* Gleason 7 (4 + 3 = 7).
- *Grade Group 4:* Gleason 8 (4 + 4 = 8; 3 + 5 = 8 or 5 + 3 = 8).
- *Grade Group 5:* Gleason 9 or 10 (4 + 5 = 9; 5 + 4 = 9 or 5 + 5 = 10).

### 2.8.6 Histopathological and Molecular Classification

Prostate epithelium is formed by basal, intermediate, luminal, and neuroendocrine cells. The most common histology found in prostate cancer is called adenocarcinoma. Other, less common histologic types include neuroendocrine prostate cancer and small cell prostate cancer. These rare variants tend to be more aggressive, produce much less PSA, and spread outside the prostate earlier [66, 69].

#### 2.8.6.1 Molecular Classification

Although new microdissection techniques and laser capture microscopy of individual neoplastic lesions, and also cell classification techniques have emerged, prostate cancer is still cytogenetically poorly characterized, partly due to technical limitations and the reduction in the number of radical prostatectomies, the main source for obtaining material for analysis. Prostate neoplastic lesions are multifocal, that is, samples from nearby regions can be genetically different (non-clonal), suggesting that lesions may evolve independently and hinder the definition of disease progression mechanisms [66].

*BRCA1* and *BRCA2* genes are linked to an increased risk of breast and ovarian cancers in some families. Inherited mutations of the *BRCA1* or *BRCA2* genes can increase prostate cancer risk in men (especially mutations in *BRCA2*) [62].

## 2.9 Stomach

### 2.9.1 Introduction and Epidemiology

Stomach cancer is slow developing, rarely causing symptoms in the early stages, and so, screening is justified only in populations with a history of high incidence of the disease. This cancer develops from changes in the stomach mucosa, and its location is essential to plan therapy; for example, a tumor in the gastroesophageal junction can be staged and treated as esophageal cancer [71].

This is the fifth most common cancer in the world, and its survival varies greatly as it spreads. The localized tumor has a 5-year survival of 70%, while the metastatic tumor has only 6% survival. The most common type is adenocarcinoma, which accounts for 95% of cases. Other types of tumors that are found in this organ are lymphomas and sarcomas, gastrointestinal stromal tumors (GIST), and carcinoid. Other rarer types are squamous cell carcinoma, leiomyosarcoma, and small cell carcinoma [71].

### 2.9.2 Risk Factors

- 2 times more incidents in men and usually affects individuals over 60 years.
- Diet is largely responsible for the development of the disease, including the consumption of salted, smoked, and pickled foods, alcohol, and tobacco.
- *H. pylori* infection.
- Previous stomach surgery.
- Pernicious anemia.
- Obesity.
- Achlorhydria.
- Family history of the disease.
- Ethnicity: Higher incidence in Hispanics, blacks, and Asians [72, 73].

- Elderly with atrophic gastritis or pernicious anemia, patients with sporadic gastric adenomas, familial adenomatous polyposis, or hereditary nonpolyposis colon cancer are more likely to develop stomach cancer. As well as immigrant populations from high-incidence regions, workers in the rubber and coal industry also have an increased predisposition [74].

### 2.9.3 Signs and Symptoms

The disease signs are:

- Lack of appetite, with abdominal pain and discomfort and a feeling of fullness in the upper abdomen after a light meal
- Heartburn or poor digestion
- Episodes of nausea and vomiting
- Diarrhea or constipation
- Swelling or accumulation of fluid in the abdomen

In more advanced stages the patient has symptoms of weakness, weight loss, anemia, and blood in vomiting or stool [72, 73].

### 2.9.4 Detection

For the disease diagnosis it is recommended to elaborate the medical history and perform imaging tests such as endoscopy, and if necessary, biopsy guided by endoscopy or tomography. Other tests such as x-ray, CT scanning, endoscopic ultrasound, PET-scan, MRI scanning, and laparoscopy help to confirm the diagnosis [75].

Laboratory tests such as blood count (presence of anemia) with platelet counts, blood test in the feces, and liver and kidney function tests are added to the imaging tests. Determine, if possible, the Siewert classification of the tumor of the gastroesophageal junction. Other tests that can be used are echoendoscopy, PET-CT, and laparoscopy with peritoneal lavage cytology [75, 76].

### 2.9.5 Staging

According to 2018 AJCC, the TNM system is used [77], where T means the primary tumor extension, with the evolution assessed through the stomach wall layers (mucosa, submucosa, muscular, subserosa, and serosa); N indicates the involvement of regional lymph nodes; and M indicates metastases in liver and lungs [78, 79, 80].

Stages 0 to IB: cancer has not spread to nearby lymph nodes or distant parts of the body

**Stage 0**

- *Tis N0 M0:* There is high grade dysplasia in the stomach lining, or there are cancer cells only in the innermost layer of the stomach, that have not grown into deeper layers of tissue such as the lamina propria.

**Stage IA**

- *T1 N0 M0:* The main tumor has grown from the top layer of cells of the mucosa into the next layers below such as the lamina propria, the muscularis mucosa, or submucosa.

**Stage IB**

- *T1 N1 M0:* The main tumor has grown from the top layer of cells of the mucosa into the next layers below, such as the lamina propria, the muscularis mucosa, or submucosa, and cancer has spread to 1–2 nearby lymph nodes.
- *T2 N0 M0:* The main tumor is growing into the muscularis propria layer. Cancer has not spread to nearby lymph nodes.

- *Stages IIA to III C*: Cancer has not spread to distant parts of the body.

**Stage IIA**

- *T1 N2 M0:* The main tumor has grown from the top layer of cells of the mucosa into the next layers below, such as the lamina propria, muscularis mucosa, or submucosa, and cancer has spread to 3–6 nearby lymph nodes.

- *T2 N1 M0:* The main tumor is growing into the muscularis propria layer, and cancer has spread to 1–2 nearby lymph nodes.
- *T3 N0 M0:* The main tumor is growing into the subserosa layer. Cancer has not spread to nearby lymph nodes.

**Stage IIB**

- *T1 N3a M0:* The main tumor has grown from the top layer of cells of the mucosa into the next layers below such as the lamina propria, muscularis mucosa, or submucosa, and cancer has spread to 7–15 nearby lymph nodes.
- *T2 N2 M0:* The main tumor is growing into the muscularis propria layer, and cancer has spread to 3–6 nearby lymph nodes.
- *T3 N1 M0:* The main tumor is growing into the subserosa layer (T3), and cancer has spread to 1–2 nearby lymph nodes.
- *T4a N0 M0:* The main tumor has grown through the stomach wall into the serosa, but it has not grown into any of the nearby organs or structures. Cancer has not spread to nearby lymph nodes.

**Stage IIIA**

- *T2 N3a M0:* The main tumor is growing into the muscularis propria layer, and cancer has spread to 7–15 nearby lymph nodes.
- *T3 N2 M0:* The main tumor is growing into the subserosa layer, and cancer has spread to 3–6 nearby lymph nodes.
- *T4a N1 M0:* The main tumor has grown through the stomach wall into the serosa, but it has not grown into any of the nearby organs or structures. Cancer has spread to 1–2 nearby lymph nodes.
- *T4a N2 M0:* The main tumor has grown through the stomach wall into the serosa, but it has not grown into any of the nearby organs or structures. Cancer has spread to 3–6 nearby lymph nodes.
- *T4b N0 M0:* The main tumor has grown through the stomach wall and into nearby organs or structures. Cancer has not spread to nearby lymph nodes.

**Stage IIIB**

- *T1 N3b M0:* The main tumor has grown from the top layer of cells of the mucosa into the next layers below such as the lamina propria, the muscularis mucosa, or submucosa, and cancer has spread to 16 or more nearby lymph nodes.
- *T2 N3b M0:* The main tumor is growing into the muscularis propria layer, and cancer has spread to 16 or more nearby lymph nodes.
- *T3 N3a M0:* The main tumor is growing into the subserosa layer, and cancer has spread to 7–15 nearby lymph nodes.
- *T4a N3a M0:* The main tumor has grown through the stomach wall into the serosa, but it has not grown into any of the nearby organs or structures, and cancer has spread to 7–15 nearby lymph nodes.
- *T4b N1 M0:* The main tumor has grown through the stomach wall and into nearby organs or structures. Cancer has spread to 1–2 nearby lymph nodes.
- *T4b N2 M0:* The main tumor has grown through the stomach wall and into nearby organs or structures. Cancer has spread to 3–6 nearby lymph nodes.

**Stage IIIC**

- *T3 N3b M0:* The main tumor is growing into the subserosa layer, and cancer has spread to 16 or more nearby lymph nodes.
- *T4aN3bM0:* The main tumor has grown through the stomach wall into the serosa, but it has not grown into any of the nearby organs or structures, and cancer has spread to 16 or more nearby lymph nodes.
- *T4b N3a M0:* The main tumor has grown through the stomach wall and into nearby organs or structures, and cancer has spread to 7–15 nearby lymph nodes.
- *T4b N3b M0:* The main tumor has grown through the stomach wall and into nearby organs or structures, AND cancer has spread to 16 or more nearby lymph nodes.

**Stage IV**

- *Any T Any N M1:* Cancer might or might not have grown into any of the layers of the stomach wall, and it might or might not have spread to nearby lymph nodes. Cancer has spread to distant organs such as the liver, lungs, brain, or the peritoneum.

**Note**

- *TX:* Main tumor cannot be assessed due to lack of information.
- *T0:* No evidence of a primary tumor.
- *NX:* Regional lymph nodes cannot be assessed due to lack of information.

### 2.9.6 Histopathological and Molecular Classification

The 2010 WHO classification recognizes four major histologic patterns of gastric cancers: tubular, papillary, mucinous, and poorly cohesive (including signet ring cell carcinoma), plus uncommon histologic variants [81].

#### 2.9.6.1 Molecular Classification

Stomach cancer is related to:

- Presence of Epstein Barr Virus.
- Detection of microsatellite instability (MSI) (high level, low level, or stable).
- Defect in a mismatch repair gene (dMMR).
- Tumor mutational burden (TMB).
- NTRK genes, protein p53, CMET, HER2, EGFR, VEGR [77, 82].
- Presence of HER2 protein (immunohistochemistry or FISH).
- PD-L1 has been important for the therapeutic decision [77].

## 2.10 Thyroid Cancer

### 2.10.1 Introduction and Epidemiology

Thyroid nodules are a common clinical problem; epidemiological studies show the worldwide prevalence of palpable nodules in approximately 5% of women and in 1% of men living with sufficient iodine. In contrast, a high-resolution ultrasound can detect nodules in 19–68% of randomly selected individuals, with a higher frequency in older women. In the United States approximately 63,000 new cases of cancer were diagnosed early in 2014, compared to 37,200 cases in 2009 when the last ATA Guideline (*American Thyroid Association*) was published; annual incidence was tripled from 4.9 per 100,000 in 1975 to 14.3 per 100,000 in 2009 [83]. GLOBOCAN estimated 586,202 new cases (3%) and 43,646 new deaths (0.4%) related to thyroid cancer in 2020 [84].

### 2.10.2 Risk Factors

The incidence of large tumors and mortality related to thyroid cancer has increased slightly, suggesting some factors, such as:

- Radiation exposure
- Thyroid carcinoma in first-degree relatives
- Iodine intake
- Obesity
- Diabetes
- Estrogen
- Reproductive factors
- Hashimoto's thyroid
- Lifestyle

### 2.10.3 Signs and Symptoms

Thyroid cancer can cause the following signs and symptoms:

- Swelling and lump in the neck, sometimes with rapid growth

- Pain in the front of the neck, sometimes even in the ears
- Hoarseness or constant change of voice (which does not disappear)
- Difficulty swallowing and breathing
- Constant cough that is not due to a cold
- Fatigue
- Appetite changes
- Weight changes

Many of these symptoms can be caused by other health conditions or even by other types of cancers in the neck area. Thyroid nodules are usually benign, but when one of these symptoms or signs appear, the patient should seek medical care for the identification and treatment of the cause [85].

### 2.10.4 Detection

The diagnosis of thyroid cancer should initially be made through clinical examination to evaluate the extent and site of the disease and distant manifestations of the tumor, such as tracheal and/or esophageal compression, or bone, pulmonary and cerebral metastases [86].

The initial detection of the nodule may be through palpation and/or an imaging examination. Thyroid nodule assessment includes TSH (thyroid stimulating hormone), ultrasound, and ultrasound-guided fine needle aspiration biopsy (FNAB) of the nodule. Cervical lymph node biopsy should also be performed, and in this case the thyroglobulin dosage in the sampled material increases the diagnosis sensitivity [87].

### 2.10.5 Staging

The TNM classification is also used for the staging of thyroid cancer according to 5 stages, from stage 0 to stage IV. In addition to the TNM system, papillary and follicular subtypes are also staged based on the patient age. Staging can be clinical or pathological; the clinical staging is based on the results of tests performed prior to surgery, which may include physical examination and imaging tests; and pathological staging is based on what was found during surgery, including biopsy [88].

**Classification (T): Primary Tumor** [88]

- *TX:* Primary tumor cannot be assessed.
- *T0:* No evidence of tumor.
- *T1:* Tumor has ≤2 cm and is limited to the thyroid.
- *T1a:* Tumor is ≤1 cm.
- *T1b:* Tumor has >1 cm but <2 cm.
- *T2*: Tumor has >2 cm but <4 cm and is limited to the thyroid.
- *T3*: Tumor is >4 cm, but the tumor does not extend beyond the thyroid.
- *T4*: Tumor has any size and extends beyond the thyroid.
- *T4a:* Tumor spreads beyond the thyroid to nearby soft tissues (larynx, trachea, esophagus, or recurrent laryngeal nerve).
- *T4b:* Tumor spreads beyond the regions mentioned in *T4a*.

**Classification (N): Regional Lymph Nodes** [88]

- *NX:* Regional lymph node cannot be assessed.
- *N0:* No evidence of cancer in regional lymph node.
- *N1*: Cancer spreads through the lymph nodes.
- *N1a*: Cancer spreads through the lymph nodes around the thyroid (central compartment).
- *N1b:* Cancer spreads through the central compartment.

**Classification (M): Distant Metastasis** [88]

- *MX:* Distant metastasis cannot be assessed.
- *M0*: Cancer has not spread to other parts of the body.
- *M1*: Cancer has spread to other parts of the body.

**Papillary or Follicular Thyroid Cancer in Individuals Under 55 Years of Age**

- *Stage I*: Tumor of any T, spread or not to the lymph node of any N and without distant metastasis.
- *Stage II:* Tumor of any T, with or without metastasis (M1), regardless of having spread to the lymph nodes (any N).

**Papillary or Follicular Thyroid Cancer in Individuals Aged 55 or More.**

- *Stage I* – T1N0M0.
- *Stage II* – (T2 or T3) N0M0.
- *Stage III* – T3 without spreading to the lymph nodes and without metastasis; or localized tumor (T1, T2, or T3) that spread to the central compartment of the lymph nodes (N1a) and without distant metastasis (M0).
- *Stage IVA* – T4a, regardless of whether it spread to the lymph nodes (any N) and without distant metastasis (M0), or localized tumor (T1, T2 or T3) that spread to the central compartment of the lymph nodes (N1b) and without distant metastasis (M0).
- *Stage IVB* – Tumor that has spread to nearby structures, regardless of whether it spreads to the lymph nodes (any N) and without distant metastasis (M0).
- *Stage IVC* – All tumors (any T and any N) when there is evidence of metastasis (M1).

**Medullary Thyroid Cancer**

- *Stage I:* T1N0M0.
- *Stage II:* (T2 or T3) N0M0.
- *Stage III*: Large and localized tumor (T2 or T3) that spreads through the central compartment of the lymph nodes (N1) and without metastasis (M0).
- *Stage IVA:* T4a, regardless of spreading through the lymph nodes (any N) and without distant metastasis (M0) or (T1, T2 or T3) spread throughout the central compartment of the lymph nodes (N1b) and without distant metastasis (M0).
- *Stage IVB:* T4b, regardless of spreading through the lymph nodes (any N) and without distant metastasis (M0).
- *Stage IVC:* Tumor with evidence of metastasis (any T and any N and M1).

**Anaplastic Thyroid Cancer**

- *Stage IV:* All anaplastic tumors are classified as stage IV, regardless of tumor size, location, or metastasis.

- *Stage IVA:* T4a, regardless of spreading to lymph nodes (any N) and without distant metastasis (M0).
- *Stage IVB:* T4b, regardless of spreading to lymph nodes (any N) and without distant metastasis (M0).
- *Stage IVC:* Tumor with evidence of metastasis (any T, any N and M1).
- *Recurrence:* Recurrent cancer occurs when the disease comes back after treatment; there will be another sequence of tests to assess the extent of this recurrence. These tests and imaging tests are often similar to those performed during the first diagnosis [6]

### 2.10.6 Histopathological and Molecular Classification

Papillary thyroid cancer accounts for 80–90% of all types of thyroid cancer, in women:men rate of 3:1. Follicular thyroid cancer, including Hürthle cell variant, accounts for about 10% of thyroid cancers, and is more malignant than papillary, with hematogenous dissemination. Medullary cancer is about 4% of thyroid tumors, composed of parafollicular cells (C cells), which produce calcitonin, caused by a mutation of the proto-oncogene RET. Anaplastic cancer is of undifferentiated type, which corresponds to about 1% of thyroid tumors and has a characteristic of rapid and painful growth [89].

Thyroid nodules are a common problem with the total prevalence of the population between 3% and 8% and most nodules are benign. Approximately 5% of nodules are malignant and generally have a good prognosis [90]. Ultrasound and fine needle biopsy (FNB) diagnoses correctly classify most cases. But when the cytological result is indeterminate (fundamentally Bethesda classification of Bethesda III and IV), the patient often undergoes surgery.

#### 2.10.6.1 Molecular Classification

Molecular markers are genetic mutations that show malignant thyroid cells that can be analyzed in fine needle biopsy fragments of thyroid tissue biopsy using molecular techniques. In papillary thyroid carcinoma, the best known is the BRAF mutation, present in 40–45% of cases, followed by RAS and RET/PTC in approximately 20% of cases. In follicular cancer, the RAS mutation is found in 40 to 50% of cases, followed by PAX8/PPARy translocation in 30 to 35% of cases [90].

## References


1. American Cancer Society Journals – ACS Journals register. https://acsjournals.onlinelibrary.wiley.com/doi/full/10.3322/caac.21660. Accessed on 10 Feb 2021.
2. American Cancer Society. Breast Cancer Facts & Figures 2019-2020. Atlanta: American Cancer Society, Inc 2019. Accessed on 31 Mar 2021.
3. International Agency for Research on Cancer register. https://gco.iarc.fr/today/fact-sheets-cancers. Accessed on 10 Feb 2021.
4. Instituto Nacional do Câncer-INCA register. https://www.inca.gov.br/tipos-de-cancer/cancer-de-mama/profissional- de-saude . Accessed on 10 Feb 2021.
5. BMJ Best Practice. Câncer de mama invasivo primário - Sintomas, diagnóstico e tratamento . https://bestpractice.bmj.com/topics/pt-br/716. Accessed on 10 Feb 2021.
6. SociedadeBrasileira de OncologiaClínica. https://sboc.org.br/images/diretrizes/lote-7/B/Diretrizes_SBOC_2020_-_Mama_adjuvante.pdf. Accessed on 12 Feb 2021.
7. American Cancer Society – The American Cancer Society register. https://www.cancer.org/cancer/breast-cancer/understanding-a-breast-cancer-diagnosis/stages-of-breast-cancer.html. Accessed on 12 Feb 2021.
8. Cancer.Net–American Society of Clinical Oncology register. www.cancer.net/cancer-types/breast-cancer/stages Accessed on 10 Feb 2021.
9. Breastcancer.org. Breast Cancer Stages. www.breastcancer.org/symptoms/diagnosis/staging. Accessed on 10 Feb 2021.
10. Cancer.Net–American Society of Clinical Oncology register.https://www.cancer.net/cancer-types/breast-cancer/introduction. Accessed on 10 Feb 2021.
11. Felix AS, Brinton LA. Cancer Progress and priorities: uterine Cancer. Cancer Epidemiol Biomarkers Prev. 2018;27(9):985–94. https://doi.org/10.1158/1055-9965.EPI-18-0264.
12. American Cancer Society Journals – ACS Journals register. https://acsjournals.onlinelibrary.wiley.com/doi/full/10.3322/caac.21660. Accessed on 18 Apr 2021.

13. Mayo Clinic – The Mayo Clinic register. www.mayoclinic.org/diseases-conditions/endometrial-cancer/symptoms-causes/syc-20352461. Accessed 04 Mar 2021.
14. Cancer.Net–American Society of Clinical Oncology register. www.cancer.net/cancer-types/uterine-cancer/risk-factors-and-prevention. Accessed on 3 Mar 2021.
15. The Memorial Sloan Kettering Cancer Center. The Memorial Sloan Kettering Cancer Center register. www.mskcc.org/cancer-care/types/uterine-endometrial/symptoms. Accessed on 3 Mar 2021.
16. American Cancer Society – The American Cancer Society register. www.cancer.org/cancer/endometrial-cancer/detection-diagnosis-staging/how-diagnosed.html.Accessed on 5 Mar 2021.
17. University of Rochester Medical Center – The University of Rochester Medical Center register. www.urmc.rochester.edu/encyclopedia/content.aspx?contenttypeid=34&contentid=17123-1.Accessed on 5 Mar 2021.
18. Katz A, Marques R, Novism Y et al. Câncer de Endométrio –In: Oncologia Clínica – Terapia Baseadaem Evidências, Editores: Artur Katz, Ricardo Marques, Yana Novism, Vanderson Rocha, Frederico P. Costa, Gustavo Dias dos S. Fernandes, Claudio Ferrari, Paulo M.G. Hoff- (Centro de Oncologia do Hospital SírioLibanês) 2ª 2014 (São Paulo) 350–353).
19. Pathology Outilines.com – The PathologyOutilines.com register. www.pathologyoutlines.com/topic/uterusendometrialcarc.html.Accessed on 6 Mar 2021.
20. Cancer.Net – American Society of Clinical Oncology register. https://www.cancer.net/cancer-types/colorectal-cancer. Accessed on 9 Mar 2021.
21. Arnold M, Sierra MS, Laversanne M, Soerjomataram I, Jemal A, Bray F. Global patterns and trends in colorectal cancer incidence and mortality. Gut. 2017;66(4):683–91. https://doi.org/10.1136/gutjnl-2015-310912.
22. National Cancer Institute register. https://www.cancer.gov/types/colorectal/hp. Accessed on 9 Mar 2021.
23. Weiser MR. AJCC 8th edition: colorectal Cancer. Ann Surg Oncol. 2018;25:1454–5. https://doi.org/10.1245/s10434-018-6462-1. Accessed on 9 Mar 2021.
24. Weisenberg E. Staging-carcinoma. PathologyOutlines.com website. https://www.pathologyoutlines.com/topic/colontumorstaging8ed.html. Accessed on 9 Mar 2021.
25. Up To Date. https://uptodate.com/contents/pathology-and-prognostic-determinants-of-colorectal-cancer. Accessed on 21 Apr 2021.
26. SociedadeBrasileira de Patologia. http://www.sbp.org.br/mdlhisto/sistema-digestivo-colon-reto-neoplasias/. Accessed on 21 Apr 2021.
27. BMJ Best Practice. Carcinoma de célulasrenais - Sintomas, diagnóstico e tratamento. Accessed on 31 Mar 2021.

28. American Cancer Society – The American Cancer Society register. https://www.cancer.org/cancer/kidney-cancer/about/key-statistics.html. Accessed on 31 Mar 2021.
29. Câncer de Rim. https://www.pfizer.com.br/sua-saude/oncologia/cancer-de-rim. Accessed on 27 Mar 2021.
30. American Cancer Society – The American Cancer Society register. https://www.cancer.org/cancer/kidney-cancer/causes-risks-prevention/risk-factors.html. Accessed on 27 Mar 2021.
31. Clevelandclinic.org. Kidney Cancer: Causes, Symptoms, Diagnosis & Treatments. https://my.clevelandclinic.org/health/diseases/9409-kidney-cancer-overview. Accessed on 31 Mar 2021.
32. Mayo Clinic – The Mayo Clinic register. https://www.mayoclinic.org/diseases-conditions/kidney-cancer/symptoms-causes/syc-20352664. Accessed on 31 Mar 2021.
33. Câncer renal - Distúrbiosrenais e urinários - Manual MSD VersãoSaúde para a Família register. https://www.msdmanuals.com/pt/casa/dist%C3%BArbios-renais-e-urin%C3%A1rios/c%C3%A2nceres-do-rim-e-do-trato-geniturin%C3%A1rio/c%C3%A2ncer-renal. Accessed on 31 Mar 2021.
34. National Kidney Foundation. Kidney Cancer - Symptoms, causes, and treatment. https://www.kidney.org/atoz/content/what-kidney-cancer. Accessed on 31 Mar 2021.
35. American Cancer Society – The American Cancer Society register. https://www.cancer.org/cancer/kidney-cancer/detection-diagnosis-staging/staging.html. Accessed on 31 Mar 2021.
36. UCLA Health. Kidney Cancer. Types of Kidney Cancer https://www.uclahealth.org/urology/types-of-kidney-cancer. Accessed on 31 Mar 2021.
37. Cancer.Net – American Society of Clinical Oncology register. https://www.cancer.net/cancer-types/kidney-cancer/introduction. Accessed on 30 Apr 2021.
38. William G. Kaelin Jr. Kidney Cancer pp 31-57.Molecular Biology of Kidney Cancer. https://link.springer.com/chapter/10.1007/978-3-319-17903-2_3. Accessed on 30 Apr 2021.
39. Cancer.Net-American Society of Clinical Oncology register. https://www.cancer.net/cancer-types/liver-cancer/introduction. Accessed on 15 Apr 2021.
40. Instituto Nacional do Câncer-INCA register. https://www.inca.gov.br/tipos-de-cancer/cancer-de-figado. Accessed on 15 Apr 2021.
41. Yang JD, Hainaut P, Gores GJ, Amadou A, Plymoth A, Roberts LR. A global view of hepatocellular carcinoma: trends, risk, prevention and management. Nat Rev Gastroenterol Hepatol. 2019;16(10):589–604. https://doi.org/10.1038/s41575-019-0186-y. Accessed on 15 Apr 2021.

42. The Global Cancer Observatory. Source: Globocan 2020. 40-All-cancers-excluding-non-melanoma-skin-cancer-fact-sheet.pdf. Accessed on 15 Apr 2021.
43. Singal AG, Lampertico P, Nahon P. Epidemiology and surveillance for hepatocellular carcinoma: new trends. J Hepatol. 2020;72(2):250–61. https://doi.org/10.1016/j.jhep.2019.08.025. Accessed on 19 Apr 2021.
44. Villanueva A. Hepatocellular Carcinoma. N Engl J Med. 2019;380:1450–62. https://doi.org/10.1056/NEJMra1713263. Accessed on 19 Apr 2021.
45. American Cancer Society – The American Cancer Society register.https://www.cancer.org/cancer/liver-cancer/detection-diagnosis-staging/staging.html. Accessed on 19 Apr 2021.
46. Curley SA, Jr Barnett CC, Abdalla EK. Staging and prognostic factors in hepatocellular carcinoma. UpToDate, Inc. All Rights Reserved. ©2021. Accessed on 19 Apr 2021.
47. Lee JS. The mutational landscape of hepatocellular carcinoma. Clin Mol Hepatol. 2015;21(3):220–9. https://doi.org/10.3350/cmh.2015.21.3.220. Accessed on 19 Apr 2021.
48. World Health Organization. International Agency for Research on Cancer. Cancer Today. https://gco.iarc.fr/today/home. Accessed on 31 Mar 2021.
49. American Cancer Society. Cancer Information and Resources. Lung. Key statistics. https://www.cancer.org/cancer/lung-cancer/about/key-statistics.html. Accessed on 31 Mar 2021.
50. American Cancer Society. Cancer Information and Resources. Lung Cancer. Causes and Risk Prevention. https://www.cancer.org/cancer/lung-cancer/causes-risks-prevention/risk-factors.html. Accessed on 31 Mar 2021.
51. National Health Service. Lung Cancer. Causes. https://www.nhs.uk/conditions/lung-cancer/causes/.Accessed on 31 Mar 2021.
52. National Health Service. Lung Cancer. Symptoms. https://www.nhs.uk/conditions/lung-cancer/symptoms/. Accessed 31 Mar 2021.
53. American Cancer Society. Lung Cancer. Detection and Diagnostic and staging. https://www.cancer.org/cancer/lung-cancer/detection-diagnosis-staging.html. Accessed on 31 Mar 2021.
54. National Comprehensive Cancer Network. Clinical Practice Guidelines in Oncology. Non-small cell lung cancer. Version 2.2021 – December 15, 2020. https://www.nccn.org/professionals/physician_gls/pdf/nscl.pdf. Accessed on 31 Mar 2021.
55. Araujo LH, Grupo Brasileiro de OncologiaTorácica, et al. Câncer de pulmão no Brasil. J Bras Pneumol [online]. 2018;44(1):55–64. ISSN 1806-3756. https://doi.org/10.1590/s1806-37562017000000135.
56. Cancer.Net – American Society of Clinical Oncology register. https://www.cancer.net/cancer-types/melanoma. Accessed on 1 Mar 2021.

57. Cancer.Network – Home of the journal *Oncology*. https://www.cancer-network.com/view/report-provides-latest-incidence-and-survival-statistics-melanoma. Accessed on 1 Mar 2021.
58. National Cancer Institute – Surveillance, Epidemiology, and End Results Program. https://seer.cancer.gov/statfacts/html/melan.html. Accessed 1 Mar 2021.
59. National Cancer Institute register. https://www.cancer.gov/types/skin/hp. Accessed on 1 Mar 2021.
60. Keung EZ, Gershenwald JE. The eighth edition American joint committee on Cancer (AJCC) melanoma staging system: implications for melanoma treatment and care. Expert Rev Anticancer Ther. 2018;18(8):775–84. https://doi.org/10.1080/14737140.2018.1489246.
61. Ward WH, Farma JM. Cutaneous melanoma: etiology and therapy [online]. Brisbane (AU): Codon Publications; 2017.
62. Cancer.Net - American Society of Clinical Oncology. Prostate Cancer. https://www.cancer.net/cancer-types/prostate-cancer. Accessed on 25 Apr 2021.
63. American Cancer Society. Prostate Cancer. https://www.cancer.org/cancer/prostate-cancer/about/what-is-prostate-cancer.html. Accessed on 25 Apr 2021.
64. The Global Cancer Observatory. Source: Globocan 2020. 40-All-cancers-excluding-non-melanoma-skin-cancer-fact-sheet.pdf. Accessed on 25 Apr 2021.
65. Siegel RL, Miller KD, Fuchs H, Jemal A. Cancer statistics, 2021. CA Cancer J Clin. 2021;71:7–33. https://doi.org/10.3322/caac.21654.
66. Grozescu T, Popa F. Prostate cancer between prognosis and adequate/proper therapy. J Med Life. 2017;10(1):5–12.
67. Sociedade Brasileira de Oncologia Clínica. Diretrizes do tratamentooncológico. SBOC 2021. Available at https://sboc.org.br/diretrizes-publicas/2021. Accessed on 25 Feb 2021.
68. American Cancer Society. Prostate Cancer - Early detection, diagnosis, and staging. https://www.cancer.org/cancer/prostate-cancer/detection-diagnosis-staging/staging.html. Accessed on 25 Apr 2021.
69. Cancer Research UK. Prostate Cancer - Stages, types, and grades. https://www.cancerresearchuk.org/about-cancer/prostate-cancer/stages. Accessed on 2 May 2021.
70. Humphrey PA. Histopathology of prostate Cancer. Cold Spring Harb Perspect Med. 2017;7(10):a030411.
71. American Cancer Society. Stomach Cancer. What is stomach cancer. https://www.cancer.org/cancer/stomach-cancer/about/what-is-stomach-cancer.html. Accessed on 31 Mar 2021.
72. American Cancer Society. Stomach Cancer. Risk Factors. https://www.cancer.net/cancer-types/stomach-cancer/risk-factors. Accessed on 31 Mar 2021.

73. National Health System. Stomach Cancer. Causes. https://www.nhs.uk/conditions/stomach-cancer/causes/ Accessed on 31 Mar 2021.
74. National Cancer Institute. Stomach Cancer. Stomach (Gastric) Cancer Prevention. Health Professional Version.https://www.cancer.gov/types/stomach/hp/stomach-prevention-pdq. Accessed on 31 Mar 2021.
75. American Society of Clinical Oncology. Stomach Cancer: Diagnosis. https://www.cancer.net/cancer-types/stomach-cancer/diagnosis. Accessed on 31 Mar 2021.
76. National Comprehensive Cancer Network. Clinical Practice Guidelines in Oncology. Stomach Cancer. Version 2.2021 – December 15, 2020. https://www.nccn.org/professionals/physician_gls/pdf/nscl.pdf. Accessed on 31 Mar 2021.
77. American Cancer Society. Stomach Cancer. Early Detection, Diagnosis, and Staging. Stomach Cancer Stages. https://www.cancer.org/cancer/stomach-cancer/detection-diagnosis-staging/staging.html Accessed on 31 Mar 2021.
78. American Society of Clinical Oncology. Stomach Cancer: Stages. https://www.cancer.net/cancer-types/stomach-cancer/stages. Accessed on 31 Mar 2021.
79. Sociedade Brasileira de Oncologia Clínica. Diretrizes de tratamentosoncológicosrecomendados pela SociedadeBrasileira de OncologiaClínica. Estômago: doençalocalizada. Estadiamento. https://sboc.org.br/images/diretrizes/lote-8/Estomago_Localizado_2020-Modelo%208.pdf. Accessed on 31 Mar 2021.
80. Barchi LC, et al. Brazilian gastric cancer association guidelines (part 1): an update on diagnosis, staging, endoscopic treatment, and follow-up. Arq Bras Cir Dig. 2020;33(3):e1535. São Paulo. Epub Dec 18, 2020. https://doi.org/10.1590/0102-672020200003e1535.
81. Canadian Cancer Society. Stomach Cancer. Grading and classifying stomach cancer. https://www.cancer.ca/en/cancer-information/cancer-type/stomach/grading/?region=on#:~:text=The%20Lauren%20classification%20is%20based,stomach%20cancer%2C%20look%20and%20behave. Accessed on 31 Mar 2021.
82. Ramos MFKP. Caracterização dos subtiposmoleculares do cancer gástrico por expressãogênica e proteica. São Paulo: Programa de CiênciasemGastroenterologia. Tese de doutorado. Faculdade de Medicina da Universidade de São Paulo; 2019. https://www.teses.usp.br/teses/disponiveis/5/5168/tde-03072019-152538/publico/MarcusFernandoKodamaPertilleRamos.pdf. Accessed on 31 Mar 2021.
83. Liebert MA. 2015 American Thyroid Association Management Guidelines for adult patients with thyroid nodules and differentiated Thyroid Cancer. Thyroid. 2016;26(1):1–33. [a] American Thyroid Association [a], Inc. https://doi.org/10.1089/thy.2015.0020.

84. American Cancer Society Journals – ACS Journals register: https://acs-journals.onlinelibrary.wiley.com/doi/full/10.3322/caac.21660. Accessed on 18 Apr 2021.
85. American Cancer Society. The American Cancer register. https://www.cancer.org/cancer/thyroid-cancer/detection-diagnosis-staging/siptom. Accessed on 15 Feb 2021.
86. Laura Fugazzolaa, Rossella Eliseic, Dagmar Fuhrerd, Barbara Jarzabe, Sophie Leboulleuxf, Kate Newboldg, Jan Smith. European thyroid association guidelines for the treatment and follow-up of advanced radioiodine-refractory thyroid cancer. Eur Thyroid J. 2019 (8):227–245 https://doi.org/10.1159/000502229.
87. Katz A, Marques R, Novism Y et al. Câncer de Tireóide – In: Oncologia Clínica – Terapia Baseadaem Evidências, Editores: Artur Katz, Ricardo Marques, Yana Novism et al. (Centro de Oncologia do Hospital SírioLibanês) 2ª edição. 2014: 87–88. São Paulo – Brazil.
88. Cancer.Net – American Society of Clinical Oncology register. https://www.cancer.net/cancer-types/thyroid-cancer/stages#:~:text=Medullary%20thyroid%20cancer,and%20no%20metastasis%20(M0). (2021). Accessed on 22 Feb 2021.
89. Cancer Research UK – The Cancer Research UK register: https://www.cancerresearchuk.org/about-cancer/thyroid-cancer/stages-types/types. Accessed on 18 Apr 2021.
90. Sociedade Brasileira de Patologia – The Sociedade Brasileira de Patologia register. http://www.sbp.org.br/mdlhisto/tireoide-neoplasias/?gclid=EAIaIQobChMI4Ki%2D%2DbyQ7wIVj4ORCh3S0QCdEAAYASAAEgIWffD_BwE (2021). Accessed on 22 Feb 2021.

# Hematological Diseases

# 3

Rafael Duarte Paes,
Douglas Coutinho Ribeiro da Costa,
Joyce Ferreira Viana,
and Hebe Mizuno Watanabe

## 3.1 Leukemias

Leukemia is a clonal proliferation of hematopoietic stem cells in the bone marrow. It is a common malignancy in children and adults that occurs when alterations in normal cell regulatory processes lead to uncontrolled proliferation of hematopoietic stem cells in the bone marrow [1, 2].

Leukemias can be divided into acute and chronic varieties, both of which have a myelocytic and lymphocytic type. Acute leukemias differ from chronic leukemias in that the former are characterized by an arrest at an early stage of maturation. The leukemia cells proliferate rapidly and have a prolonged reproductive life span. The presence of these cells inhibits normal hemopoiesis, resulting in granulocytopenia, thrombocytopenia, and anemia [1]. In adolescent and young adult populations, acute

R. D. Paes (✉)
Oncoclínicas, Sao Paulo, Brazil

D. C. R. da Costa
Hospital Samaritano, João Pessoa, PB, Brazil

J. F. Viana
Clínica São Germano Oncologia, São Paulo, SP, Brazil

H. M. Watanabe
Hospital Beneficência Portuguesa de São Paulo, São Paulo, SP, Brazil



C. W. P. Schmidt, K. M. Otoni (eds.), *The Golden Guide to Oncologic Pharmacy*, https://doi.org/10.1007/978-3-030-98596-7_3

leukemias are the most prevalent, with chronic myeloid leukemia being infrequently seen [3].

The acute leukemias are characterized by aberrant differentiation and proliferation of malignantly transformed hematopoietic stem cells. These cells accumulate within the bone marrow and lead to suppression of the growth and differentiation of normal blood cells [4].

In acute leukemia, abnormal blood cells remain immature and cannot perform proper functions, which causes the number of cancerous cells, and the disease progression, to increase quickly [5]. While in chronic leukemia, present cancerous cells are mature and retain their normal functions, which lead to a slow progression of the disease.

According to a review performed between 1990 and 2017, globally, while the number of newly diagnosed leukemia cases increased from 354.5 thousand in 1990 to 518.5 thousand in 2017, the age-standardized incidence rate (ASIR) decreased by 0.43% per year during the same period. The leukemia ASIR was higher in males than in females, whereas females experienced a more pronounced decrease in ASIR during the study period when compared to males [6].

For the sake of clarity, here we will divide leukemias classes, highlighting their differences.

## 3.2 Chronic Lymphocytic Leukemia (CLL)

### 3.2.1 Introduction and Epidemiology

Chronic lymphocytic leukemia (CLL) is the most common leukemia among adults in the Western world. CLL (and the corresponding nodal entity small lymphocytic lymphoma, SLL) is classified as a lymphoproliferative disorder characterized by the relentless accumulation of mature B-lymphocytes showing a peculiar immunophenotype in the peripheral blood, bone marrow, lymph nodes, and spleen. CLL clinical course is very heterogeneous: most patients follow an indolent clinical course with no or delayed treatment need and with a prolonged survival, while others experience aggressive disease requiring early treatment followed by frequent relapses [7].

Chronic lymphocytic leukemia (CLL) is the most frequent (30%) leukemia in the Western world. The median age at diagnosis is 70 years and there is a 2:1 male/female ratio.

### 3.2.2 Risk Factors

Etiology of CLL is unknown. No specific risk factors have been identified [8]. Several of the epidemiological studies aimed at identifying risk factors for CLL/SLL occurrence, but no acquired causative factors leading to CLL development have been identified so far. A genetic predisposition to disease development (family history of hematological malignancies – CLL and/or non-Hodgkin lymphomas, NHL) has been ascertained, and it is supported by several lines of evidence [7].

### 3.2.3 Signs and Symptoms

About 50–70% CLL patients are asymptomatic. The most frequent presentation is painless symmetrical lymphadenopathy. Other presenting features include systemic symptoms of weight loss, night sweats, tiredness, and features of bone marrow failure. Autoimmune complications especially hemolytic anemia and immune thrombocytopenia can occur. Infections are common due to hypogammaglobulinemia (Ajithkumar, T & Hatcher, H, 2011). Ten percent of patients can undergo transformation to a more aggressive tumor, most commonly diffuse large B-cell lymphoma, called Richter's syndrome [8].

### 3.2.4 Diagnosis

CLL is a proliferative disorder of monoclonal CD5+ B lymphocytes. The diagnostic consists of hematopathology review of the lymph node or bone marrow biopsy, flow cytometry of blood to check the presence of monoclonal B lymphocytes (≥5 × 10 [9]/L in peripheral blood), and the absolute monoclonal B lymphocyte count [9].

A direct Coombs test and serum immunoglobulin estimation is needed. Bone marrow examination helps to establish the extent and pattern of marrow involvement and to evaluate response to treatment [8].

### 3.2.5 Staging

Two staging systems are currently applied in CLL patients to define disease burden and treatment indication: Rai and Binet staging system. These two systems have many advantages as they are easy to define, being based only on complete blood cell count (CBC) and physical examination, and they have been shown to be powerful prognostic indicators [7]. The Rai staging system is based on progressively shorter overall survival, while Binet staging system is based on the number of lymphoid sites involved at physical exam (cervical, axillary, and inguinal nodes, hepatomegaly, splenomegaly) and the CBC values [10, 11].

## 3.3 Chronic Myeloid Leukemia (CML)

### 3.3.1 Introduction and Epidemiology

Chronic myeloid leukemia (CML) is characterized by progressive replacement of the normal elements of the marrow with mature myeloid cells no longer responsive to mechanisms that govern proliferation of normal myeloid cells. This results in an ever-increasing ratio of leukemic to normal myeloid cells [12].

Chronic myeloid leukemia (CML) accounts for 20% of leukemia. The median age at diagnosis is 55 years, and males are affected more frequently than females (male/female ratio of 1.3:1) [8].

### 3.3.2 Risk Factors

The only recognized risk factor for CML is prior radiation exposure.

### 3.3.3 Signs and Symptoms

The symptoms of CML result from the hypermetabolic state and splenomegaly associated with the huge expansion of myelopoiesis. Symptoms include weight loss, fever, sweats, and fatigue. Splenomegaly is present in the majority of patients at diagnosis. The total blood granulocyte pool is usually 10–100 times higher than normal. Myeloid cells of all levels of maturation are present in the blood; the number of primitive cells in the marrow tend to be higher. CML is also characterized by an increase in the number of eosinophils, basophils, monocytes, and lymphocytes in the blood. Thrombocytopenia at presentation should lead to suspicion that another diagnosis is required or that blastic phase of the disease is present. Anemia, if present, is mild. Circulating nucleated red blood cells are common [1].

The bone marrow aspirate is markedly hypercellular with the hyperplasia of all stages and classes of myeloid cells. The myeloid/erythroid ratio is markedly elevated with megakaryocytic hyperplasia. The proportion of immature myeloid elements (blast cells, promyelocytes, myelocytes) is increased relative to that of normal marrow. Focal myelofibrosis is present in the marrow of most patients at diagnosis [1].

Fifty percent of CML patients are asymptomatic and are diagnosed following an abnormal blood count. The remainder presents with non-specific symptoms of weight loss, excessive sweating, spontaneous bleeding, and pain due to splenic enlargement and hyperviscosity. Some patients with hyperuricemia present with a gout-like arthritis. Symptoms of advanced stage include general cachexia, fever, bone marrow failure, and bone pain [8].

### 3.3.4 Diagnosis

CML is characterized by the Philadelphia chromosome (Ph), which results from a reciprocal translocation between chromosomes 9 and 22. The translocation results in two fusion genes. One, on chromosome 22, consists of the proximal region of the BCR gene and the distal region of the ABL gene, which has moved from chromosome 9. A fusion gene that consists of the proximal portion of the ABL gene and the distal portion for BCR gene is also produced. Whereas the latter gene is expressed in some patients, the biologic significance of its expression is unknown. The normal ABL gene has tyrosine kinase activity and is probably involved in signal transduction. The BCR-ABL fusion gene product has increased tyrosine kinase activity and is capable of autophosphorylation, conferring to chronic myelogenous leukemia (CML) cells a proliferative advantage over the normal hemopoietic elements. That occurs in about 90–95% patients with CML [1, 8].

Patients with CML but without Ph chromosome may still have BCR-ABL rearrangement, which will behave similar to Ph + disease. Patients without Ph chromosome and BCR-ABL molecular abnormalities are classed as atypical CML, and they often need a different treatment approach [1].

Other Ph-negative patients with CML do not have CML but have a different myeloproliferative or myelodysplastic disorder. These patients tend to be older, and their course is more rapid than that of patients with CML; patients with Ph-negative CML often die in less than 1 year [1].

### 3.3.5 Staging

CML occurs in three different phases (chronic, accelerated, and blast phase) and is usually diagnosed in the chronic phase in the developed world. Untreated chronic phase CML (CP-CML) will eventually progress to accelerated phase CML (AP-CML) or blast phase (BP-CML) in 3–5 years on average [11].

### 3.3.6 Histological and Molecular Classification

In CML, the genetic and cytogenetic changes play important roles in prognosis and treatment process. Philadelphia chromosome (Philadelphia (Ph) translocation t(9;22)(q34;q11)) is an important characteristic in CML. This translocation plays an important role not only in CML pathogenesis, but also in diagnosis since it is considered as a prognostic biomarker in this disease [13].

## 3.4 Acute Lymphoblastic Leukemia (ALL)

### 3.4.1 Introduction and Epidemiology

ALL is more common in men than in women and has a variable prevalence in different ethnic groups, being highest in the Hispanic population [3].

### 3.4.2 Risk Factors

For ALL, the topic of exposures and their role remains contentious. Some studies considered ionizing and non-ionizing (e.g., electromagnetic field [EMF]) radiation an established causal exposure for childhood ALL, as evidenced by the impact of the 1945 atomic bombs in Japan and by the modestly but significantly elevated risk caused by X-ray pelvimetry during pregnancy. Meta-analysis suggests a modestly elevated risk at high levels (>0.2μT), 15, but the reliability of this finding is uncertain. It is impossible to prove that EMF never causes ALL, but at most, it might be involved in only a small minority of cases.

Infection was the first suggested causal exposure for childhood ALL and remains the strongest candidate. Two specific hypotheses have been proposed, and both postulate that ALL results from an abnormal response to a common infection. It is important to continue exploring the possible biological mechanisms of infectious promotion of ALL, as they could eventually lead to prophylactic interventions [14].

### 3.4.3 Signs and Symptoms

The acute leukemia symptoms result from varying degrees of anemia, neutropenia, and thrombocytopenia or from infiltration into tissues. Although virtually any organ system may become involved once leukemia cells enter the peripheral blood, the lymph nodes, liver, spleen, central nervous system (CNS), and skin are the most common sites detected clinically [4].

### 3.4.4 Diagnosis

The diagnosis of ALL generally requires demonstration of more than 20% of bone marrow lymphoblastic, which includes flow cytometric immunophenotyping for molecular characterization of leukemic clone and minimal/measurable residual disease (MRD), morphologic assessment, and karyotyping. For stratification and treatment planning, the diagnosis requires testing for specific recurrent genetic abnormalities using FISH and RT-PCR testing BCR-ABL1 [11].

### 3.4.5 Histological and Molecular Classification

The FAB classification of ALL includes three subtypes (L1–L3), which are differentiated based on morphology, including cell size, prominence of nucleoli, and the amount and appearance of cytoplasm.

## 3.5 Acute Myeloid Leukemia (AML)

### 3.5.1 Introduction and Epidemiology

Acute myeloid leukemia (AML) is the most common acute type in adults [14, 15]. Although acute myeloid leukemia can occur in any age group, it is a predominant disease in older adults, with a median age at diagnosis of 68 years. The incidence of AML is rising, partly due to an increasing prevalence of therapy-related

AML as more patients with cancer treated with cytotoxic chemotherapy are cured of their primary malignancy [14, 15].

### 3.5.2 Risk Factors

AML reportedly is associated with exposure to chemotherapy and ionizing radiation, and also to chemicals that include petroleum products and organic solvents (benzene), herbicides, and pesticides (organophosphates) [8, 16]. The degree of risk depends on age, dose of radiation, and duration of exposure [5].

Many inherited conditions predispose children to the development of AML. Among these are Down syndrome, Fanconi anemia, severe congenital neutropenia (Kostmann syndrome), neurofibromatosis type 1, dyskeratosis congenita, and familial platelet disorder with a predisposition to AML [16].

### 3.5.3 Signs and Symptoms

The presentation of childhood AML reflects signs and symptoms that result from leukemic infiltration of the bone marrow and extramedullary sites. Replacement of normal bone marrow hematopoietic cells results in neutropenia, anemia, and thrombocytopenia. Children commonly present with signs and symptoms of pancytopenia, including fever, fatigue, pallor, bleeding, bone pain, and infections. Infiltration of extramedullary sites can result in lymphadenopathy, hepatosplenomegaly, chloromatous tumors (myeloblastomas and granulocytic sarcomas), disease in the skin (leukemia cutis), orbit, and epidural space, and, rarely, testicular involvement [16].

### 3.5.4 Diagnosis

The diagnosis of AML is made by the presence of more than 20% blasts in the peripheral blood or in the bone marrow, or through the presence of unique genetic abnormalities found in the bone marrow regardless of blast count [t(8;21), inv. [16], or t(15;17)]. In addition to morphological assessment of peripheral blood and bone marrow, immunophenotyping by flow cytometry is used at the time of diagnosis to confirm the myeloid origin of malignant blast populations and to aid in further categorization of acute myeloid leukemia subtype. Cytogenetic analysis and screening for commonly occurring gene mutations and rearrangements should also be done [15, 17].

### 3.5.5 Histological and Molecular Classification

In 1970, the French-American-British (FAB) classification of AML was developed by a group of French, American, and British leukemia experts. This group divided AML into subtypes, M0 through M7, based on the type of cell the leukemia develops from and how mature the cells are. According to the FAB classification, the subtypes M0 to M5 start in precursors of white blood cells, M6 AML originates in very early forms of red blood cells, and M7 AML starts in early forms of cells that form platelets [18].

In 2016, the World Health Organization updated the guidelines and distinguished in six groups of AML: AML with recurrent genetic abnormalities, AML with myelodysplasia-related changes, therapy-related myeloid neoplasms, AML not otherwise specified, myeloid sarcoma, and myeloid proliferations related to Down syndrome.

AML is further classified into three prognostic risk groups: favorable, intermediate, and adverse [1]. These are based on both cytogenetics and relatively recent recognition of molecular diseases subsets that are distinct from the contribution of cytogenetic risk. These newly recognized molecular subsets have different responses to standard therapeutics [17].

## 3.6 Lymphomas

### 3.6.1 Hodgkin Lymphoma

#### 3.6.1.1 Disease Overview

Hodgkin lymphoma (HL) is a type of lymphoma in which cancer originates from a specific type of white blood cells called lymphocytes. HL was recognized as a unique illness almost two centuries ago (1832 by Thomas Hodgkin). In 1898 and 1902, respectively, Carl Sternberg and Dorothy Reed independently described the cytogenetic features of the malignant cells of Hodgkin lymphoma, now called Reed–Sternberg cells; detailed descriptions of the typical microscopic appearance allowed confident separation of this type of lymphoma from other diseases causing similar symptoms and lymphadenopathy. Finally, and most importantly in terms of making clear the need for definite identification of the disease, curative treatments, initially with radiation therapy, and later multiagent chemotherapy, became available more than 50 years ago. Thus, Hodgkin lymphoma has been sufficiently, dependably, and accurately diagnosed that its specific patterns of presentation and clinical behavior are well understood [19, 20].

#### 3.6.1.2 Introduction and Epidemiology

Hodgkin lymphoma is an uncommon disorder with an annual incidence around 83,000 new cases (Globocan 2020) in the world according to International Agency for Research on Cancer (IARC). HL shows a bimodal distribution with a first peak in the third decade and a second peak after the age of 50. Men are affected by HL slightly more often than women among all subtypes, except for the nodular sclerosing subtype that occurs slightly more often in young females than in male patients. Among the group of young adults, the most common subtype is nodular-sclerosing (NS) HL occurring at a higher frequency than the mixed-cellularity (MC) subtype. The frequency of MC increases with age, while that of NS reaches a plateau in the group >30 years of age [21, 22].

#### 3.6.1.3 Risk Factors

The exact cause of Hodgkin lymphoma is unknown, but the following factors may raise a person's risk of developing Hodgkin lymphoma:

- Age: People between the ages of 15 and 40 and people older than 55 are more likely to develop Hodgkin lymphoma.
- Gender: In general, men are slightly more likely to develop Hodgkin lymphoma than women, although the nodular sclerosis subtype is more common in women (see epidemiology).

- Family history: Brothers and sisters of people with Hodgkin lymphoma have a higher chance of developing the disease, although the increase in risk is small.
- Virus exposure: The Epstein-Barr virus (EBV) causes infectious mononucleosis. Nearly all adult Americans and many others around the world have an EBV infection. About 20–25% of people with Classic HL in the United States have lymphoma cells that test positive for EBV. People with HIV also have a higher risk of developing Hodgkin lymphoma, particularly lymphocyte-depleted Hodgkin lymphoma [23].

#### 3.6.1.4 Signs and Symptoms

Common symptoms or signs caused by Hodgkin lymphoma include:

- Painless swelling of lymph nodes in the neck, underarm, or groin area that does not go away within a few weeks.
- Unexplained fever that does not go away.
- Unexplained weight loss.
- Night sweats, usually drenching.
- Pruritus, a generalized itching that may be severe.
- Fatigue.
- Pain in the lymph nodes triggered by drinking alcohol.
- Shortness of breath, cough, or chest discomfort may be caused if lymph nodes in the chest are affected.

Some of these symptoms described above are called "B symptoms" and helps describe disease in progress:

- Unexplained weight loss of more than 10% of original body weight during the 6 months before diagnosis.
- Unexplained fever, with temperatures above 100.4 °F (38 °C).
- Drenching night sweats. Many people with Hodgkin lymphoma say their nightclothes or the sheets on the bed were so wet they needed to be changed during the night. Sometimes, heavy sweating occurs during the day [23, 24].

#### 3.6.1.5 Diagnosis

The following tests may be used to help diagnose Hodgkin lymphoma. Not all tests listed below will be used for every person:

- Medical history and physical examination – detailed questions about medical history and a physical examination, which can identify whether the person has experienced some typical symptoms of Hodgkin (see Sect. 3.6.2.4).
- Biopsy or core needle biopsy – affected tissue lymph node. Biopsy of cHL usually has Reed–Sternberg cells. For people with nodular lymphocyte-predominant Hodgkin lymphoma, the Reed–Sternberg cells often look different and are called "LP" cells.

**Immunohistochemistry Evaluation**

Typical immunophenotype for cHL – CD15+, CD30+, PAX 5 + (weak), CD3-, CD20-(majority), CD45-, CD79a- .

Typical immunophenotype for NLPHL – CD20+, CD45+, CD79a+, BCL6+, PAX 5+, CD3-, CD15-, CD30-.

Laboratory tests: Blood tests may include a complete blood count (CBC) and an analysis of the different types of white blood cells, in addition to the erythrocyte sedimentation rate (ESR or "sed rate") and liver and kidney function tests. Blood tests alone cannot detect Hodgkin lymphoma.

Some factors that are considered less favorable and lead to a poorer prognosis include:

Age 45 and older; low blood albumin levels defined as less than 4 g/L; low hemoglobin, defined as less than 10.5 g/dL; white blood cell count that is more than 15,000 per cubic millimeter (mm3); lymphocyte count that is less than 600 per mm3; less than 8% of the total white blood cell count, or both; and a higher erythrocyte sedimentation rate especially for early-stage Hodgkin lymphoma.

**HIV and Hepatitis B/C Testing**

Computed tomography scan and magnetic resonance imaging (MRI). A mediastinal lymph node mass, located in the center of the chest, that is larger than 10 cm is associated with a poorer prognosis. Small mediastinal masses are not associated with a poorer prognosis. Having a high number of involved lymph node sites is associated with a poorer prognosis too.

Positron emission tomography (PET) or PET-CT scan. PET-CT scanning has become the standard for assessment of response in most lymphomas. For HL and fluorodeoxyglucose (FDG)-avid NHL subtypes, PET and PET-CT improve the accuracy of staging compared with CT scans for nodal and extranodal sites. PET-CT leads to change in stage in 10–30% of patients, more often upstaging, although alteration in management occurs in fewer patients, with no demonstrated impact on overall outcome. However, improving staging accuracy ensures that fewer patients are undertreated or overtreated.

*Some tests may be done if a person's treatment plan includes chemotherapy.*

Lung function tests: test of the diffusing capacity of the lungs for carbon monoxide (DLCO); a DLCO threshold of ≥60% is acceptable for use of bleomycin.

Heart evaluation: A heart evaluation, including an echocardiogram (ECHO) or a multigated acquisition (MUGA) scan (important for anthracycline-based chemotherapy).

Pregnancy test: for women of childbearing age.

Counseling for fertility: (fertility preservation), smoking cessation, and psychosocial [25–27].

### 3.6.1.6 Types of Hodgkin Lymphoma

The American Joint Committee on Cancer (AJCC) and World Health Organization (WHO) classifications recognize two major categories of Hodgkin lymphoma: classic Hodgkin lymphoma and nodular lymphocyte-predominant Hodgkin lymphoma.

### 3.6.1.7 Classification of Hodgkin Lymphoma

#### Classic Hodgkin Lymphoma (cHL)

Classic HL is the most common type of Hodgkin lymphoma. More than 90% of cases of Hodgkin lymphoma are within the cHL category. cHL is diagnosed when certain abnormal lymphocytes, known as Reed–Sternberg cells, are found. cHL is divided into four subtypes according to the cellular composition of the background infiltrate; this type of cells are typically positive for CD30 (an activation marker) and for CD15 (an antigen associated with the granulocyte and monocyte lineages), while they usually lack expression of CD45 and of molecules characteristic of the B- and T-cell lineages.

Genetic – mutations in genes *STAT6*, *SOCS1*, *PDL1/PDL2* alterations, *CIITA* rearrangements.

Nodular sclerosis Hodgkin lymphoma: In addition to Reed–Sternberg cells, there are bands of connective tissue (called fibrosis) found in the lymph node. This type of lymphoma often affects the lymph nodes in the central part of the chest, called the mediastinum.

Lymphocyte-rich classic Hodgkin lymphoma: It usually affects areas other than the mediastinum. In addition to Reed–Sternberg cells, the lymph node tissue contains many normal lymphocytes.

Mixed cellularity Hodgkin lymphoma: This subtype sometimes develops in the abdomen and carries many different cell types, including large numbers of Reed–Sternberg cells.

Lymphocyte-depleted Hodgkin lymphoma: is the least common subtype of cHL. Only about 1% of people with cHL have this subtype. It is most common in older adults; people with the human immunodeficiency virus (HIV), and people in non-industrialized countries. The lymph node contains almost all Reed–Sternberg cells.

### Nodular Lymphocyte-Predominant Hodgkin Lymphoma

Nodular lymphocyte-predominant Hodgkin lymphoma is more similar to B-cell non-Hodgkin lymphoma. People with this type of Hodgkin lymphoma have large cells in the affected area called "popcorn cells" or "LP cells" that have a marker called CD20 on their surface and different of cHL these cells lack CD30 and CD15.

Genetic – mutations in genes *DUSP2, JUN, SGK1, SOCS1, BCL6* rearrangements [23, 28].

#### 3.6.1.8 Hodgkin Lymphoma Staging

The staging system used for Hodgkin lymphoma is the Lugano classification, which is based on the older Ann Arbor system. It has four stages, labeled I, II, III, and IV; the stage of Hodgkin lymphoma describes the extent of the spread of the tumor. As explained in Symptoms and Signs, each stage may also be further divided into "A" and "B" categories, based on whether or not the person is experiencing specific symptoms.

Bulky disease – this term is used to describe tumors in the chest that are at least 1/3 as wide as the chest, or tumors in other areas that are at least 10 cm (about 4 in) across. It's usually labeled by adding the letter X to the stage. It's especially important for stage II lymphomas, because bulky disease may require more intensive treatment.

- Stage I: The lymphoma is found in one lymph node region. Or, the lymphoma has invaded one extralymphatic organ or site (identified using the letter "E") but not any lymph node regions (stage IE); this is rare in Hodgkin lymphoma.
- Stage II: Any of the following conditions applies:
- Stage II: The lymphoma is in two or more lymph node regions on the same side of the diaphragm.
- Stage IIE: The lymphoma involves one organ and its regional lymph nodes (lymph nodes located near the site of the lymphoma), with or without lymphoma in other lymph node regions on the same side of the diaphragm.
- Stage II bulky: Either stage II or stage IIE applies; plus there is a mass in the chest. The mass is either larger than one-third the diameter of the chest or larger than 10 centimeters (cm). A centimeter is roughly equal to the width of a standard pen or pencil.
- Stage III: There is lymphoma in lymph node areas on both sides of the diaphragm, meaning above and below it.
- Stage IV: The lymphoma has spread to one or more organs beyond the lymph nodes. Hodgkin lymphoma usually spreads to the liver, bone marrow, or lungs [29, 30].

## 3.6.2 Non-Hodgkin Lymphoma

### 3.6.2.1 Disease Overview

In 1865, Thomas Hodgkin was immortalized by his peer, Samuel Wilks, in the annals of medical literature through the eponymous use of the term "Hodgkin's disease." Consequently, it must have seemed logical for the medical community of the time to name the other, more heterogeneous group of neoplastic lymph node enlargements as non-Hodgkin lymphoma (NHL). NHL is not a single disease but rather a group of several closely related cancers, called lymphoid neoplasms. The most recent 2016 revision of the World Health Organization classification of lymphoid neoplasms estimates that there are at least 86 types of NHL. Although the various types of NHL share many common characteristics, they differ in certain features, including their appearance under the microscope, their molecular features and growth patterns, their impact on the body, and how they respond to different types of treatment [31].

### 3.6.2.2 Introduction and Epidemiology

Non-Hodgkin lymphoma (NHL) is the most common hematological malignancy worldwide, accounting for nearly 3% of cancer diagnoses and deaths, annual incidence around 545,000 new cases (Globocan 2020) in the world according to the International Agency for Research on Cancer (IARC). NHL is the seventh most prevalent cancer and has the sixth highest mortality among cancers in the USA. NHL accounts for 4% of US cancer diagnoses, and incidence has increased to 168% since 1975 (while survival has improved to 158%). NHL is more common among men, those >65 years old, and those with autoimmune disease or a family history of hematological malignancies. According to the latest World Health Organization (WHO) classification, the most common NHL in Western countries is DLBCL, accounting for around 31% of adult cases. Other common aggressive B-cell subtypes include mantle cell lymphoma (MCL) (6% of cases) and BL (2% of cases). Among indolent B-cell NHL, FL accounts for 22% of cases in the Western world, followed by marginal zone lymphoma

(MZL) (8% of cases), chronic lymphocytic leukemia/small-cell lymphocytic lymphoma (CLL/SLL) (6% of cases), and lymphoplasmacytic lymphoma (LPL) (1% of cases). Common T-cell lymphomas make up only 10–15% of NHL diagnoses and include peripheral T-cell lymphoma (PTCL) (6% of cases) and cutaneous T-cell lymphoma (CTCL) (4% of cases) [21].

#### 3.6.2.3 Risk Factors

The exact cause of NHL is not known; however, the following factors may raise a person's risk of developing NHL.

Age: 60s and 70s.

- Gender: Men are very slightly more likely to develop NHL than women.
- Bacterial infections: For example, mucosa-associated lymphoid tissue (MALT) lymphoma of the stomach is thought to be caused by an infection with bacteria called *Helicobacter pylori*.
- Viruses: the Epstein–Barr virus (EBV) is associated with some types of NHL (e.g., Burkitt lymphoma). Hepatitis C infection has been associated with an increased risk of marginal zone lymphomas of the spleen.
- Immune deficiency disorders: Immune system disorders, such as HIV/AIDS, increase the risk of NHL, especially the aggressive B-cell lymphomas.

  Autoimmune disorders

- Organ transplantation: Drugs that reduce immune system function in order to protect the transplanted organ from rejection raise the risk of NHL.
- Previous cancer treatment. Previous treatment with certain drugs for other types of cancer may increase the risk of NHL.
- Chemical exposure: Exposure to certain chemicals may increase the risk of NHL. This may include pesticides, herbicides (like Agent Orange), and petrochemicals.

- Genetic factors: These possible risks are being studied in ongoing research.
- Breast implants: Having breast implants can increase the risk of breast lymphomas.
- Exposure to ionizing radiation: This can include exposure to radiation from atomic bombs, nuclear reactor accidents, and medical radiation therapy.
- Diet/weight: There is some inconclusive evidence that being overweight or having a diet filled with fatty foods or red meat may slightly increase the risk of lymphoma [32].

#### 3.6.2.4 Symptoms and Signs

General symptoms:

- Enlarged lymph nodes in the abdomen, groin, neck, or underarms
- Enlarged spleen or liver
- Fever that cannot be explained by an infection or other illness
- Weight loss with no known cause
- Sweating and chills
- Fatigue

Examples of symptoms related to a specific tumor location:

- A tumor in the abdomen can cause a stretched belly or pain in the back or abdomen.
- An enlarged spleen may cause back pain and a feeling that the stomach is full.
- A tumor in the groin may cause swelling in the legs.
- A tumor in the underarms may cause swelling in the arms.
- If the lymphoma spreads to the brain, there may be symptoms similar to those of a stroke.
- A tumor in the center of the chest may press on the trachea and cause coughing, chest pain, difficulty breathing, or other respiratory problems.

Like we see in HL, in NHL some symptoms described above are called "B symptoms," but according to 2014 Lugano Classification, these symptoms not necessarily change the way the lymphoma is treated.

- Unexplained weight loss of more than 10% of original body weight during the 6 months before diagnosis.
- Unexplained fever, with temperatures above 100.4 °F (38 °C).
- Drenching night sweats: Many people with Hodgkin lymphoma say their nightclothes or the sheets on the bed were so wet they needed to be changed during the night. Sometimes, heavy sweating occurs during the day [33].

#### 3.6.2.5 Diagnosis

- Medical history and physical examination – detailed questions about medical history and a physical examination with performance status, which can identify whether the person has experienced some typical symptoms of lymphoma (see Symptoms and Signs). Attention to node-bearing areas, including Waldeyer's ring, and to size of liver and spleen.
- Biopsy. Having enough tissue in the biopsy sample is very important in making a diagnosis. Needle biopsy samples are rarely big enough to make a definite diagnosis of lymphoma. In most cases, a core biopsy or surgical biopsy is needed to correctly diagnose and classify the lymphoma.
- Computed tomography (CT or CAT) scan.
- Magnetic resonance imaging (MRI). MRI can be used to measure the tumor's size.
- Positron emission tomography (PET) or PET-CT scan.
- Bone marrow aspiration and biopsy. Lymphoma often spreads to the bone marrow, so looking at a sample of the bone marrow can be important for diagnosing lymphoma and determining the stage. With certain types of lymphoma, these procedures may not be required if a PET scan has been done.
- Testing of the tumor. There are several types of molecular and genetic testing:

- Cytogenetics and/or fluorescent in situ hybridization (FISH) studies healthy and abnormal chromosomes in dividing cancer cells (e.g., T(14;18) rearrangement of BCL6, deletion 1p36 present in follicular lymphoma; translocation of MYC, BCL 2, and BCL6 present in diffuse large B-cell lymphoma (DLBCL)).
- Immunohistochemistry (IHC) is a special staining process to look at proteins on the surface of or inside the cancer cell (e.g., Panel: CD20, CD3, CD5, CD10, CD45, BCL2, BCL6, Ki 67, IRF4/MUM1, MYC, ALK, HHV8, SOX11 used in DLBCL).
- Polymerase chain reaction (PCR) detects specific DNA sequences that occur in some cancers.
- Extended molecular profiling is used to evaluate changes in specific genes in the tumor cells (e.g., next-generation sequencing (NGS)).
- Lumbar puncture: for patient at risk for CNS involvement.
- Laboratory tests: Blood tests may include a complete blood count (CBC) and an analysis of the different types of white blood cells, metabolic panel, uric acid, and lactate dehydrogenase (LDH).
- HIV and hepatitis B/C testing.

Some tests may be done if a person's treatment plan includes chemotherapy.

Heart evaluation: a heart evaluation, including an echocardiogram (ECHO) or a multigated acquisition (MUGA) scan (important for anthracycline-based chemotherapy).

Pregnancy test: for women of childbearing age.

Counseling for fertility: fertility preservation, smoking cessation, and psychosocial [34].

#### 3.6.2.6 Non-Hodgkin Lymphoma Types

In the 2017 WHO classification, more than 80 mature lymphoma entities are recognized, grouped into three major categories: B-cell neoplasms, T-cell, and NK-cell neoplasms. Non-Hodgkin lymphoma is further classified by other factors, including whether it is aggressive (fast-growing) or indolent (slow-growing).

Aggressive lymphomas include:

- Diffuse large B-cell lymphoma
- Anaplastic large-cell lymphoma
- Burkitt lymphoma
- Lymphoblastic lymphoma
- Mantle cell lymphoma
- Peripheral T-cell lymphoma

Indolent lymphomas include:

- Follicular lymphoma
- Cutaneous T-cell lymphoma
- Lymphoplasmacytic lymphoma
- Marginal zone B-cell lymphoma
- MALT lymphoma
- Small-cell lymphocytic lymphoma

**Subtypes of B-Cell Lymphoma**

Diffuse large B-cell lymphoma (DLBCL): DLBCL is the most common form of lymphoma. About 30% of NHL in the USA is DLBCL. It is an aggressive form of NHL that involves organs other than the lymph nodes about 40% of the time. There are different types of DLBCL, including germinal center and activated B cells (ABC).

- Primary mediastinal B-cell lymphoma is often found in the mediastinum, the area of the chest cavity between the lungs. This type of lymphoma, which is more common in young women, may produce fast-growing tumors that may encompass the mediastinum cavity and press on the airways and blood vessels.
- Primary central nervous system (CNS) lymphoma originates in the brain or spinal cord and may be found in patients with acquired immunodeficiency syndrome (AIDS) or those whose immune systems may be compromised, including organ transplant patients. When primary CNS lymphoma originates in the eye, it is called ocular lymphoma.

Double hit/triple hit lymphoma: This is a highly aggressive subtype, accounting for about 5% of cases. Rarely, low-grade follicular lymphoma may also transform into double hit lymphoma. Double hit lymphomas have changes in the *MYC* gene and in either the *BCL2* or *BCL6* gene. Double hit lymphoma is often diagnosed in older adults. Triple hit lymphomas have changes in the *MYC*, *BCL2*, and *BCL6* genes.

Follicular lymphoma: Follicular lymphoma is the second most common form of lymphoma in the USA and Europe. About 20% of people with NHL have this subtype. It usually begins in the lymph nodes, is most often indolent, and grows very slowly.

Mantle cell lymphoma: About 5–7% of people with NHL have mantle cell lymphoma. It most often appears in people older than 60 and is much more common in men than in women. It usually involves the bone marrow, lymph nodes, spleen, and gastrointestinal system, which includes the esophagus, stomach, and intestines. Mantle cell lymphoma is identified by a protein called cyclin D1 or by a genetic change within the lymphoma cells involving chromosomes 11 and 14.

Extranodal marginal zone B-cell lymphoma of MALT: This type of lymphoma most commonly occurs in the stomach. However, it may also occur in the lung, skin, thyroid, salivary gland, or in the orbit, adjacent to the eye, or in the bowel. Patients with this type of lymphoma sometimes have a history of autoimmune disease, such as lupus, rheumatoid arthritis, or Sjögren syndrome. When MALT occurs in the stomach, it is sometimes caused by a bacteria called *Helicobacter pylori*.

Nodal marginal zone B-cell lymphoma: This rare type of indolent lymphoma involves the lymph nodes. About 1% of people with lymphoma have this subtype.

Lymphoplasmacytic lymphoma: This is an indolent form of lymphoma, and 1% of people with NHL have this subtype. This form of lymphoma often involves the bone marrow, sometimes lymph nodes, and spleen. In many patients, this lymphoma produces a protein, called an “M protein,” that is found in the blood. When this occurs, the condition is called Waldenstrom’s macroglobulinemia (WM).

Burkitt lymphoma/Burkitt cell leukemia: This is a very rare and aggressive form of lymphoma. There are three forms of Burkitt lymphoma (endemic, sporadic, and immunodeficiency-related lymphoma).

The endemic subtype occurs most commonly in Africa, appears most often in the jawbones of children, and is usually associated with infection with EBV. It can also be associated with HIV. In the USA, Burkitt lymphoma sometimes appears with a mass in the abdomen, but it can affect many other parts of the body. Because this type of lymphoma spreads quickly, it needs immediate treatment. This subtype often has abnormalities involving the MYC gene, which can contribute to cancer growth.

## Subtypes of T-Cell and NK-Cell Lymphoma

Anaplastic large cell lymphoma, primary cutaneous type: This subtype of lymphoma only involves the skin. It is often indolent, although aggressive subtypes of the disease are possible.

Anaplastic large cell lymphoma, systemic type: This form makes up about 2% of all lymphomas and about 10% of all childhood lymphomas. In people with this subtype, an increased amount of the ALK-1 protein may be found in the cancer cells.

Peripheral T-cell lymphoma, not otherwise specified (NOS): This is an aggressive form of lymphoma. It is most common in people older than 60 and makes up about 6% of all lymphomas in the USA and Europe.

Angioimmunoblastic T-cell lymphoma: This is an aggressive form of lymphoma with specific symptoms (enlarged, often tender, lymph nodes, fever, weight loss, rash, high levels of immunoglobulins in the blood). Patients with angioimmunoblastic lymphoma have lowered immune system functions, so infections are also common.

Adult T-cell lymphoma/leukemia (human T-cell lymphotropic virus type I positive): This type of lymphoma is caused by a virus called the human T-cell lymphotropic virus type I. It is an aggressive disease that often involves the bone and skin.

Extranodal NK/T-cell lymphoma, nasal type: This is an aggressive type of lymphoma that is very rare in the USA and Europe in general, but more common in Asian and Hispanic communities. It can occur in children or adults, most often involving the nasal area and sinuses. It can also involve the gastrointestinal tract, skin, the testicles, or other areas in the body.

Enteropathy-associated T-cell lymphoma: This type of lymphoma is rare in the USA but is more common in Europe. It is an aggressive form of T-cell lymphoma that involves the intestines.

Hepatosplenic T-cell lymphoma: This is an aggressive form of peripheral T-cell lymphoma that involves the liver and spleen. The disease occurs most often in teenaged and young men.

Mycosis fungoides: This is a rare T-cell lymphoma that primarily involves the skin. It often has a very long and indolent course but may become more aggressive and spread to lymph nodes or internal organs [28, 32, 35].

#### 3.6.2.7 Non-Hodgkin Lymphoma Staging

The same staging system used for Hodgkin lymphoma is used to NHL, the Lugano classification, which is based on the older Ann Arbor system. It has four stages, labeled I, II, III, and IV; the stage of Hodgkin lymphoma describes the extent of the spread of the tumor, but the suffixes A or B for symptoms will not be included for NHL (see Hodgkin Lymphoma Staging) [27, 36].

### 3.6.3 Multiple Myeloma

#### 3.6.3.1 Introduction and Epidemiology

Multiple myeloma (MM) is the abnormal proliferation of clonal plasma cells within the bone marrow, known as plasma cells. Plasma cells are white blood cells, derived from B lymphocytes; it is responsible for the production and secretion of immunoglobulins (Ig) G, A, D, E, or M protein (M for monoclonal) or part of these, the light chains k (kappa) and l (lambda) [37–39].

Abnormal proliferation leads to accumulation of M protein in the bone marrow, with IgG (50%) and IgA (20%) being more frequent. The buildup reduces the normal production of blood elements, and then it causes bone destruction and pain by invading adjacent structures. Excess immunoglobulins in peripheral blood reduce blood viscosity and fluidity, which causes hyper viscosity. The evolution of the disease leads to anemia, kidney failure, bone damage, and an increased risk of infections due to reduced immunity [38–41].

It is an incurable disease which accounts for approximately 1% of oncological diseases and approximately 10% of malignant hematological diseases worldwide. According to the US Surveillance, Epidemiology, and End Results (SEER), in 2020 they estimate 32,270 new cases of multiple myeloma in the USA, corresponding to 1.8% of all new cancer cases, with an annual incidence of approximately 7 per 100,000 men and women, with a relative survival of 53.9% at 5 years. There are about 176,000 cases and 117,000 deaths per year attributed to the MM worldwide [42, 43].

Multiple myeloma has a greater predominance in blacks, due to the higher prevalence of monoclonal gammopathy of undetermined significance (MGUS) in this ethnicity and in males, with a mean age at diagnosis of 66 years and with only 2% of patients aged less than 40 years at diagnosis and so far, no reports in pediatrics [38, 40, 41, 44].

Delay in the diagnosis of MM is common, partially due to nonspecific initial symptoms, which can lead to complications before treatment and increased risk of treatment failure, disease progression, and death [45, 46].

#### 3.6.3.2 Pathogenesis and Risk Factors

Multiple myeloma (MM) is believed to have evolved from MGUS, which is an asymptomatic premalignant condition of clonal proliferation of plasma cells. This condition is present among 3–4% of the population over 50 years of age, with a progression rate to MM or other malignant disease around 1% per year, making MGUS a risk factor for MM. The cause of the development of MGUS remains unclear, but it is believed that it occurs through cytogenetic anomaly which is probably caused by the response of plasma cells under antigenic stimulation [39, 47].

Other related risk factors are also reported such as heredity (risk 3.7 times increased if they have first-degree relatives with myeloma), chronic infectious antigenic stimulation caused by

HIV (human immunodeficiency virus), HCV (the virus of the hepatitis C) and HHV8 (Herpes Virus 8), exposure to ionizing radiation, occupational exposure of rural workers (not associated with benzene), nutritional factors (higher risk with a diet rich in liver and butter), and obesity. However, these related factors are conflicting, and there is a lack of significant data in literature, since most patients diagnosed with MM do not have any known risk factors [48].

#### 3.6.3.3 Signs and Symptoms

MM can present considerable signs and symptoms, the most common being abbreviated in the acronym "CRAB" which stands for hypercalcemia, renal dysfunction, anemia, and bone lesions [37, 44, 49].

Bone pain is one of the most reported symptoms at the time of MM diagnosis, with an incidence of 50–90% of patients, being generally located in the patient's back and chest. Due to bone infiltration by malignant plasma cells, pathological fractures are present in 80% of patients at the time of diagnosis. The increase in tumor mass causes an increase in the production of osteoclast activating factors (lymphotoxin, tumor necrosis factor, hematopoietic growth factor, interleukins among others), leading to increased osteoclastogenesis and bone resorption, which in turn leads to increased serum calcium.

Anemia is present in 70% of patients at diagnosis due to the physical displacement of erythrocyte precursors and the specific inhibition of erythropoiesis by cytokines in the microenvironment. Anemia may be important with symptoms of fatigue, angina, and dyspnea, or asymptomatic, detected through laboratory tests. Multiple myeloma anemia has normochromic and normocytic features, but it may present mild macrocytosis on blood count [39, 49, 50].

Hypercalcemia occurs in 13–30% of patients at the time of diagnosis and may cause confusion, polydipsia, disorientation, constipation, polyuria, nausea, irritability, and muscle weakness. Alternative causes of hypercalcemia should be discarded through laboratory tests for intact parathyroid hormone (PTH) and PTH-related peptide assays in order to exclude paraneoplastic hypercalcemia. Suppressed PTH levels should raise the possibility and investigation for multiple myeloma [49, 50].

Renal failure is present in 20–40% of patients due to hypercalcemia or light chain deposition in the distal renal tubules. Detection occurs due to an asymptomatic elevation of serum creatinine, and rarely due to the presence of oliguria or uremia [49, 50].

Infection is one of the main causes of morbidity and mortality in patients with MM at diagnosis and during the course of the disease as a result of the impairment of the immune system [39].

#### 3.6.3.4 Diagnosis

MM diagnosis is laborious due to the variety of symptoms and their similarity in several other diseases, the presence of unexplained symptoms such as bone fracture and/or bone pain in young people, hypercalcemia with normal PTH, anemia without the presence of bleeding, and renal failure without a previous history of diabetes or autoimmune diseases; it should raise awareness of a possible diagnosis of MM [49].

The initial assessment of the MM diagnostic asks for a complete blood count, serum albumin, β2-microglobulin, serum calcium, renal function tests, serum and urinary protein electrophoresis with immunofixation, C-reactive protein, lactate dehydrogenase, serum monoclonal free light chains (FLC), 24-hour protein collection with protein quantification, and bone marrow and image exam (computed tomography and/or magnetic resonance) to detect possible bone lesions [50–52].

Fluorescent in situ hybridization (FISH) analysis occurs after selection of CD138 plasma cells including at least t(4;14) and del17p, with t(14;16), 1q21 gain, and del (1p32) analysis also recommended [51, 52].

The evaluation of the monoclonal component, through laboratory tests, allows to verify the presence, type of abnormal protein, and amount present in the serum and/or urine, providing help in the diagnosis and evaluation of the response to treatment [37, 53].

For years, the diagnosis of MM required the presence of lesions in target organs, known as CRAB criteria (hypercalcemia, renal dysfunction, anemia, and bone lesions). In 2014, the International Myeloma Working Group (IMWG) re-evaluated the criteria for diagnosis and included three biomarkers: clonal plasma cells in bone marrow greater than or equal to 60%, free light chain ratio (FLC) kappa or lambda greater than or equal to 100, as long as the FLC level is 100 mg/L or higher or focal lesion on MRI. This allowed diagnosis in patients without CRAB features and initiation of treatment before severe organ damage. Computed tomography (CT) and proton emission tomography (PET-CT) were also included to help in diagnosis [41, 50, 54].

#### 3.6.3.5 Staging and Prognosis

The outcome of MM depends on biological differences, global burden of disease, and clinical status of the patient. To assess the individual prognosis of each patient, clinical scoring systems were developed, the first of which was the staging system by Salmon and Durie (1975), which used as biomarkers the degree of anemia, renal failure, serum calcium, component monoclonal, and bone involvement, correlating with the tumor mass. Afterward, it was found that the system was not able to adequately assess overall survival and disease-free time. With this, the International Staging System (ISS) emerged in 2005, which included the levels of β2-microglobulin, albumin, C-reactive protein, and the proliferative activity of multiple myeloma cells as prognostic factors. Fluorescent in situ hybridization (FISH) and conventional karyotyping are also used for risk stratification [44, 51].

The Salmon and Durie, ISS, and R-ISS (revised ISS) systems are used in staging, and in the last two systems, β2-microglobulin, and albumin levels reflect the tumor burden, the presence of renal failure, the rate of turnover, and the nutritional and performance status of patients. The IMWG (International Myeloma Working Group) updated the ISS score to include high-risk cytogenetics [t (4; 14), t (14; 16), del17p, and serum lactate dehydrogenase. These risk factors are relevant for early progression after autologous bone marrow transplantation. Conversely, the ISS and R-ISS provide prognostic information in the diagnosis of MM and not in cases of relapsed or refractory MM [51].

#### 3.6.3.6 Drug-Related Biomarkers

Drug-related biomarkers are being studied to predict treatment response, seeking efficacy, and reducing unnecessary toxicities. Recent pharmacogenomics studies revealed that genes could predict clinical outcomes after treatments with immunomodulatory drugs or bortezomib. The expression of the cereblon protein, an intracellular binding partner of immunomodulatory drugs, has been studied as a biomarker [51].

The studies used quantitative real-time PCR analysis, gene expression profiling, or immunohistochemistry to quantify cereblon expression, and the results showed that loss of cereblon expression was associated with resistance to immunomodulatory drugs. However, new analyses described mutations in the cereblon, causing limitations in the trials. When evaluating predictors for responses to daratumumab, higher expression of CD38 was found in patients who were responsive to treatment. However, good responses were also seen in patients with low CD38 expression, concluding that the level of CD38 expression was not predictive of response in advanced MM. Despite this result, attempts to evaluate agents that maintain increased CD38 upregulation are maintained, such as the use of trans-retinoic acid and histone deacetylase inhibitors [51].

The expression of BCL-2, BCL-XL, or MCL-1, which are anti-apoptotic proteins, measured by quantitative real-time PCR, predicts pharmacological responses to venetoclax, a BCL-2 inhibitor, which is active mainly in patients with translocations t [11, 14]. Although this is not a routine test for defining treatment, fluorescent in situ hybridization for t(11;14) should be requested if venetoclax is a treatment option. The evaluation of biomarkers, such as cereblon and CD38 protein expression, despite their prognostic and predictive value, is not routinely evaluated in the treatment of multiple myeloma [51].

#### 3.6.3.7 Response Assessment

Correct evaluation of the MM can indicate the patient's prognosis. Patients who have a complete response after induction have improved progression-free survival and overall survival after treatment. In 2011, the IMWG updated the MM response criteria to include two new categories: strict full response and very good partial response [51].

Before the start of each treatment cycle, patients should be evaluated for their response to the proposed therapy. For patients with intact immunoglobulins, the recommended method of monitoring is serum and urinary M protein quantification. The interval between the evaluation of all serum and urinary parameters is at the physician's discretion, taking into account the aggressiveness of the disease, organ involvement, and other relevant clinical factors [51].

Complete response to treatment is considered when the patient presents normalization of SFLC (serum free light chain) values, absence of plasma cell infiltration in the bone marrow, and negative immunofixation in serum and urine samples [51, 55].

Recurrence occurs when the patient who previously responded completely to the treatment presents the reappearance of the MM, while the progression refers to patients with an increasing burden of disease when compared to the diagnosis or persistent residual disease. Progression can be determined biochemically (an increase of an existing monoclonal peak) or through radiological and clinical examinations. The evaluation of the response can be challenging, especially after treatment and response with the use of monoclonal antibodies, as these can interfere with the quantification of the M protein, requiring more specific assays for the evaluation [51].

#### 3.6.3.8 Minimum Residual Disease

The treatment for MM has evolved in recent years due to the introduction of drugs with different mechanisms of action, better understanding of the disease, and improved diagnostic criteria, leading to longer patient survival [55].

Despite the evolution in survival with the introduction of drug combinations, bone marrow transplantation, post-transplant consolidation, and prolonged maintenance, most patients present relapse, showing a persistent disease that requires new methods to detect and quantify the level of disease minimum residual (DRM) [44].

MM often relapses due to residual MM cells, drug resistance, and/or persistence of resistant dormant subclones. MRD can be detected through multipara flow cytometry, polymerase chain reaction (PCR), or state-of-the-art sequencing to identify clonal cells [51].

Flow cytometry can identify malignant plasma cells and abnormally expressed cell surface markers in up to 90% of patients by analyzing a bone marrow sample. Technical advances have increased the sensitivity of cytometry to the range 10–6. The biggest challenges of this MRD analysis using flow cytometry are the heterogeneous infiltration of the biopsy and the dilution of peripheral blood, which can make the sample unfeasible [51].

By PCR, DRM analysis detects residual tumor cells by amplifying a tumor-specific molecular marker, with IGH (immunoglobulin heavy chain gene) being used in various B cell diseases. Allele-specific oligonucleotide PCR with primers complementary to the heavy chain variable sequence is a sensitive approach to detect residual malignant plasma cells. However, it becomes a laborious and time-consuming method as it requires patient-specific primers and probes for quantitative PCR, which are not always available [51].

Next-generation sequencing of IGH segments allows evaluating the functioning of the B lineage with consensus primers. The B lineage repertoire includes a malignant plasma cell clone, allowing next-generation IGH sequencing to quantitatively determine MRD without patient customization, provided the malignant clone has been identified in a diagnostic or collection sample performed with the active disease. The lack of standardization and limited commercial availability are the main restrictions for this procedure [51].

The third approach to assessing MRD is PET-CT and MRI imaging. The studies showed that patients with negative PET-CT after induction treatment and autologous stem cell transplantation had better progression-free and overall survival when compared to patients with positive PET-CT (52 versus 38 months and 5-year estimates of 90% versus 71%, respectively). The advantage of PET-CT compared to other approaches is its ability to assess MRD outside the bone marrow. Disadvantages are high cost, insufficient standardization, and reduced tracer uptake capacity in some patients [51].

DRM testing is not recommended for routine follow-up of patients with MM, but will likely be included in the standard response and progression assessment soon. Current alternatives for evaluating MRD are next-generation flow cytometry (bone marrow cells) or next-generation sequencing (molecular analysis), which can be combined with imaging evaluation [51].

In the future, DRM could be used to guide treatments and probably as a marker for progression-free survival and overall survival [51].

### 3.6.4 Myelodysplastic Syndrome

#### 3.6.4.1 Introduction and Epidemiology

During formation, some cells can be abnormal, and this process is called "dysplastic," while the term "myelodysplastic" was used for the first time by a French–American–British (FAB) group to describe abnormalities during the formation of myeloid cell. Myelodysplastic syndrome (MDS) represents a very heterogeneous group of myeloid disorders and increased risk of transformation to acute myelogenous leukemia (AML) [56, 57]. MDS main characteristics include clonal stem cell proliferation, recurrent genetic abnormalities, myelodysplasia, ineffective hematopoiesis, and peripheral blood cytopenia [58].

It can be clinically classified based on the underlying cause. Primary MDS occurs when MDS is diagnosed, and its cause cannot be related to treatment, or the patient has no history of cytotoxic therapy or radiotherapy. On the other hand, secondary MDS is when the cause of the disease is related to prior cancer treatment, and it was included in WHO classification as therapy-related myeloid neoplasms (t-MN) [59].

t-MN cover many malignant disorders previously described as therapy-related myelodysplastic syndrome (t-MDS) or therapy-related acute myeloid leukemia (t-AML). It is characterized by a result of complication based on exposure to cytotoxic agents, in special by alkylating agents and topoisomerase-II inhibitors [60].

MDs frequently affects more males than females and is rare among children/adolescents and young adults, with an incidence rate of 0,1 per 100,00 people per year in those age groups, and the risk increases with aging. The average age of patients is 70 years, with crude incidence between 4 and 5 cases per 100,000 seniors per year, and it will likely be higher due to underreporting records [59, 61].

#### 3.6.4.2 Risk Factors

The exposure to some risk factors may lead the pathologies development. Here we identify some of those literature described factors which may be related to the MDS development.

Age: aging is one of the most important risk factors for a lot of pathologies, and it is not different for MDS, once the prevalence in young people (less than 50 years) is uncommon and most cases are found in elderly (more than 70 years). Over the years, we accumulate somatic mutations, and these molecular changes can co-operate with some pathology's genesis [62].

Sex: MDS affects more men than women. Even though the mechanism remains unclear, the increased risk in men may be related to lifestyle and exposure to certain chemicals in the past.

Cancer treatment: Patients who have been treated with some chemotherapy drugs have an increased probability to develop secondary MDS. Procarbazine, chlorambucil, cyclophosphamide, ifosfamide, etoposide, teniposide, and doxorubicin are some drugs that can lead to MDS. These drugs can cause DNA mutations that isolated may not lead to secondary MDS carcinogenesis, however this factor associated with previous chemotherapy and the accumulated doses that were given to the patient over the years can contribute to the develop of a t-MN [60].

Genetic syndromes: The advent of easy access to molecular panels made easier to know how hereditary predisposition can lead to the development of MDS. People who carry some inherited syndromes are more willing to develop MSD. These syndromes may present mutation in one or more well-described genes *loci* that can affect the outcome of primary MDS patient [63]. Examples of syndromes include:

- Fanconi anemia (FA)
- Shwachman–Diamond syndrome (SDS)
- Diamond–Blackfan anemia (DBA)
- Familial platelet disorder with a propensity to myeloid malignancy
- Severe congenital neutropenia
- Dyskeratosis congenita

Familial MDS: In some families it is difficult to understand the cause of MDS; sometimes a gene mutation in a family can be related to the MDS, but in other cases, this relationship is not clear. Some guidelines have proposed screening newly diagnosed myeloid malignancy for further referral for genetic counseling and genetic testing.

Smoking: We already know that smoking can cause cancer almost anywhere in our body even though these parts are not directly in contact with the smoke, as it could happen to passive smokers (secondary smokers). Smoking in MSD is not different; a lot of substances are absorbed by blood as it passes through the lungs and can directly affect these cells. People who are in contact with the burning of a cigarette as well as the people who inhale the breathed-out smoke from smoker can be classified as secondary smokers, and these people are liable to suffer DNA mutation and consequently development of a tumor [64].

Environmental exposures: The exposure to some environmental factors, such as benzene and ionizing radiation, suggests that they may be involved in the development of MDS. Other types of exposure, such as pesticides and solvents, should be analyzed since some professional categories, as agricultural and textile workers, have more probability to develop MDS [65, 66].

#### 3.6.4.3 Signs and Symptoms

It is important to know that signs and symptoms can vary from patient to patient, and even other pathologies can present signs and symptoms similar to MDS.

The signs and symptoms tend to reflect the lineage most affected and may include:

- Fatigue.
- Weakness.
- Easy bruising or bleeding.
- Bone pain.
- Fever.
- Shortness of breath.
- Frequent infections.

#### 3.6.4.4 Detection

Nowadays we know that some medications and viral infections may cause morphologic chances in marrow cells, leading these cells to be like MDS cells. To be more assertive in the MDS diagnosis, the physician must carefully evaluate some features like count and peripheral blood smear, marrow morphology, cytogenetics, duration of abnormal blood counts, causes of cytopenia, and concomitant illness.

To maintain a pattern during the MDS diagnosis, an international working group (IWG) defined minimal diagnostic criteria for this disease that includes two prerequisites: [1] constant cytopenia (it should last more than 6 months in at least one of the following lineages: erythroid cells, neutrophil granulocytes, and platelets; in case of bilineage dysplasia or specific karyotype, only 2 months of stable cytopenia are needed) and [2] exclusion of other factors that can lead the patient to have cell dysplasia and abnormal blood cell count.

Beyond the prerequisites, the diagnosis of MDS requires one of the following decisive criteria:

1. Dysplasia (≥10% in more than one major bone marrow lineages).
2. Blast cell count of 5–19%.
3. Abnormality in typical cytogenetic of MDS.

Other co-criteria may be used in patients with MDS features, but they show questionable results (chromosome aberration, borderline percentage of dysplasia, and blast count). This complementary test may include mutation analysis, flow cytometer, gene chip analysis, and others [61, 67]. If these tests are not available or results are negative, the diagnosis of MDS should not be established, and the standard recommendation for this situation is to repeat diagnostic tests after some time interval.

**Diagnostic problems in MDS**

Since the diagnostic factors are guided by morphological aspects, patients who have questionable results can be misclassified as MDS, and this situation directly affects patients' treatment and outcome.

For patients who have cytopenia, it is recommended other tests that allow the right diagnostic of cytopenia. If other diagnoses were already discarded, it is not possible to identify the cause, and the patient does not have dysplasia, it can be classified as idiopathic cytopenia of undetermined significance (ICUS). Part of these patients have cytogenetic abnormalities and may carry somatic mutations [68]. Patients in this context of cytopenia and somatic mutations can be considered a clonal cytopenia of undetermined significance (CCU).

Differently of ICU and CCU, patients without evidence of hematological disorder but with somatic mutations on blood cells can be classified as clonal hematopoiesis of undetermined potential (CHIP). Thus, an isolated identification of a cytogenetic alteration without cytopenia and dysplastic changes in bone marrow should be interpreted with caution as it does not necessarily represent a pre-MDS or leukemia phase [69].

For some authors, the classification above is considered as a precursor of MDS, once approximately 25% of patients with ICU may develop MDS or AML and the probability gets higher when it involves somatic mutations, mainly in the presence of highly predictive mutation patterns [70, 71].

#### 3.6.4.5 Staging and Differentiation

To propose an adequate treatment for MDS patient, it is necessary to correctly stratify the patient based on the sum of disease and patient-related particularities. Finding the correct algorithm for the patient can often be an arduous task that can take time and effort. Knowing the evolution of classification system and their nuances is necessary for the correct clustering of the patient and establish score system that can predict patient's prognosis.

In 1982 was born the first useful classification system; that was proposal for the French-American-British (FAB) cooperative group, and their classification was mainly based on morphologic features [72].

Over time, other criteria were needed to explain some events, and it is in this context that WHO updated the FAB classification, including some issues and excluding others. Nowadays WHO system recognizes six main types of MDS:

- MDS with multilineage dysplasia (MDS-MLD): Cytopenia in at least one blood cell, dysplasia in at least 10% of cells in two or more lineages in the bone marrow, less than 15% of sideroblasts or less than 5% of sideroblasts in bone marrow (if the cells are mutated in SF3B1 gene), and less than 5% of blast in bone marrow.
- MDS with single lineage dysplasia (MSD-SLD): Cytopenia in one or two blood cells, dysplasia in at least 10% of cells in one lineage in the bone marrow, less than 15% of sideroblasts or less than 5% of sideroblasts in bone marrow (if the cells are mutated in SF3B1 gene), and less than 5% of blast in bone marrow.
- MDS with ring sideroblasts (MDS-RS): Cytopenia in one or two blood cells, more than 15% of erythroid precursor with ring sideroblasts in bone marrow or more than 5% of erythroid precursor with ring sideroblasts in the bone marrow (if the cells are mutated in SF3B1 gene). This condition can be divided into two types based on the number of cell types that are affected by dysplasia:
  - MDS-RS with single lineage dysplasia (MDS-RS-SLD): Dysplasia in one cell type
  - MDS-RS with multilineage dysplasia (MDS-RS-MLD): Dysplasia in more than one cell type
  - MDS with excess blasts (MDS-EB): Cytopenia in at least one blood cell, dysplasia in at least 10% of cells in one or

more lineage in the bone marrow (some cases dysplasia may not happen). This condition has blasts in peripheral blood or bone marrow; because of this it can be divided in two types based on the count and blast location:
  - MDS-EB1: 5–9% of blasts in bone marrow or 2–4% in the blood
  - MDS-EB2: 10–19% of blasts in bone marrow or 5–19% in the blood
- MDS with isolated del(5q): Cytopenia in at least one blood cell, dysplasia in at least 10% of cells in one or more lineages in the bone marrow, less than 5% of blast in bone marrow, and this condition is characterized by the bone marrow cells showing a missing part of chromosome 5.
- MDS unclassifiable (MDS-U): Cytopenia in at least one blood cell, dysplasia in at least 10% of cells in one or more lineage in the bone marrow and less than 5% of blasts in bone marrow [73].

The types of MDS were classified based on the number of dysplastic lineage, number of lineage with cytopenia, ring sideroblasts in erythroid elements of bone marrow, percentage of blasts, and cytogenetics.

#### 3.6.4.6 Risk Stratification

The prognosis of MDS patients is heterogeneous, and prognostic tools are necessary, helping physicians in stratifying patients' risk and to choose the appropriate therapy, consequently improving outcomes.

The International Prognostic Scoring System (IPSS) is a tool created in 1997 that presents high reproducibility, is very easy to use, and has a fundamental importance once it allowed patient's prognostic for many decades [74], being widely used to indicate allogenic bone marrow transplantation. With the evolution of MDS, some limitations were identified, mainly the prognostic of low-risk patients. It leads to a tool update in 2012, when the Revised International Prognostic Score (IPSS-R) was launched, with different cut off for many features and attributing better weights for cytogenetics based on the last version. Both versions were developed for primary MDS patients, limiting the use of the tool.

IPSS-R consider the following factors:

- Cytogenetics: poor prognosis is associated to high risk or multiple abnormalities.
  - Very good, e.g., del(11q)
  - Good, e.g., del(5q), del(12p)
  - Intermediate, e.g., del(7q), +8, +19
  - Poor, e.g., – 7, inv. [3]/t(3q)/del(3q)
  - Very poor, more than 3 abnormalities
- Percentage of blast in bone marrow: worse prognosis for greater count of blasts.
- Cytopenia: poor prognosis associated with hemoglobin <8 g/dL (< 80 g/L), platelets count <50.000/mcL (< 50 × 10 [9]/L), and absolute neutrophil count (ANC) < 800/mcL (0,8 × 10 [9]/L) [75, 76].

Trying to overcome IPSS and IPSS-R limitations, MD Anderson Cancer Center developed the global MDACC model (adding patient's age and performance status), allowing the evaluation of all patients that are considered as MSD at any time of disease natural course [77], and MDACC MDS lower risk prognostic model that may improve prognostication in patients with low risk MDS [57, 78]. Moreover, WHO developed the WHO prognostic Scoring System (WPSS) that incorporates WHO classification as well as the presence or not of transfusion dependence [79].

All the described tools have limitations and may not correctly stratify a determined population. Due to this fact other criteria have been studied to be incorporated in these tools.

The selection criteria for the tool will depend on the variables available at the moment of patient stratification as well as clinical practice of each physician.

#### Allogenic Stem-Cell Transplantation

Despite the fact transplantation is a high-risk mortality treatment and not all the patients are eligible for this kind of treatment, allogenic stem-cell transplantation can offer a curative option for MDS patients [80, 81], in comparison with other therapies that may prolong survival [82].

During diagnosis and risk stratification phase, physicians must analyze patient's eligibility for transplantation. Some authors consider patients stratified as high risk MDS with good performance status e no or few coexisting conditions as the best candidates for transplantation, while patients with low risk, poor performance status and coexisting comorbidities should consider other therapies [83].

### 3.6.4.7 Molecular Considerations

As we already saw in this chapter, gene sequencing improves diagnostic and prognostic process. The literature shows some studies describing the mutational landscape of MDS and its potential prognostic and therapeutic implications. Genes frequently mutated in MDS, grouped based on their cell's role, include:

- Signal transduction: JAK2, KRAS, CBL.
- DNA methylation: DNMT3A, TET2, IDH1/2.
- Transcriptional regulation: EVI1, RUNX1, GATA2.
- Chromatin modification: EZH2, ASXL1.
- RNA splicing: SF3B1, U2AF1, SRSF2, and ZRSR2 [84].

Mutations in genes RUNX1, TP53, and EZH2 have been associated with poor prognosis [84–89], while mutations on SF3B1 are associated with favorable outcomes [84–86, 89]. Thus, during the treatment choice, analysis of the cytogenetic and molecular profiling has been shown crucial. For example, patients with mutation on TP53 gene were recently associated with high response rate to decitabine protocol, while mutations on TET2 have shown higher responses on azacytidine protocols [85, 90, 91].

## References


1. Preisler HD. The leukemias. Disease-a-month. 1994;40:525–79.
2. Davis AS, Viera AJ, Mead MD. Leukemia: an overview for primary care. Am Family Phys. 2014;89:731–8.
3. Juliusson G, Hough R. Leukemia. Prog Tumor Res. 2016;43:87–100. https://doi.org/10.1159/000447076.
4. Devine SM, Larson RA. Acute leukemia in adults: recent developments in diagnosis and treatment. CA Cancer J Clin. 1994;44:326–52. https://doi.org/10.3322/canjclin.44.6.326.
5. Jin MW, Xu SM, An Q, et al. A review of risk factors for childhood leukemia. Eur Rev Med Pharmacol Sci. 2016;20:3760–4.
6. Dong Y, Shi O, Zeng Q, et al. Leukemia incidence trends at the global, regional, and national level between 1990 and 2017. Exp Hematol Oncol. 2020;9:14. https://doi.org/10.1186/s40164-020-00170-6.
7. Scarfò L, Ferreri AJ, Ghia P. Chronic lymphocytic leukaemia. Crit Rev Oncol Hematol. 2016;104:169–82. https://doi.org/10.1016/j.critrevonc.2016.06.003.
8. Ajithkumar TV, Hatcher HM. 21 – Cancers of the haematopoietic system. In: Ajithkumar TV, Hatcher HM, editors. Specialist training in oncology. Mosby, 2011, pp.298–319.
9. Network NCC. Chronic myeloid leukemia (version 03.2021). 2021. https://www.nccn.org/professionals/physician_gls/pdf/cml.pdf. Accessed 02 05 2021.
10. Network NCC. Chronic Lymphocytic leukemia/small lymphocytic lymphoma (version 04.2021). 2021. Accessed 02 05 2021.
11. Network NCC. Acute lymphoblastic leukemia (version 02.2021). 2021. https://www.nccn.org/professionals/physician_gls/pdf/all.pdf. Accessed 02 05 2021.
12. Pejovic T, Schwartz PE. Leukemias. Clin Obstet Gynecol. 2002;45:866–78. https://doi.org/10.1097/00003081-200209000-00033.
13. Asnafi AA, Deris Zayeri Z, Shahrabi S, et al. Chronic myeloid leukemia with complex karyotypes: prognosis and therapeutic approaches. J Cell Physiol. 2019;234:5798–806. https://doi.org/10.1002/jcp.27505.
14. Inaba H, Greaves M, Mullighan CG. Acute lymphoblastic leukaemia. Lancet. 2013;381:1943–55. https://doi.org/10.1016/s0140-6736(12)62187-4.
15. Short NJ, Rytting ME, Cortes JE. Acute myeloid leukaemia. Lancet. 2018;392:593–606. https://doi.org/10.1016/s0140-6736(18)31041-9.
16. Rubnitz JE, Gibson B, Smith FO. Acute myeloid leukemia. Hematol Oncol Clin North Am. 2010;24:35–63. https://doi.org/10.1016/j.hoc.2009.11.008.
17. Pelcovits A, Niroula R. Acute myeloid leukemia: a review. Rhode Island Med J (2013). 2020;103:38–40.

18. Bennett JM, Catovsky D, Daniel MT, et al. Proposals for the classification of the acute leukaemias. French-American-British (FAB) co-operative group. Br J Haematol. 1976;33:451–8. https://doi.org/10.1111/j.1365-2141.1976.tb03563.x.
19. Stone MJ. Thomas Hodgkin: medical immortal and uncompromising idealist. Proc (Bayl Univ Med Cent). 2005;18:368–75. https://doi.org/10.1080/08998280.2005.11928096.
20. Connors JM. Clinical manifestations and natural history of Hodgkin's lymphoma. Cancer J (Sudbury, Mass). 2009;15:124–8. https://doi.org/10.1097/PPO.0b013e3181a282d8.
21. Sung H, Ferlay J, Siegel RL, et al. Global cancer statistics 2020: GLOBOCAN estimates of incidence and mortality worldwide for 36 cancers in 185 countries. CA Cancer J Clin. 2021;71:209–49. https://doi.org/10.3322/caac.21660.
22. Thomas RK, Re D, Zander T, et al. Epidemiology and etiology of Hodgkin's lymphoma. Ann Oncol. 2002;13 Suppl 4: 147–52. https://doi.org/10.1093/annonc/mdf652.
23. Oncology ASoC. Lymphoma – Hodgkin: introduction. 2020. https://www.cancer.net/cancer-types/lymphoma-hodgkin/introduction. Accessed 02 05 2021.
24. Oncology ASoC. Lymphoma – Hodgkin: symptoms and signs. 2021. https://www.cancer.net/cancer-types/lymphoma-hodgkin/symptoms-and-signs. Accessed 02 05 2021.
25. Oncology ASoC. Lymphoma – Hodgkin: diagnosis. 2020. https://www.cancer.net/cancer-types/lymphoma-hodgkin/diagnosis. Accessed 02 05 2021.
26. Network NCC. Hodgkin Lymphoma (version 04.2021). 2021. https://www.nccn.org/professionals/physician_gls/pdf/hodgkins.pdf. Accessed 02 05 2021.
27. Cheson BD, Fisher RI, Barrington SF, et al. Recommendations for initial evaluation, staging, and response assessment of Hodgkin and non-Hodgkin lymphoma: the Lugano classification. J Clin Oncol. 2014;32:3059–68. https://doi.org/10.1200/jco.2013.54.8800.
28. de Leval L, Jaffe ES. Lymphoma classification. Cancer J (Sudbury, Mass). 2020;26:176–85. https://doi.org/10.1097/ppo.0000000000000451.
29. Oncology ASoC. Lymphoma – Hodgkin: stages. 2020. https://www.cancer.net/cancer-types/lymphoma-hodgkin/stages. Accessed 02 05 2021.
30. Society AC. Hodgkin lymphoma stages. 2021. https://www.cancer.org/cancer/hodgkin-lymphoma/detection-diagnosis-staging/staging.html. Accessed 02 05 2021.
31. Foundation LR. What is lymphoma. 2021. https://lymphoma.org/aboutlymphoma/nhl/. Accessed 02 05 2021.

32. Oncology ASoC. Lymphoma – non-Hodgkin: subtypes. 2019. https://www.cancer.net/cancer-types/lymphoma-non-hodgkin/subtypes. Accessed 02 05 2021.
33. Oncology ASoC. Lymphoma – non-Hodgkin: symptoms and signs. 2019. https://www.cancer.net/cancer-types/lymphoma-non-hodgkin/symptoms-and-signs. Accessed 02 05 2021.
34. Oncology ASoC. Lymphoma – non-Hodgkin: diagnosis. 2019. https://www.cancer.net/cancer-types/lymphoma-non-hodgkin/diagnosis. Accessed 02 05 2021.
35. America CTCo. Non-Hodgkin lymphoma types. 2021. https://www.cancercenter.com/cancer-types/non-hodgkin-lymphoma/types. Accessed 04 06 2021.
36. Oncology ASoC. Lymphoma – non-Hodgkin: stages. 2019. https://www.cancer.net/cancer-types/lymphoma-non-hodgkin/stages. Accessed 04 06 2021.
37. Hungria VT, Crusoe EQ, Quero AA, et al. Guidelines on the diagnosis and management of multiple myeloma treatment: Associação Brasileira de Hematologia e Hemoterapia e Terapia Celular Project guidelines: Associação Médica Brasileira – 2012. Rev Bras Hematol Hemoter. 2013;35:201–17. https://doi.org/10.5581/1516-8484.20130050.
38. Usmani SZ, Hoering A, Cavo M, et al. Clinical predictors of long-term survival in newly diagnosed transplant eligible multiple myeloma – an IMWG Research Project. Blood Cancer J. 2018;8:123. https://doi.org/10.1038/s41408-018-0155-7.
39. Almeida JRCd. Farmacêuticos Em Oncologia – uma Nova Realidade. Atheneu: São Paulo; 2010.
40. Massumoto C-S, Fernanda de Oliveira. Manual de Onco-Hematologia – TMO e Práticas Assistenciais Interdisciplinares. 1st ed. Triall: São Paulo; 2017.
41. Rajkumar SV, Kumar S. Multiple myeloma: diagnosis and treatment. Mayo Clin Proc. 2016;91:101–19. https://doi.org/10.1016/j.mayocp.2015.11.007.
42. Institute NC. Cancer Stat Facts: Myeloma. 2021. https://seer.cancer.gov/statfacts/html/mulmy.html. Accessed 04 June 2021.
43. Eslick R, Talaulikar D. Multiple myeloma: from diagnosis to treatment. Aust Family Phys. 2013;42:684–8.
44. Bruce A, Chabner DLL. Manual de Oncologia de Harrison. 2nd ed. Artmed: Porto Alegre; 2015.
45. Lyratzopoulos G, Saunders CL, Abel GA, et al. The relative length of the patient and the primary care interval in patients with 28 common and rarer cancers. Br J Cancer. 2015;112 Suppl 1:S35–40. https://doi.org/10.1038/bjc.2015.40.
46. Kariyawasan CC, Hughes DA, Jayatillake MM, et al. Multiple myeloma: causes and consequences of delay in diagnosis. QJM. 2007;100:635–40. https://doi.org/10.1093/qjmed/hcm077.
47. Landgren O, Kyle RA, Pfeiffer RM, et al. Monoclonal gammopathy of undetermined significance (MGUS) consistently precedes multiple

myeloma: a prospective study. Blood. 2009;113:5412–7. https://doi.org/10.1182/blood-2008-12-194241.
48. Katz A, Ricardo M; Novis Y, Rocha V, Costa FP, Fernandes GS, Ferrari CLS, Hoff PMG. Oncologia Clínica: Terapia Baseada em Evidências. 2nd ed. Hospital Sírio Libanês: São Paulo; 2014.
49. Zago Maf, Roberto Passetto; Pasquini, Ricardo. Hematologia: fundamentos e prática. Atheneu: São Paulo; 2001.
50. Rajkumar SV. Prevention of progression in monoclonal gammopathy of undetermined significance. Clin Cancer Res. 2009;15:5606–8. https://doi.org/10.1158/1078-0432.CCR-09-1575.
51. Caers J, Garderet L, Kortüm KM, et al. European Myeloma Network recommendations on tools for the diagnosis and monitoring of multiple myeloma: what to use and when. Haematologica. 2018;103:1772–84. https://doi.org/10.3324/haematol.2018.189159.
52. Bird JM, Owen RG, D'Sa S, et al. Guidelines for the diagnosis and management of multiple myeloma 2011. Br J Haematol. 2011;154:32–75. https://doi.org/10.1111/j.1365-2141.2011.08573.x.
53. Hungria VTM, Maiolino A. Mieloma Múltiplo: progressos e desafios. Rev Bras Hematol Hemoter. 2007;29:1–2. https://doi.org/10.1590/S1516-84842007000100002.
54. Rajkumar SV. Updated diagnostic criteria and staging system for multiple myeloma. American Society of Clinical Oncology educational book American Society of Clinical Oncology Annual Meeting 2016; 35: e418–23. https://doi.org/10.1200/edbk_159009.
55. Kumar S, Paiva B, Anderson KC, et al. International Myeloma Working Group consensus criteria for response and minimal residual disease assessment in multiple myeloma. Lancet Oncol. 2016;17:e328–46. https://doi.org/10.1016/s1470-2045(16)30206-6.
56. Feld J, Belasen A, Navada SC. Myelodysplastic syndromes: a review of therapeutic progress over the past 10 years. Expert Rev Anticancer Ther. 2020;20:465–82. https://doi.org/10.1080/14737140.2020.1770088.
57. Montalban-Bravo G, Garcia-Manero G. Myelodysplastic syndromes: 2018 update on diagnosis, risk-stratification and management. Am J Hematol. 2018;93:129–47. https://doi.org/10.1002/ajh.24930.
58. Arber DA, Orazi A, Hasserjian R, et al. The 2016 revision to the World Health Organization classification of myeloid neoplasms and acute leukemia. Blood. 2016;127:2391–405. https://doi.org/10.1182/blood-2016-03-643544.
59. Cazzola M. Myelodysplastic syndromes. N Engl J Med. 2020;383:1358–74. https://doi.org/10.1056/NEJMra1904794.
60. Larson RA. Therapy-related myeloid neoplasms. Haematologica. 2009;94:454–9. https://doi.org/10.3324/haematol.2008.005157.
61. Greenberg PL, Stone RM, Al-Kali A, et al. Myelodysplastic syndromes, version 2.2017, NCCN Clinical Practice Guidelines in Oncology. Journal of the National Comprehensive Cancer Network JNCCN. 2017;15:60–87. https://doi.org/10.6004/jnccn.2017.0007.

62. Steensma DP, Bejar R, Jaiswal S, et al. Clonal hematopoiesis of indeterminate potential and its distinction from myelodysplastic syndromes. Blood. 2015;126:9–16. https://doi.org/10.1182/blood-2015-03-631747.
63. Bannon SA, DiNardo CD. Hereditary predispositions to myelodysplastic syndrome. Int J Mol Sci. 2016;17 https://doi.org/10.3390/ijms17060838.
64. National Center for Chronic Disease P, Health Promotion Office on S and Health. Reports of the Surgeon General. The health consequences of smoking—50 years of progress: a report of the surgeon general. Atlanta: Centers for Disease Control and Prevention (US); 2014.
65. Lewis EB. Leukemia and ionizing radiation. Science. 1957;125:965–72. https://doi.org/10.1126/science.125.3255.965.
66. Nisse C, Haguenoer JM, Grandbastien B, et al. Occupational and environmental risk factors of the myelodysplastic syndromes in the North of France. Br J Haematol. 2001;112:927–35. https://doi.org/10.1046/j.1365-2141.2001.02645.x.
67. Valent P, Horny HP, Bennett JM, et al. Definitions and standards in the diagnosis and treatment of the myelodysplastic syndromes: Consensus statements and report from a working conference. Leukemia Res. 2007;31:727–36. https://doi.org/10.1016/j.leukres.2006.11.009.
68. Kwok B, Hall JM, Witte JS, et al. MDS-associated somatic mutations and clonal hematopoiesis are common in idiopathic cytopenias of undetermined significance. Blood. 2015;126:2355–61. https://doi.org/10.1182/blood-2015-08-667063.
69. Jawad MD, Shi M, Oliveira JL, et al. Clinical course of patients with incidental finding of 20q- in the bone marrow without a morphologic evidence of myeloid neoplasm. Am J Hematol. 2016;91:556–9. https://doi.org/10.1002/ajh.24347.
70. Hansen JW, Westman MK, Sjö LD, et al. Mutations in idiopathic cytopenia of undetermined significance assist diagnostics and correlate to dysplastic changes. Am J Hematol. 2016;91:1234–8. https://doi.org/10.1002/ajh.24554.
71. Malcovati L, Gallì A, Travaglino E, et al. Clinical significance of somatic mutation in unexplained blood cytopenia. Blood. 2017;129:3371–8. https://doi.org/10.1182/blood-2017-01-763425.
72. Bennett JM, Catovsky D, Daniel MT, et al. Proposals for the classification of the myelodysplastic syndromes. Br J Haematol. 1982;51:189–99.
73. Hong M, He G. The 2016 revision to the World Health Organization classification of myelodysplastic syndromes. J Transl Int Med. 2017;5:139–43. https://doi.org/10.1515/jtim-2017-0002.
74. Greenberg P, Cox C, LeBeau MM, et al. International scoring system for evaluating prognosis in myelodysplastic syndromes. Blood. 1997;89:2079–88.
75. Greenberg PL, Tuechler H, Schanz J, et al. Revised international prognostic scoring system for myelodysplastic syndromes. Blood. 2012;120:2454–65. https://doi.org/10.1182/blood-2012-03-420489.

76. Schanz J, Tüchler H, Solé F, et al. New comprehensive cytogenetic scoring system for primary myelodysplastic syndromes (MDS) and oligoblastic acute myeloid leukemia after MDS derived from an international database merge. J Clin Oncol. 2012;30:820–9. https://doi.org/10.1200/jco.2011.35.6394.
77. Kantarjian H, O'Brien S, Ravandi F, et al. Proposal for a new risk model in myelodysplastic syndrome that accounts for events not considered in the original International Prognostic Scoring System. Cancer. 2008;113:1351–61. https://doi.org/10.1002/cncr.23697.
78. Garcia-Manero G, Shan J, Faderl S, et al. A prognostic score for patients with lower risk myelodysplastic syndrome. Leukemia. 2008;22:538–43. https://doi.org/10.1038/sj.leu.2405070.
79. de Swart L, Crouch S, Hoeks M, et al. Impact of red blood cell transfusion dose density on progression-free survival in patients with lower-risk myelodysplastic syndromes. Haematologica. 2020;105:632–9. https://doi.org/10.3324/haematol.2018.212217.
80. Stern M, de Wreede LC, Brand R, et al. Sensitivity of hematological malignancies to graft-versus-host effects: an EBMT megafile analysis. Leukemia. 2014;28:2235–40. https://doi.org/10.1038/leu.2014.145.
81. Porter DL, Antin JH. Donor leukocyte infusions in myeloid malignancies: new strategies. Best Pract Res Clin Haematol. 2006;19:737–55. https://doi.org/10.1016/j.beha.2006.05.003.
82. Fenaux P, Mufti GJ, Hellstrom-Lindberg E, et al. Efficacy of azacitidine compared with that of conventional care regimens in the treatment of higher-risk myelodysplastic syndromes: a randomised, open-label, phase III study. Lancet Oncol. 2009;10:223–32. https://doi.org/10.1016/s1470-2045(09)70003-8.
83. de Witte T, Bowen D, Robin M, et al. Allogeneic hematopoietic stem cell transplantation for MDS and CMML: recommendations from an international expert panel. Blood. 2017;129:1753–62. https://doi.org/10.1182/blood-2016-06-724500.
84. Papaemmanuil E, Gerstung M, Malcovati L, et al. Clinical and biological implications of driver mutations in myelodysplastic syndromes. Blood. 2013;122:3616–27. https://doi.org/10.1182/blood-2013-08-518886.
85. Bejar R, Stevenson KE, Caughey BA, et al. Validation of a prognostic model and the impact of mutations in patients with lower-risk myelodysplastic syndromes. J Clin Oncol. 2012;30:3376–82. https://doi.org/10.1200/jco.2011.40.7379.
86. Haferlach T, Nagata Y, Grossmann V, et al. Landscape of genetic lesions in 944 patients with myelodysplastic syndromes. Leukemia. 2014;28:241–7. https://doi.org/10.1038/leu.2013.336.
87. Takahashi K, Patel K, Bueso-Ramos C, et al. Clinical implications of TP53 mutations in myelodysplastic syndromes treated with hypomethylating agents. Oncotarget. 2016;7:14172–87. https://doi.org/10.18632/oncotarget.7290.

88. Nazha A, Narkhede M, Radivoyevitch T, et al. Incorporation of molecular data into the Revised International Prognostic Scoring System in treated patients with myelodysplastic syndromes. Leukemia. 2016;30:2214–20. https://doi.org/10.1038/leu.2016.138.
89. Malcovati L, Karimi M, Papaemmanuil E, et al. SF3B1 mutation identifies a distinct subset of myelodysplastic syndrome with ring sideroblasts. Blood. 2015;126:233–41. https://doi.org/10.1182/blood-2015-03-633537.
90. Welch JS, Petti AA, Miller CA, et al. TP53 and decitabine in acute myeloid leukemia and myelodysplastic syndromes. N Engl J Med. 2016;375:2023–36. https://doi.org/10.1056/NEJMoa1605949.
91. Itzykson R, Kosmider O, Cluzeau T, et al. Impact of TET2 mutations on response rate to azacitidine in myelodysplastic syndromes and low blast count acute myeloid leukemias. Leukemia. 2011;25:1147–52. https://doi.org/10.1038/leu.2011.71.

# Drugs Used in Chemotherapy 4

Samanta Oliveira da Silva
and Ellen Mayara Corrêa

## 4.1 Introduction

Chemotherapy is one of the treatment modalities for cancer. It can be used with *curative intent* (aiming at eradicating the tumor), *disease control* (aiming at preventing the tumor from growing and developing, providing greater quality and life expectancy to the patient), or *palliative* (aiming at greater control of symptoms and a better quality of life to the patient).

Cancer cells differ from healthy cells by their ability to grow fast and disorderly, bypassing stages of cell cycle control (Fig. 4.1). These stages are checkpoints that repair the damage that has occurred or induce the cell to apoptosis if the error is irreparable [1].

Cytotoxic chemotherapeutic agents act by disrupting the cell cycle through various mechanisms. They can have specific action at some stage of the cell cycle, or not be phase-specific. Due to its systemic action, it also affects healthy cells that grow rapidly such as nail, hair, and mucous membrane cells [1]. From this mechanism, we can understand the toxicity caused by this class of drugs.

S. O. da Silva (✉)
Guarulhos, SP, Brazil

E. M. Corrêa
São Caetano do Sul, SP, Brazil



C. W. P. Schmidt, K. M. Otoni (eds.), *The Golden Guide to Oncologic Pharmacy*, https://doi.org/10.1007/978-3-030-98596-7_4

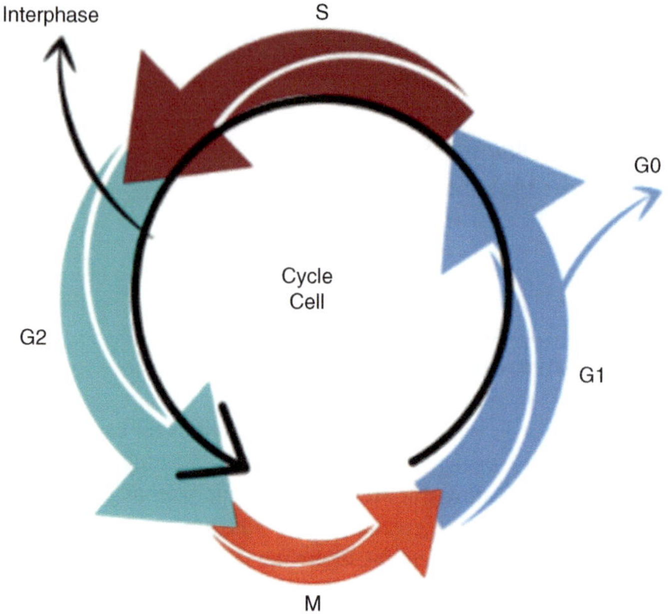


**Fig. 4.1** Cell cycle. *Interphase:* The longest phase of the cell cycle. Cell grows in size and copies its DNA. In G0 the cell is at rest; in G1 there are a cell growth, RNA, proteins, and organelle synthesis; in S there is a division of genetic material and DNA duplication; in G2 there is reorganization of cell content and preparation for mitosis. *Mitosis (M):* DNA separation and cytoplasm division, with consequent formation of two new cells

Chemotherapy can be *adjuvant* (when it is used after some previous treatment, such as surgery, aimed at reducing relapse due to micro-metastatic disease) or *neoadjuvant* (when it is performed before surgery, aiming at reducing the size of the tumor for a more conservative surgery and better recovery) [1].

In this chapter we will talk about the drugs used in this therapeutic modality. Fig. 4.1 is a representation of the cell cycle and each of its phases.

## 4.2 Alkylating Agents

Alkylating agents were discovered in 1942 through the mustard gas used during World War I and World War II. At that time it was noticed that this substance caused leukopenia in soldiers who had contact with this gas, and from then onwards, its mechanism of action, toxicities began to be better studied, and several drugs for the treatment of cancer were developed [2].

It is a class of drugs that cause DNA damage by promoting its alkylation. They are non-specific cell cycle agents [2, 3].

Due to DNA damage, although it rarely occurs, the use of alkylating agents can cause leukemia. The risk is dose-dependent, that is, the higher the total dose, the higher the risk [3].

Currently, they are used as conditioning for hematopoietic stem cell transplantation, in addition to the treatment of various types of cancer, such as lung, breast, ovary, multiple myeloma, and sarcoma [3].

We will see below its subclasses and representatives.

### 4.2.1 Nitrogen Mustards

- Bendamustine: It acts by crosslinking DNA strands, resulting in their degradation. It is active against resting and dividing cells. It has moderate emetogenic potential. It can cause severe myelosuppression and anaphylactic reactions, in addition to tumor lysis syndrome, which usually occurs in the first course of treatment. It is recommended not to be used in patients with ClCr<40 mL/min [4–6].
- Cyclophosphamide: It forms crosslinks with the DNA of tumor cells, causing an imbalance in the RNA and protein synthesis, inducing cell death. It is metabolized by the liver and has urinary and partially fecal excretion if administered orally. It has moderate emetogenic potential at doses less than or equal to 1500 mg/m$^2$, and high emetogenic potential at doses higher

than 1500 mg/$m^2$. It is a drug with potent immunosuppressive action, which it has been used in several protocols for bone marrow transplants after stem cell infusion [4–6].

One of the main reactions that should be monitored with the use of cyclophosphamide is hemorrhagic cystitis. This occurs due to the accumulation of acrolein, a toxic metabolite of cyclophosphamide, which accumulates in the urinary tract. To avoid this reaction, it is necessary to use mesna, a detoxifying agent that reduces the deposition of acrolein in the bladder [7]. Intense hydration should also be used to prevent this reaction, which is considered only in patients with a need for fluid restriction.

High doses of cyclophosphamide can cause cardiotoxicity and cardiac dysfunction (CHF, cardiac necrosis, hemorrhagic myocarditis, pericardial effusion, acute heart failure that can manifest from 1 to 10 days of treatment), in addition to pulmonary fibrosis [4, 5].

- Chlorambutil: Oral medicine. It acts by forming crosslinks with DNA, inhibiting its synthesis and functionality. It is metabolized by the liver, excreted in urine, and is not dialysable. Its chronic use can cause myelocytic leukemia and secondary malignancies. It is important to monitor liver function tests, blood count, and uric acid level during treatment. It has low emetogenic potential and high myelosuppressive potential. It is suggested that it be ingested on an empty stomach [4–6].
- Ifosfamide: It acts after being activated by hepatic microsomal enzymes. It destroys and blocks DNA synthesis, causing its strands to break. It is a synthetic analogue of cyclophosphamide, so it can also cause hemorrhagic cystitis and cardiotoxicity. Neurotoxicity, encephalopathy, confusion, and coma due to CNS toxicity may also be associated with therapy. It has hepatic metabolism (acrolein is one of its metabolites), renal excretion, and moderate emetogenic potential [4–6].
- Mechlorethamine: It inhibits DNA and RNA synthesis through the formation of carbon ions; it causes changes in DNA strands

(inter- and intra-strand cross-linking) promoting coding breakage and replication failure. It has rapid and extensive metabolism, and urinary excretion. Some adverse effects are coagulation disorders, hyperuricemia, and dermatitis. It has high emetogenic potential [4–6].

- Melphalan: Derived from mechlorethamine. It has fecal and urinary excretion, and the half-life time for intravenous administration is approximately 75 minutes, while for oral presentation is 60–120 minutes. It is not dialyzable and has moderate emetogenic potential. Some of the adverse effects are myelosuppression and mucositis [4–6].

Cryotherapy is widely used to reduce the incidence and duration of oral mucositis caused by the use of melphalan; patients suck ice or ice cream or put cold water in their mouths before, during, and after infusion of the medication [8, 9]..

### 4.2.2 Nitrosureas

They are alkylating drugs with known action in the central nervous system, as they cross the blood-brain barrier. Therefore, they are effective for the treatment of some brain tumors [3].

The representatives of this class are:

- Fotemustine: It acts by inhibiting DNA synthesis and has a chelating and carbamylating effect. It has low emetogenic potential at doses above 150 mg/m$^2$, and minimal at doses below this; it has easy tissue penetration and high plasma clearance. Some of its most common reactions are paresthesia, anemia, leukopenia, thrombocytopenia, and elevated transaminases [4, 6].
- Streptozocin: It acts by inhibiting DNA synthesis. It is believed to present some specificity for endocrine cells from pancreatic tumors. It has liver metabolism and urinary excretion. It often causes severe nausea, nephrotoxicity, and neurological reactions (confusion, lethargy, depression). There are also reports

of changes in glucose metabolism in some patients. It has high emetogenic potential [4–6].

- Lomustine: It alkylates DNA strands, generating inhibition of DNA, RNA, and proteinsynthesis, in addition to amino acid carbamylation. It has hepatic metabolism, 50% renal excretion, and < 5% fecal. It is recommended that pulmonary function tests be performed before starting therapy, and that this should be repeated frequently, as this may cause late pulmonary toxicity; it is contraindicated for patients with pulmonary fibrosis. It is an oral medication, which should be administered on an empty stomach, and you should ingest food/drinks about 2 hours after administration. It has moderate to high emetogenic potential [4–6].
- Carmustine: its action occurs through its metabolites, which inhibit several enzymes involved in the formation of DNA. Furthermore, it also interferes with the synthesis of DNA, RNA, and proteins by breaking down their strands. In high-dose therapies, it can cause hypotension due to the alcohol contained in its composition as a diluent; in addition, pulmonary toxicity is dose dependent, that is, the risk increases with cumulative doses >1400 mg/m$^2$. Some adverse reactions are myelosuppression, reversible increases in liver parameters (bilirubin, alkaline phosphatase, and AST), seizures, and hemiplegia. It has urinary excretion [4, 5].

### 4.2.3 Triazenes

- Dacarbazine: It's a non-classic alkylating. It causes double-strand DNA breaks, leading to apoptosis of the cell. It has hepatic metabolism, and its excretion is approximately 40% in the urine. Its emetogenic potential is high. There is recommendation for dose adjustment for renal dysfunction and monitoring of liver function. Hematological toxicity is the most common toxicity [4–6].
- Temozolomide: It is an imidazotetracene, chemically transformed in the systemic circulation at physiological pH, forming the active compound MTIC (monomethyl-triacenoimidazole-

carboxamide), which has cytotoxic activity. Its excretion is via urine, and women may have approximately 5% lower temozolomide clearance (adjusted for body surface area) than men [10]. It has moderate/high emetogenic potential when used at doses above 75 mg/m$^2$, and low when used in doses below 75 mg/m$^2$. It can cause severe hepatotoxicity and viral infections, mainly due to *Pneumocystis jirovecii* pneumonia, with a higher proportion in patients using corticosteroids. It is an oral medicine, and it is suggested to take away from meals or at bedtime to reduce emetogenic effects [4–6].

### 4.2.4 Alkyl Sulfonate

- Busulfan: Interferes with normal DNA function by alkylation and crosslinking of DNA strands. It reacts with the N-7 position of guanosine and interferes with DNA replication and RNA transcription. Busulfan has a more prominent effect on myeloid cells than on lymphoid cells [10]. Low emetogenic potential. The high doses used in conditioning for hematopoietic stem cell transplantation can cause tonic-clonic epileptic seizures that can occur up to 24 hours after the last dose of Busulfan. Therefore, there is an indication for the use of prophylactic anticonvulsant therapy (phenytoin, levetiracetam, benzodiazepines, or valproic acid), which should be started 24 hours before the first dose of Busulfan and maintained for at least 24 hours after the last dose. Other important aspects are attention to hypoalbuminemia, monitoring of liver function, and signs/symptoms of veno-occlusive disease, due to the increased risk of VOD due to its use [4–6].

### 4.2.5 Platinum Coordination Complexes

- Cisplatin: composed of a heavy metal complex containing a central platinum atom. It acts through bonds between the strands (intra and interstrand) of DNA, altering its synthesis, function, and inhibiting transcription. Its excretion is urinary

(90%) and fecal (10%). It poses a risk of cumulative nephrotoxicity, especially if used concomitantly with aminoglycoside antibiotics; intense pre-hydration (1 to 2 L intravenously associated with magnesium sulfate), and mannitol is used to stimulate diuresis. It has a high emetogenic potential [4–6].

- Carboplatin: part of a more modern generation of platinum analogues. Its mechanism is by changing the structure of DNA, through crosslinks in its strands. It is structurally similar to cisplatin, with a central platinum atom, but it has less renal, neurological, and gastrointestinal toxicity [4]. It has moderate emetogenic potential [6]. In some protocols, when the patient does not tolerate the use of cisplatin (e.g., cases of limiting renal toxicity), carboplatin can be assessed and also prescribed [4–6].
- Oxaliplatin: its mechanism of action is through the inhibiting of DNA synthesis and replication, in addition to interfering with the synthesis of RNA and cellular proteins. Just like cisplatin, it produces covalent bonds that lead to the formation of interfilament and intrafilament bridges in DNA. It has moderate emetogenic potential, urinary excretion, and is not dialyzable. Some of the most common reactions are peripheral neuropathy, anemia, fatigue, thrombocytopenia, and fever; some reactions to a lesser extent, but which should be considered are cardiovascular toxicity, posterior reversible leukoencephalopathy syndrome, and rhabdomyolysis [4–6].

### 4.2.6 Other Alkylating Agents

- Estramustine: Its mechanism of action is not yet fully elucidated. It combines the effects of estradiol and nitrogen mustard, in addition to having characteristics of a microtubular agent because it binds to proteins associated with microtubules, preventing the normal function of tubulin. It promotes a reduction in plasma testosterone levels and an increase in estrogen levels. It has moderate/high emetogenic potential. It has hepatic metabolism and fecal excretion. Some of the most common adverse reactions are edema, breast tenderness, gastrointestinal reactions, and dyspnea. Its administration is orally, and the capsule should be ingested away from meals, as absorption is decreased when administered with meals, with milk or calcium-rich medicines [4–6].

- Lurbinectedin: An agent that selectively inhibits the RNA polymerase II enzyme, affecting the active transcription of encoding genes and inducing cell apoptosis. It is believed to cause dysregulation of cytokine synthesis associated with tumor growth by preventing oncogenic transcription in macrophages. It is hepatically metabolized by CYP3A4 and excreted by feces (89%) and urine (6%). There is a strong recommendation for the use of pre-medicating the patient with antiemetics. It can cause severe hepatotoxicity; therefore it is suggested that liver function tests be performed before prior to initiation of treatment and during use as needed. Some of the most common adverse reactions are myelosuppression, fatigue, increased blood glucose, and dyspnea. It may cause peripheral neuropathy (11%). Extreme caution should be exercised with drug interactions with inhibitors and inducers of CYP3A4, due to the increase and decrease, respectively, of systemic exposure of lurbinectedin [4, 5].
- Procarbazine: Oral alkylating agent, derived from methylhydrazine. It acts by inhibiting the synthesis of proteins, DNA, and RNA; it can suppress mitosis and directly damage DNA. It has hepatic and renal metabolism, and urinary excretion. It has moderate/high emetogenic potential, and some of its adverse effects are myelosuppression, neurotoxicity (CNS and peripheral neuropathy), and liver dysfunction. It can be given as a single dose or divided into 2 or 3 daily doses. It is important to monitor adherence to treatment, and guide the patient to avoid consumption of alcohol and foods rich in tyramine (procarbazine has MAO-inhibiting activity) [4–6].
- Treosulfan: An alkylating agent similar to Busulfan, differing from it by the presence of two hydroxyl groups in its structure. It acts by enzymatic conversion to an active epoxide compound that reacts with the nucleophilic centers in the DNA via alkyla-

tion. It has active epoxide L-diepoxybutane metabolism and urinary excretion. As more serious adverse events, it can cause cardiomyopathy, alveolitis, and pulmonary fibrosis [4].

- Thiotepa: It is pharmacologically similar to mechlorethamine. It reacts with phosphate groups to inhibit the synthesis of proteins, DNA, and RNA, as it produces chromosomal alterations and blocks the synthesis of nucleoproteins. It has hepatic metabolism, urinary excretion, and is dialyzable. It can be used intravesically to treat bladder cancer and intrathecally in cases of leptomeningeal metastases. It may cause reactions such as rash, asthenia, fatigue, fever, stomatitis, and myelosuppression [4–6, 10].
- Trabectedin: It causes changes in the cell cycle after its binding to DNA, which forms a cascade of signals that affect transcription factors, DNA-binding proteins, and repair pathways. It has moderate hepatic metabolism and emetogenic potential. It is not recommended for patients with CrCl<30 mL/min e CPK > 2.5 × LSN (due to the high risk of rhabdomyolysis). It can cause reactions such as hand-foot syndrome, stomatitis, fatigue, and myelosuppression. It is recommended to pay attention to drug interactions inhibitors and inducers of CYP3A4, due to the increase and decrease, respectively, in the systemic exposure of trabectedin [4–6].

## 4.3 Antimetabolites

A class of specific cell cycle drugs, with S-phase action, which act on the metabolism of proliferating cells, by replacing the normal building blocks of DNA and RNA, performing a biochemical blockage in DNA synthesis. Thus, they interfere with cell division [3, 11, 12]..

The agents of this group, in their subclasses, and some of their characteristics are:

### 4.3.1 Folate Analogues

- Methotrexate: It inhibits dihydrofolate reductase (DHFR), preventing the conversion of dihydrofolic acid to tetrahydrofolic acid, which is essential for the production of thymines and purines. It binds with thymidylate synthase (TS), causing inhibition of purine and synthesis of thymidylic acid [4]. It is indicated for a wide variety of pathologies, from onco-hematological diseases to solid tumors. It has an immunosuppressive action, and is used in several allogeneic bone marrow transplant protocols after stem cell infusion as prevention of graft-versus-host disease, and in the treatment of autoimmune diseases. It has hepatic and intracellular metabolism, and urinary excretion [5]. It may cause alopecia, photosensitivity, thrombocytopenia, increased liver enzymes, and mucositis. Its use should be avoided in patients with ascites, pleural effusion, or significant peripheral edema, as toxicity can be increased in these situations. For doses above 500 mg/m$^2$, calcium folinate rescue should be used [4].
- Pemetrexed: It acts by disrupting the folate-dependent metabolic process, essential for cell replication, in addition to inhibiting thymidylate synthase, DHFR, and glycinamide ribonucleotide formyl transferase (GARFT), folate-dependent enzymes for new biosynthesis of thymidine and purine nucleotides. Its metabolism is minimal, and its excretion is renal. Treatment can cause severe kidney toxicity. It is not recommended for patients with ClCr<45 mL/min; therefore it is necessary to monitor creatinine clearance before each dose. It is recommended to pre-medicate with dexamethasone, 4 mg by mouth, 12/12 h, for 3 days, starting 1 day before administration. Administer folic acid (0.4 to 1 mg by mouth, 1×/day) for at least 5 days before and continue throughout the treatment and until 21 days after the last dose. Administer vitamin B12 1000 mcg in a single dose 1 week before the start of treatment and repeat every 9 weeks. It has low emetogenic potential [4–6].

- Pralatrexate: DHFR inhibitor and competitive inhibitor for polyglutamylation by the enzyme folylpolyglutamate synthase. This inhibition causes depletion of thymidine and other biological molecules on which a single carbon transfer depends. It has negligible hepatic metabolism, and renal excretion. It is recommended to administer low dose of folic acid orally (start 10 days before the first cycle, continue throughout the treatment and for 30 days after the last dose) and vitamin B12 1000 mcg IM (start within 10 weeks before the first cycle and then every 8–10 weeks). It can cause severe mucositis, kidney failure, dermatological reactions, and fatigue. It has minimal emetogenic potential [4–6].
- Raltitrexed: inhibitor of thymidylate synthase, which causes DNA fragmentation and cell death. It suffers intense cell metabolism (there seems to be no systemic metabolism). Its excretion is 50% renal and 15% fecal. Some reactions it can cause are nausea, vomiting, diarrhea, asthenia, anemia, fever, and leukocytopenia [4].

### 4.3.2 Purine Analogues

- Cladribina: Prodrug activated by phosphorylation and converted into the active part, Cd-ATP. This active form inserts itself into the DNA and promotes its strand break and interruption of its synthesis and repair. This also results in a depletion of the nicotinamide adenine dinucleotide and adenosine triphosphate (ATP). It destroys dividing or resting lymphocytes and monocytes, malignant or not, which have a large amount of deoxycytidine kinase but a small amount of deoxynucleotides. It has minimal emetogenic potential. Excretion is urinary, and its most common adverse reactions are fever, myelosuppression, and fatigue. For patients with a high tumor burden, prophylaxis for tumor lysis syndrome is recommended [4–6, 10].
- Clofarabine: It acts by interfering in DNA synthesis by reducing the deoxyribonucleotide triphosphate pools, by

inhibiting ribonucleotide reductase through the termination of DNA chain elongation and by competing with DNA polymerase for incorporation into the DNA chain, inhibiting cell repair. It can also promote mitochondrial-mediated apoptosis. It has hepatic metabolism (0.2%) and renal excretion. It can cause reactions such as severe and prolonged myelosuppresion, tumor lysis syndrome, increased liver parameters (AST, ALT, and bilirubins), and nephrotoxicity. Monitor and discontinue if sinusoidal obstruction syndrome is suspected [4, 5, 10].

- Fludarabine: Prodrug resistant to deamination by adenosine deaminase. Fluorinated nucleotide analogous to the antiviral agent vidarabine. It inhibits DNA synthesis by inhibiting DNA polymerase and ribonucleotide reductase; it also inhibits DNA primase and DNA ligase I. It has low/minimal emetogenic potential, hepatic metabolism, and renal excretion. It can cause reactions such as myelosuppression, asthena, cough, fatigue, fever, and tremors. Use prophylaxis for patients at risk of tumor lysis syndrome. At high doses it can cause irreversible or fatal neurotoxicity, which manifests 21 to 60 days after use [4–6].
- Mercaptopurine: It blocks DNA and RNA synthesis; inside the cell, it is converted into an active form that competes for an enzyme necessary for purine synthesis. Its metabolism is hepatic and in the gastrointestinal mucosa, and excretion is urinary. It's not dialyzable. It has low/minimal emetogenic potential and can cause reactions such as hyperuricemia, hypoglycemia-induced seizure, and hepatotoxicity. It is given orally, and should be ingested on an empty stomach. Oral hydration of at least 2 L/day is recommended to prevent uric acid nephropathy [4–6].
- Nelararabine: is a prodrug of the analogue deoxyiguanosineara-G. It is demethylated by adenosine deaminase (ADA) in ara-G and then intracellularly phosphorylated by deoxyguanosine and deoxycytidine kinases in its 5′-monophosphate metabolite. The monophosphate metabolite is subsequently converted into active form 5′-triphosphate,

ara-GTP. The accumulation of ara-GTP in DNA leads to inhibition of its synthesis and cell death. In vitro, T cells are more sensitive than B cells to their cytotoxic effects. The main metabolic pathway is O-demethylation by adenosine deaminase to form the ara-G, and its excretion is partially urinary. It has minimal emetogenic potential. It is administered intravenously and must not be diluted during preparation. The dose to be used should be transferred to PVC, EVA, or glass bags and administered for 2 h in adults and within 1 h in children. Neurotoxicity is dose-limiting, and neurological events are often not reversible even after discontinuation of the drug, so continuous monitoring of signs and symptoms (such as altered mental status, drowsiness, seizures, peripheral neuropathy, paralysis) should be carried out. It is recommended that the patient be hydrated in an endovenous route and that the use of allopurinol should be considered in patients at risk for tumor lysis syndrome [4–6].

- Pentostatin: Pentostatin is a purine antimetabolite that inhibits adenosine deaminase, preventing the deamination of adenosine in inosine. The accumulation of deoxyadenosine (dAdo) and deoxyadenosine 5′-triphosphate (dATP) leads to a reduction in purine metabolism that blocks DNA synthesis and leads to cell death. It has hepatic metabolism, renal excretion, and minimal emetogenic potential. It is recommended to perform intravenous hydration before and after administration of the drug. It may cause nausea, vomiting, stomatitis, myelosuppression, fatigue, and fever. Concomitant use with fludarabine can cause fatal lung toxicity [4–6, 10].
- Thioguanine: Analogue of mercaptopurine which, after being converted into its active form, inhibits the synthesis of purines, blocking the formation of DNA. Its metabolism is hepatic; excretion is urinary and not dialyzable. It has minimal emetogenic potential. It is an oral chemotherapy that can be administered with or without food. Some reactions that may occur are hyperuricemia, stomatitis, myelosuppression, and hepatotoxicity [4, 6, 10].

### 4.3.3 Pyrimidine Analogues

- Fluorouracil: F-UMP (an active metabolite) binds to RNA to replace uracil and inhibit cell growth; the active metabolite F-dUMP, inhibits thymidylate synthase (TS), depleting thymidine triphosphate (a necessary component of DNA synthesis). It has low emetogenic potential; its metabolism is hepatic and urinary excretion. For hemodialysis patients, administer 50% of the dose after this procedure. It is contraindicated in patients with DPD deficiency (dihydropyrimidine dehydrogenase, an enzyme encoded by the DPYD gene). Some of the main adverse effects are myelosuppression, hand-foot syndrome, loss of appetite, headache, mucositis, and alopecia [4–6, 10].
- It can also cause cardiotoxicity associated with complications of coronary vasculature, such as angina, which has a higher incidence of continuous infusion when compared in bolus infusions, with an incidence reported in the literature ranging from 1 to 45% and onset during infusion or up to 72 h, in addition to acute coronary syndrome, hypotension, and heart failure [13–15].
- Capecitabine: It is a prodrug of 5-fluorouracil, metabolized in the liver into 5-deoxy-5-fluorouridine and converted in vivo in 5-fluorouracil by the enzyme thymidine phosphorylase, expressed at higher levels in tumors than in normal tissues. Capecitabine is an oral drug with minimal/low emetogenous potential. It has hepatic metabolism, renal excretion and is dialyzable. It is contraindicated in patients with DPD deficiency, and as the toxicity in this patient profile is severe, there may be fatal neutropenia, mucositis, and diarrhea; nevertheless, as it is a rare mutation, screening for the mutation before starting treatment is not necessarily performed [4–6].

One of its most common reactions is hand-foot syndrome (54–63%), characterized by painful erythema, edema, dysesthesia (abnormal burning sensation, tingling, or pain), desquamation, blistering, and ulcers in the palmar and plantar regions [16]. It can also cause edema, diarrhea, stomatitis, myelosuppression, and cardiotoxicity. It is essential to evaluate the degree of toxicity of the reactions presented, to perform the management and dose modifications whenever necessary. It should be administered within 30 minutes after breakfast and dinner, with water, and without breaking or chewing the tablets [4].

- Cytarabine: Within cells, cytarabine is converted into azacitidine triphosphate, its active compound, which blocks the DNA synthesis and function and inhibits DNA polymerase. It also inhibits the enzyme ribonucleotide reductase by reducing levels of deoxyribonucleotides, essential for DNA synthesis and function. It is metabolized to a greater extent by the liver and to a lesser extent by the kidneys; its excretion is urinary. It has moderate emetogenic potential at doses above 1 $g/m^2$, and low at smaller doses. It can cause reactions such as skin rash, anal inflammation, mucositis, fever, myelosuppression, and liver dysfunction [4–6].

When used in high doses, even intravenously, it can cause corneal toxicity. To avoid such a reaction, it is customary to use corticosteroid-based eye drops (e.g., dexamethasone or prednisolone) to reduce the risk [17].

- Liposomal cytarabine: Liposomal cytarabine formulation for direct administration into the CSF. It should only be used intrathecally. Some of the most common adverse events are nausea, vomiting, asthenia, headache, and fever. Monitor for immediate adverse events and neurotoxicity. It is recommended to administer dexamethasone, 4 mg 2×/day (by mouth or IV), for 5 days, starting on the day of administration of liposomal cytarabine to reduce the occurrence of chemical arachnoiditis [4].
- Floxuridine: Metabolized to fluorouracil after administration, resulting in activity similar to it. It acts by inhibiting DNA synthesis, function and repair, and RNA and protein synthesis, as well as the methylation of deoxyuridylic acid to thymidylic acid. It has hepatic metabolism and renal (10–13%) and respiratory (60% as CO2) excretion. It can cause reactions such as

liver and kidney failure, myelosuppression, gastrointestinal toxicity, and photosensitivity [4, 5].

- Gemcitabine: It acts as a false metabolite, incorporating itself into DNA and promoting cell death. It inhibits DNA synthesis through intracellular conversion into nucleoside diphosphate and triphosphate. Diphosphate inhibits ribonucleotide reductase necessary for the formation of deoxynucleosides, essential in the DNA synthesis process, and triphosphate competes with deoxynucleosides for DNA incorporation. The active metabolite, gemcitabine triphosphate, can be extracted from peripheral blood mononuclear cells. Its excretion is urinary. It has low emetogenic potential. It can cause reactions such as edema, myelosuppression, hepatotoxicity, fatigue, and ototoxicity. Use with caution in patients with kidney and liver disorders, dose adjustment may be required. If the patient is on hemodialysis, start the procedure 6 to 12 hours after gemcitabine infusion. Consider drug pneumonitis when dyspnea, fever, cough, and/or hypoxemia. Infusions over 60 minutes increase adverse events due to the accumulation of its active metabolite gemcitabine triphosphate [4–6].

### 4.3.4 Hypomethylating Agents

They are pyrimidine analogues that instill DNA methyltransferase, causing hypomethylation and cell death [4].

The representatives of its class and some features are:

- Azacitidine: It has hepatic metabolism, renal excretion (85% EV and 50%SC) and moderate emetogenic potential. It can cause reactions such as myelosuppression, chest pain, hypotension, and increased liver enzymes. Evaluate the use of prophylaxis for tumor lysis syndrome in patients with high tumor burden (the reaction can occur even with the use of allopurinol) [4–6].
- Decitabine: It has metabolism via deamination by cytidine deaminase, minimal emetogenic potential, and can cause reactions such as myelosuppression, prexia, edema, electrolyte disorders, cough, fatigue, and fever [4–6].

### 4.3.5 Other Antimetabolites

- Hydroxyurea: its mechanism of action is not yet fully elucidated. Studies support the hypothesis that hydroxyurea causes immediate inhibition of DNA synthesis by acting as an inhibitor of ribonucleotide diphosphate reductase, and inhibits the incorporation of thymidine into DNA, blocking its synthesis. It does not interfere with the production of RNA or proteins. It is metabolized in about 60% by the liver and gastrointestinal tract and excreted by urine (30–55%). It has minimal/low emetogenic potential. It's an oral medicine; if necessary, the capsules can be opened and dissolved in 100 to 120 mL of water and ingested immediately after. It should be administered on an empty stomach. It can cause reactions such as myelosuppression, headache, and genetic mutation with long-term use [4–6].
- Trifluridine/Tipiracil (TAS-102): Trifluridine is the active cytotoxic component of Trifluridine +Tipiracil; it is a thymidine-based nucleic acid analogue; the triphosphate form of Trifluridine is incorporated into DNA, interfering with DNA synthesis and inhibiting cell proliferation. Tipiracil is a thymidine phosphorylase inhibitor that prevents the rapid degradation of trifluridine, allowing an increased exposure to the drug [10, 18]. It is an oral medicine, which should be ingested 1 h after a meal in the morning and in the evening. It can cause severe myelosuppression (which can lead to dose reduction or discontinuation of treatment), nausea, fatigue, and anemia [4, 5].
- Tegafur/Uracil: Cell cycle phase specific agent (post-mitotic G-1 phase). Tegafur is a metabolic precursor of fluorouracil whose conversion takes place in vivo. Uracil is a constituent of nucleic acids that does not present isolated pharmacological activity; however, preclinical studies reveal that the combination of tegafur with uracil in a 1:4 molar ratio inhibits the catabolism of fluorouracil and selectively increases the levels of this compound in the tumor, thus increasing its efficacy. It has low/minimal emetogenic potential. It is an oral medicine that should be given on an empty stomach 1 h before or 1 h after meals. It can cause reactions such as leukopenia, thrombocytopenia, asthenia, and peripheral neuropathy [4, 6].

## 4.4 Anti-Tumor Antibiotics

Anti-tumor antibiotics differ from antibiotics used to treat infections. They are called that because they are synthetic derivatives or isolated from living microorganisms, such as varieties of *Streptomyces* [19]. They have cytotoxic properties and cause DNA damage by various mechanisms, such as DNA and RNA interleaving, DNA alkylation, and oxygen-based free radical generation to induce single- and double-strand DNA breakage [20].

### 4.4.1 Anthracyclines

This class of anti-tumor antibiotics consists of one of the most widely used chemotherapeutic categories in clinical practice for different types of tumors, both solid (such as breast cancer) and hematological (such as leukemia). They generate permanent DNA damage.

One of its main characteristics concerns the cardiotoxicity induced by its use. The exact mechanism by which this occurs is not yet fully understood, but some of the most accepted theories are anthracyclines interfere in the redox cycle, causing DNA damage by producing reactive oxygen species (ROS); the interaction of anthracyclines with type II topoisomerase can also contribute, since this enzyme can be a mediator of cardiotoxicity [21].

They have the maximum recommended cumulative dose, which can greatly limit the treatment [21].

In general, they are vesicants. Its extravasation can cause severe injuries.

Doxorubicin and daunorubicin were the first anthracyclines used in clinical practice. Epirubicin is a stereoisomer of doxorubicin, whose difference is having a larger volume of distribution and half-life time. On the other hand, idarubicin, derived from daunorubicin, differs from the former in that it is more lipophilic and has greater cellular uptake [21].

In addition to these drugs, other representatives of this class are:

- Liposomal doxorubicin: It is a form of doxorubicin encapsulated in liposomes with methoxypolyethylene glycol (MPEG),which increases the duration of the drug in the blood circulation by protecting it from the phagocytic system [4].
- Valrubicin: It is a semisynthetic analog of the doxorubicin, with negligible systemic action. Indicated for bladder carcinoma, it is used intravesically. It must be instilled through a catheter and retained in the bladder for 2 hours, and after the patient urinates [5, 10].
- Mitoxantrone: Considered an anthracenedione agent. In patients with multiple sclerosis and cancer who have used mitoxatrone, there is an increased risk of secondary acute myeloid leukemia [4, 5].

### 4.4.2 Other Anti-Tumor Antibiotics

- Mitomycin C: It acts similarly to alkylating agents, alkylating DNA, and inhibiting DNA, RNA, and protein synthesis. It is derived from cultures of *Streptomyces caespitosus*; therefore it is considered an anti-tumor antibiotic. It is mainly metabolized by the liver, but can occur in other tissues; its excretion is via the kidneys. It has low emetogenic potential. It can cause reactions such as myelosuppression, hemolytic uremic syndrome (usually associated with single doses greater than 60 mg; its symptoms can be increased by blood transfusion), and pulmonary and cardiac toxicity. It can be administered intravesically [4–6, 10].
- Bleomycin: Specific to cell cycle phase (G2 and M phases), it acts by inhibiting DNA synthesis by binding to it, causing strand breakage. It also inhibits protein and RNA synthesis. It is metabolized in several tissues, and its excretion is renal (65% approximately) and intrapleural (40% approximately). It is not dialyzable and has minimal emetogenic potential. It requires dose adjustment for renal function, and some of its

main toxicities are pneumonitis, pulmonary fibrosis (especially when used in combination with other antineoplastics drugs), hepatotoxicity, and thrombotic microangiopathy. Attention should be paid to the use of bleomycin with brentuximab due to the increased risk of pulmonary toxicity [ 4–6].

- Dactinomycin: It inhibits DNA, RNA, and protein synthesis. It binds to DNA, intercalating between guanine and cytosine base pairs, disorganizing its helix. It has minimal metabolism, fecal and urinary excretion, and moderate emetogenic potential. It can cause severe skin reactions, myelosuppression, and increase the risk of hepatic veno-occlusive disease. There is a recommendation to avoid vaccination with live viruses during treatment [4–6].

## 4.5 Topoisomerase Inhibitors

Topoisomerases are essential enzymes for cell survival, as they help to reduce the tension of DNA supertwist, promoting strand cleavage and their rebinding. They play a role in cell duplication, acting in replication, transcription, recombination, repair, and reconstruction of chromatin (a filamentous complex of DNA, RNA, and proteins present in the cell nucleus). They are divided into topoisomerase I (which induces strand DNA breakage, allowing the passage of the other strand through this space) and topoisomerase II (which promotes a breakage in both strands, allowing the passage of another double helix) [22, 23].

When the functions of topoisomerases are inhibited, the cells become vulnerable, as cell replication is hampered by impeding the repair of cleaved strands. Therefore, they are excellent targets for drug action [10, 24].

### 4.5.1 Topoisomerase I Inhibitors (Also Known as Camptothecins)

Topoisomerase I is present in high concentrations in several types of malignant neoplastic cells [4]. It is not a cell cycle-dependent enzyme [23].

The representatives of this class, and some of its characteristics, are:

- Irinotecan: Pro-drug converted into the active metabolite SN-38, which binds to the topoisomerase I-DNA complex, preventing religation of the DNA strand. It has hepatic metabolism, renal and biliary excretion, and moderate emetogenic potential. Some of the main adverse reactions are gastrointestinal (diarrhea mainly), increased bilirubin, and fever. The use of atropine should be considered as a premedication to avoid acute cholinergic symptoms and to decrease diarrhea [ 4, 6, 10].
- Liposomal Irinotecan: A form of irinotecan encapsulated in a liposome (lipid layer) that allows higher serum and plasma concentrations at lower doses [4].
- Topotecan: It inhibits the production of topoisomerase I. It has low emetogenic potential and is metabolized in plasma and liver, and its excretion is fecal and urinary. It can cause effects such as myelosuppression, neutropenic colitis, asthenia, and fatigue [ 4, 6, 10].

### 4.5.2 Topoisomerase II Inhibitors (Also Known Epipodophyllotoxins)

Caution should be exercised with rapid infusions as they can cause hypotension [4].

The representatives of this class, and some of its characteristics, are:

- Etoposide: It has hepatic metabolism, urinary and fecal excretion, and low emetogenic potential. It may cause effects such as dose-limiting myelosuppression, asthenia, fever, malaise, hepatotoxicity, cardiotoxicity, and tremors. It's not dialyzable. [4, 6, 10]
- Teniposide: It has hepatic metabolism, urinary and fecal excretion, and moderate emetogenic potential. It may cause severe

myelosuppression, mucosal inflammatory disease, and neurotoxicity (<1%). A dose adjustment may be required for patients with significant renal dysfunction. [4, 6, 10]

## 4.6 Mitotic Inhibitors

Mitotic inhibitors are a class of agents that inhibit mitosis. There are four main categories: microtubule binders, microtubule enzyme inhibitors, mitotic enzyme inhibitors, and mitosis checkpoint inhibitors. Mitotic inhibitors impede the function of the mitotic spindle and cause the mitotic arrest and cause cell death. This mitosis inhibition approach has already been validated for the treatment of non-small cell lung cancer (NSCLC), for example, paclitaxel and docetaxel, already approved by the FDA. [25, 26]

Microtubules (MTs) are protein polymers made up of alternating subunits of α and β-Tubulin, which play a fundamental role in mitosis, such as intracellular signaling and motility. Disruption of the dynamics of microtubules (MTs), inhibiting their polymerization or depolymerization, disrupts the mitotic spindle function and cell division, resulting in mitotic arrest, mitotic progression, and segregation errors during anaphase; both situations can lead to cell death. Therefore, microtubules are an intracellular target already validated in oncology treatments [25].

There are two conventional classes of agents that target MTs, those that stabilize MTs, such as taxanes (paclitaxel, nab-paclitaxel, cabazitaxel, and docetaxel) and epothilones (ixabepilone) and those that destabilize MTs, such as vinca alkaloids (vinblastine, vincristine, vinorelbine, and vinflunine) and eribulin [27].

### 4.6.1 Microtubule Binders

- Paclitaxel (PTX): It promotes the aggregation of tubulin dimers microtubules. It stabilizes MTs preventing depolymerization, affecting the cellular dynamics of MTs reorganization, essential for cell function. Furthermore, it induces the abnormal formation or bundles of MTs during the cell cycle, acting specifically in the G2 and M phases of the cell cycle. Patients with liver failure may be at increased risk of toxicity. Renal function adjustment is not necessary [4].

- Nab-Paclitaxel: is a form of paclitaxel bound to albumin, which works as an inhibitor of MTs, promoting the association of tubulin dimers and stabilization of MTs. This stabilization prevents depolymerization and inhibits cell reorganization, affecting the cells' mitotic functions. Adjustment of liver function is necessary and adjustment for renal function is not necessary [4].
- Cabazitaxel: It binds to tubulin and promotes its aggregation into microtubules, dissociating them. In this way, it causes the stabilization of MTs, which results in the inhibition of cell functions of interphase and mitosis. It should be used with caution as it can alter kidney and liver functions. The main adverse reactions it causes are hematological or kidney failure [4].
- Docetaxel: It promotes the aggregation of tubulins and stabilization of MTS, causing their dissociation, making them non-functional, blocking cell division. It acts specifically in the M phase of the cell cycle. Its use should be cautious and the need for liver function adjustment observed, while adjustment for renal function is not necessary [4].

### 4.6.2 Vinca Alkaloids

- Vinblastine: It is considered a specific agent of the M phase of the cell cycle and inhibits the formation of MTs in the mitotic spindle, resulting in the arrest of cell division in metaphase. It inhibits DNA, RNA, and protein synthesis. The need for adjustment of liver function should be noted, while adjustment for renal function is not necessary [4].
- Vincristine: it is considered a specific agent of the S and M phases of the cell cycle; it binds to the protein of cellular MTs,

promoting its rupture and blocking cell division in metaphase. The need for adjustment of liver function should be noted, while adjustment for renal function is not necessary [4].

- Vinorelbine: It interferes with the rearrangement of MTs, inhibiting the metaphase stage in mitosis. It inhibits tubulin polymerization and acts on mitotic MTs. Furthermore, it interferes with amino acid metabolism, calcium transport, cellular respiration, and nucleic acid synthesis. It is a phase M-specific agent. The need for adjustment of liver function should be noted, whereas adjustment for renal function is not necessary [4].
- Vinflunine: It binds to tubulin and inhibits the polymerization of MTs, resulting in microtubule breakdown, mitotic arrest, and cell apoptosis. The need for adjustment of renal and liver function should be noted [4].

Another important mitotic inhibitor is *eribulin.*

It inhibits the growth phase of MTs and sequesters tubulin in non-functional aggregates, blocking the G2 and M phases of the cell cycle, breaking mitotic spindles and causing cell apoptosis. The need for adjustment of renal and liver function should be noted [4].

## 4.7 Histone Inhibitors

Epigenetic dysregulation is an almost universal feature of human cancer. Rather than affecting the DNA sequence itself, like genetic alterations, epigenetic alterations work by modifying histones or DNA post-translational. Within the cell nucleus, DNA is packaged into chromatin as repeating units known as nucleosomes. Each nucleosome consists of two copies, each with four histone proteins (H2A, H2B, H3, and H4). The level of compaction and the presence or absence of post-translational modifications in histones and DNA play an important role in gene expression. Histone acetylation and methylation were the first post-translational modifications to be associated with transcription regulation [28].

Below are some histone inhibitors:

- Tazemetostat: it is an inhibitor of the EZH2 gene (Enhancer of Zest Homolog 2) and of some EZH2 function mutations. EZH2 is located on chromosome 7 and encodes a protein involved in epigenetic regulation that is deregulated and mutated in some neoplasms, leading to the development and progression of tumor cells. There is no need to adjust kidney and liver function [4].

Soon after the discovery of DNA hypomethylating agents, histone deacetylase (HDAC) inhibitors have been explored. The best activity observed was in cutaneous T-cell lymphoma refractory [28].

### 4.7.1 Histone Deacetylase Inhibitors

- Panobinostat: It inhibits the removal of acetyl groups from histone lysine residues. This inhibition results in increased histone acetylation, epigenetic alteration, causing chromatin relaxation and transcription activation, inducing cell cycle arrest or apoptosis. Adjustment for liver function is required and has not been evaluated for adjustment of renal function [4].
- Romidepsin: HDAC inhibition results in the accumulation of acetylated histones, inducing cell cycle arrest and apoptosis. It should be used with caution for patients with liver or kidney disease [4].
- Vorinostat: It is an histone deacetylase (HDAC) inhibitor that is overexpressed in tumor cells. These enzymes assist in the reactions to remove lysine acetyl groups, transcription factors, and histones. Accumulation of acetylated histones induces cell cycle blockage and leads to apoptosis. There are no conclusive data on the need for adjustment for renal and liver function [4].

## 4.8 Proteasome Inhibitors

The proteasome is a complex of multicatalytic proteins that degrade cellular proteins. Proteasome inhibitors are an important new class of drugs for the treatment of multiple myeloma and mantle cell lymphoma (MCL). Proteasome inhibitors also work as immunosuppressants and inhibit bone absorption, among other applications. The first proteasome inhibitor to be approved by the FDA was bortezomib, followed by carfilzomib and ixazomib [29].

Protein degradation is an essential cellular function. Lysosomes were considered the main cell waste elimination system, as they degrade cytoplasmic proteins and organelle degradation by autophagy; it is currently known that the proteasome pathway is responsible for degradation processes in the cell [29].

The following are some proteasome inhibitors and their particularities:

*Bortezombe*: It reversibly inhibits the activity of chymotrypsin in the 26S proteasome, an enzyme complex that degrades ubiquitinated proteins and regulates cellular protein balance. Its inhibition of proteolysis affects the activation of signaling pathways, which can lead to cell death. Dose adjustment should be performed for liver function, but not needed for renal function. Its main toxicity effect is neurotoxicity, but it can be monitored by the doctor if it occurs. [4]

*Carfilzomib*: It is a proteasome inhibitor with pro-apoptotic and anti-proliferative activities in solid and hematological tumor cells, through irreversible binding to active sites of the 20S proteasome. Dose adjustment should be made according to liver and kidney functions [4].

*Ixazomib*: It is a reversible proteasome inhibitor that induces apoptosis in vitro of multiple myeloma cell lines. It inhibits chymotrypsin in the 20S proteasome. Dose adjustment should be made according to liver and kidney functions [4].

## 4.9 Hedgehog Inhibitors

The Hedgehog (Hh) signaling pathway controls a broad spectrum of processes during embryonic development, tissue homeostasis, tissue regeneration, and maintenance in adults. Activation of Hh is triggered by the interaction of ligands, which in turn relieves the suppression of the SMO (Smoothened) transmembrane receptor. Activation of SMO promotes the dissociation of the glioma-associated oncogene (GLI) and its nuclear translocation. As final effectors of Hh signaling, GLI factors activate the expression of Hh target genes involved in the regulation of the Hh pathway, proliferation, apoptosis, angiogenesis, stem cell self-renewal, and epithelial-mesenchymal transition. In addition to the signaling cascade, GLI can be stimulated by other mechanisms that interconnect other signaling pathways, such as RAS/RAF/MEK/MAPK and PKI3/AKT/Mtor [30].

The following are some Hedgehog Inhibitors (Hh):

- Vismodegib: It is an inhibitor of the Hedgehog pathway whose signaling through SMO leads to activation and localization of nuclear transcription factors of the GLI oncogene and induction of Hh. Many of these genes are involved in proliferation, survival, and differentiation. Vismodegib binds to and inhibits the SMO protein, blocking signals for the Hh pathway. The safety and efficacy of Vismodegib have not been evaluated for patients with renal and hepatic impairment [4].
- Glasdegib and Sonidegib: it is an inhibitor of the Hh signaling pathway that binds and inhibits SMO, affecting cancer biology, interrupting cancer stem cell survival mechanisms. The need for dose adjustments for patients with renal and hepatic impairment has not been evaluated [4].

## 4.10 Enzymes

All enzymes are proteins (and, in some cases, RNA molecules) of varying functions. They catalyze reactions used in normal development to help cells to protect against and fight disease. They have important roles intra- and extracellular or even on the surface of cell membranes. Many enzymes are targets of interest from studies, but an important enzyme that has been gaining prominence in the last 30 years is the enzyme L-Asparaginase. L-Asparaginase is the first therapeutic enzyme with antineoplastic properties. Its importance is due to its antineoplastic activity. It is known as amidohydrolases (or amidases) belonging to the group of amidase enzymes and can break down the amino acid L-asparagine in aspartate and ammonia [31].

The following are some important enzymes in this context:

- L-Asparaginase: It is a macronuclear enzyme isolated from *Escherichia coli* or *Erwinia carotovora.* It hydrolyzes the amino acid asparagine, which is essential in leukemic cell division. It is an agent specific to the G1 phase of the cell cycle. No dose adjustment is necessary for kidney and liver function [4].
- Calaspargase Pegol: It is a conjugate of L-asparaginase and monomethoxy polyethylene glycol (mPEG) with a succinimidyl carbonate (SC) linker. It is based on selective killing of leukemic cells. Dosage adjustment is necessary according to liver function, but it is not necessary for renal function [4].
- Pegaspargase: is a conjugate of L-asparaginase and monomethoxy polyethylene glycol (mPEG), an enzyme that catalyzes the conversion of the amino acid L-asparagine into aspartic acid and ammonia. Leukemic cells have low levels of expression of asparagine synthetase and are dependent on serum asparagine for survival, as pegaspargase hydrolyzes asparagine, depleting its levels and then inhibiting protein, DNA, and RNA synthesis, resulting in leukemic cell death. No dose adjustment is necessary for kidney and liver function [4, 32].

## 4.11 Corticosteroids

Glucocorticoids have a wide spectrum of therapeutic indications. They are capable of inducing cell maturation, cell differentiation, and even inducing apoptosis, which allows their use in the treatment of tumors, mainly of hematopoietic lineages. They play a fundamental role in the treatment of diseases in which immune and inflammatory processes are involved, such as cancer [33]. The following are some of them used in oncology practice as antitumor aids:

- Dexamethasone: It is an adrenocorticoid with potent anti-inflammatory effects, about 25 to 30 times more potent than hydrocortisone. It has immunosuppressive, antitumor, and anti-emetic properties and little mineralocorticoid activity. Its action occurs by suppressing the migration of neutrophils, decreasing the production of inflammatory mediators and reversing the increase in capillary permeability. No dose adjustment is necessary for kidney and liver function [4].
- -Prednisone: it is a synthetic glucocorticoid with anti-inflammatory, anti-rheumatic, anti-allergic, and immunosuppressive action, all of which are powerful. It has an antitumor property and little mineralocorticoid activity. It suppresses leukocyte migration and reverses the increase in vascular permeability. Its immunosuppressive activity is characterized by reduced lymphatic system activity and volume. In high doses, it suppresses adrenal function. Its antitumor effects are associated with inhibition of glucose transport, phosphorylation, and induction of cell death in mature lymphocytes. Its antiemetic action is due to the blockage of the vomiting mechanism and inhibition of prostaglandin synthesis. No dose adjustment is necessary for kidney and liver function [4].

The following is an inhibitory agent of corticosteroid synthesis:

- Mitotane: it is an inhibitor of adrenal corticosteroid synthesis; it is suggested that it modifies the peripheral metabolism of steroids, as well as directly suppressing the adrenal cortex, altering the extra-adrenal metabolism of cortisol. It should be administered with caution to patients with liver conditions, and there is no data on the need for dose adjustment for renal function [4].

## 4.12 Hormone Therapy

### 4.12.1 The Effect of Testosterone on Prostate Cancer

The effects of androgens on the prostate and surrounding stroma are diverse. The binding of the active testosterone metabolite, 5-α-dihydrotestosterone (DHT), to androgen receptors, results in the potentiation of several cellular processes, increasing the transcription of genes affected by the androgen receptor (AR). These include increased angiogenesis due to upregulation of endothelial growth factor (EGF) and vascular endothelial growth factor (VEGF), increased epithelial proliferation, and decreased apoptosis. AR is a transcription factor activated by testosterone and DHT and regulates the expression of genes related to sexual differentiation, growth and survival of prostate cells, and consequent cancer progression [34].

### 4.12.2 Androgen Deprivation Therapies (ADT)

The main objective of ADT is to reduce the circulatory level of androgens and their associated signaling mechanisms in tissues that respond to androgens, such as the prostate [34].

For patients with localized prostate cancer, definitive therapy includes radical prostatectomy and/or radiotherapy, given with or without adjuvant androgen deprivation. Despite the success of these treatments, up to a third of patients have a biochemical recurrence characterized by an increase in PSA. For these patients, androgen deprivation therapy (ADT) is indicated [35].

When there is an evidence of metastatic prostate cancer, patients are treated with androgen deprivation with or without docetaxel chemotherapy, or with or without abiraterone, with androgen deprivation continued indefinitely. At this stage, androgen deprivation therapy may include approaches that lower serum androgen levels by orchiectomy or by gonadotropin-releasing hormone (GnRH) analogues [35].

#### 4.12.2.1 Luteinizing Hormone-Releasing Hormone (LHRH) Agonists and Antagonists

The main LHRH analogues or agonists are leuprolide, goserelin, buserelin, and triptorelin. Another option is degarelix, an LHRH antagonist that is used in the treatment of prostate cancer. These agents work to decrease luteinization and hormone production leading to decreased gonadal testosterone production. These options with GnRH antagonist or analogues may or may not be accompanied by androgen receptor blockade with non-steroidal anti-androgens, e.g., bicalutamide and flutamide [35].

GnRH agonists and antagonists are considered pharmacological alternatives to surgical castration. Despite substantially lowering serum testosterone, adrenal production of androgens may persist, and it has become clear that prostate tumors can also synthesize androgens. Therefore, other therapies are usually added to suppress signaling and androgen levels [35].

*Leuprolide or Leuprorelin*: is an analogue of GnRH that is more potent than the natural hormone; it acts as an inhibitor of gonadotropin production. It initially causes an increase in luteinizing hormone (LH, also known as lutropin and sometimes lutrophin) and follicle stimulating hormone (FSH), causing a transient increase in testosterone and DHT. DHT, also known as 5α-androstan-17β-ol-3-one, is a naturally occurring androstane steroid with a ketone group at the C3 position and a hydroxyl group at the C17β position. It is the derivative of testosterone in which the double bond between the C4 and C5 positions has been reduced or hydrogenated. Prolonged administration leads to reduced levels of LH, FSH, and sex steroids [4].

*Buserelin*: is an analogue of GnRH, and its administration leads to the release of LH and FSH, followed by suppression of gonadotropin secretion as it desensitizes the pituitary gland to the effect of GnRH. Thus, it results in decreased levels of hormones and testosterone production; this decrease is obtained at the same levels obtained with castration [4].

*Goserelin*: is an analogue of GnRH that inhibits LH secretion, leading to decreased serum testosterone concentrations in men and women. Initially, it may increase serum concentrations of testosterone and estradiol transiently, but its use for a long time will decrease the levels of these hormones. The use of goserelin extends to patients with prostate cancer and also to breast cancer, given monthly or quarterly [4].

*Triptorelin*: it is a decapeptide GnRH agonist, and after its continuous and prolonged administration, it inhibits the secretion of gonadotropins, and consequently it has a direct effect on the gonads with a decrease in the sensitivity of peripheral GnRH receptors.

The following is the main antagonist of GnRH:

*Degarelix*: is an antagonist of GnRH, and competes reversibly for GnRH receptors in the hypophysis or pituitary gland, thus rapidly reducing the release of gonadotropins, consequently decreasing testosterone secretion. Unlike GnRH agonists, the antagonists do not induce LH peak with consequent peak/decrease in testosterone and transient tumor stimulation [4].

#### 4.12.2.2 Antiandrogens

The most commonly used nonsteroidal antiandrogens today are bicalutamide, enzalutamide, apalutamide, and darolutamide. These agents bind directly to the androgen receptor (AR), also known as NR3C4 AR in order to block signaling in the ARs. Abiraterone is also a potent Cyp17A1 inhibitor antiandrogen that results in further lowering of testosterone levels by blocking the production of androgens in non-gonadal tissues. As it follows [35]:

*Bicalutamide:* It is a non-steroidal antiandrogen indicated for patients with castration-resistant prostate cancer (CRPC) with or without metastasis [36].

*Enzalutamide*: It is a non-steroidal antiandrogen indicated for patients with CRPC and also metastatic hormone sensitive (HSPC) with or without metastasis [36].

*Apalutamide and Darolutamide*: nonsteroidal antiandrogens indicated for patients with non-metastatic CRPC [36].

*Abiraterone*: is considered first-line treatment for metastatic patients with HSPC with high volume of disease and is also indicated for CRPC [36].

Other drugs used in cancer therapy for prostate cancer patients:

### 4.12.3 Hormone Therapy in Breast Cancer

Hormone therapy in the treatment of breast cancer is essential for patient survival and increased survival. They are important for reducing recurrence and mortality in early cases. Some advantages of hormone therapy, as it is for oral use, are that it improves quality of life and hospitalization savings. The main hormonal agents used in breast cancer are antiestrogens, anti-progestins, aromatase inhibitors, and hormone blockers such as GNRH agonists [37].

#### 4.12.3.1 Antiestrogens

*Fulvestrant:* It is an estrogen receptor antagonist, and its action involves the suppression of estrogen receptor protein in tumors and other target tissues. Thus, it completely blocks the trophic action of estrogen, without having any estrogen receptor agonist activity [4].

*Tamoxifen*: it is an estrogen receptor antagonist and considered an innovative drug in medical oncology because in the last four decades it has been helping to save many lives. It was the first target agent discovered for the treatment of breast cancer. It is indicated for breast cancer prevention, treatment of estrogen receptor-positive and metastatic breast cancer, adjuvant treatment of breast cancer, and for ductal breast cancer in situ. In some cases, it is indicated for endometrial cancer [4, 38].

#### 4.12.3.2 Antiprogestins

*Megestrol:* It is a progestin synthetic acetate indicated for the treatment of hormone dependent tumors. There is a probable action on pro-inflammatory cytokines, tumor necrosis factor, and interleukins 1 and 6. Its effect is believed to be a glucocorticoid helping to suppress the pituitary gland and its action and decrease cortisol levels [39].

*Aromatase Inhibitors:* Breast cancers, especially those that depend on estrogen or progesterone hormones, are the most malignant form of the disease, especially in postmenopausal women. In this scenario, strategies with modulators of estrogen receptors (ER) or inhibitors of the aromatase enzyme (AIs) are being used by researchers. Aromatase is the enzyme that converts hormones for estrogen synthesis. AIs are used to block estrogen production or to block the action of estrogen at receptors. The main AIs used in clinical practice are exemestane, anastrozole, and letrozole [40].

#### 4.12.3.3 Somatostatin Analogs

They are synthesized drugs that are the most common somatostatin analogue drugs used. Its main indications in oncology are for pancreatic and gastrointestinal neuroendocrine tumors [41].

*Lanreotide and Octreotide*: They are endogenous somatostatin synthetic analogs. Somatostatin is an inhibitory hormone found in the body. In the hypothalamus, it inhibits the release of growth hormone (GH), TSH, prolactin, and ACTH. It inhibits the secretion of insulin, glucagon, gastrin, and other peptides. It functions as a CNS inhibitory neurotransmitter, inhibiting cell proliferation. Therefore, it has a direct effect on solid tumors of the gastrointestinal tract and prolongs patient survival. Their inhibitory, antisecretory, and absorption effects are used for hormone-secreting tumors (e.g., DHT) [41].

## 4.13 Main Therapies: Target for the Treatment of Cancer

### 4.13.1 The Role of Protein Kinases (PTKs)

The knowledge of cellular and biological mechanisms that involve proliferation, differentiation, metabolism, mobility, survival, cell death, and cell cycle control has made it possible to advance specific antineoplastic therapies that aim to inhibit the activity of proteins and receptors that are involved in these cellular processes. These therapies target cell receptors, their RTK ligands, known as "growth factors" (GF) and molecules involved in signaling pathways and intracellular signal transduction, as well as the regulation of cellular activities. Dysregulation and/or overexpression of protein kinases result in inappropriate cellular responses, culminating in the establishment of cancer [42, 43].

Protein tyrosine kinases (PTKs) (PTKs) are responsible for the transfer or addition of the $\gamma$-adenosine triphosphate phosphate

(ATP) to other target proteins (e.g., threonine, serine, tyrosine) inducing chemical, structural, and transcriptional control changes in these proteins. Therefore, it results in functional alterations of these proteins and alteration of their enzymatic activities. The binding between the ligand and its receptor results in the phosphorylation of the intracellular domain of the receptor, through the reaction between ATP and tyrosine residues, causing the phosphorylation of target proteins. Intracellular phosphorylation initiates cascades of cytoplasmic reactions that result in diverse cellular responses. Activated receptors stimulate these phosphorylation cascades, occurring sequential enzymatic interactions that constitute these signaling pathways. The transduction of intracellular signals is the way in which the cell receives a certain type of signal and transmits it to different pathways, which can be transformed until reaching the effector function by changing behavior of the cell and emitting signals to divide, proliferate, or provoke cell apoptosis [42, 43].

Due to their essential role in the process of cell proliferation, glycogen metabolism, apoptosis, neurotransmission, oncogenesis, dysregulation, or overexpression of receptors in general, PTKs have been studied and researched all around the world. Because of that, the main groups of protein kinases, their characteristics, and their main activities in cell metabolism will be discussed here. There are some main types of protein kinases: protein kinase A (PKA), protein kinase C (PKC), calcium-dependent protein kinase Ca 2 / calmodulin (CaMK), cyclin-dependent protein kinase (CDK), protein kinases activated by mitogens (MAPK), tyrosine kinases (PTKs), and receptor tyrosine kinases (RTKS) [44].

## 4.14 The Main Types of Signal Transduction Pathways

### 4.14.1 Via Ras/Raf/MEK/ERK

Growth factors and mitogens use the Ras/Raf/MEK/ERK signaling cascade to transmit signals from their receptors to regulate gene expression and prevent apoptosis. This pathway is often activated in certain tumors by chromosomal translocations, such as BCR-ABL, mutations in cytokine receptors, or overexpression of wild-type or mutated receptors, for example, the EGFR. Raf/MEK/ERK is also a pathway that has profound effects on the regulation of apoptosis by post-translational phosphorylation of apoptotic molecules, and this pathway has several effects that can regulate cell cycle progression, apoptosis, or differentiation [45, 46].

The activation of this Ras/Raf/MEK/ERK pathway can occur either by mutations in growth factor receptors (GFR) or by appropriate stimulation of growth factors (GF). Furthermore, mutations can occur in intrinsic members of the pathway (Ras, Raf, MEK1) [46].

Other mechanisms activated by ras/raf/mek/erk are cell survival, motility, invasion, and proliferation, as shown in Fig. 4.2 [47]:

#### 4.14.1.1 Via PI3K/PTEN/AKT/mTOR

The PI3K/PTEN/AKT/mTOR pathway is frequently activated in several human cancers and has been considered a promising therapeutic target. Possible mechanisms by which the PI3K/PTEN/AKT/mTOR axis contributes to oncogenesis include stimulation of proliferation, survival, cell metabolism, invasion and metastasis, suppression of autophagy, and senescence [48]. Look at Fig. 4.3 where the schematic shows the operation of this pathway.

The activation of the PI3K/PTEN/AKT/mTOR pathway contributes to the development of tumors and resistance to anticancer therapies. This pathway is found unregulated in almost all human cancers, such as breast cancer, colorectal cancer, and hematologic malignancies, which demonstrates the need to explore this pathway as a potential therapeutic direction in cancer treatment. The safety and efficacy of these therapeutic approaches have been investigated in numerous preclinical and clinical studies, and it is becoming increasingly clear that PI3K inhibitors are effective in inhibiting tumor progression [49].

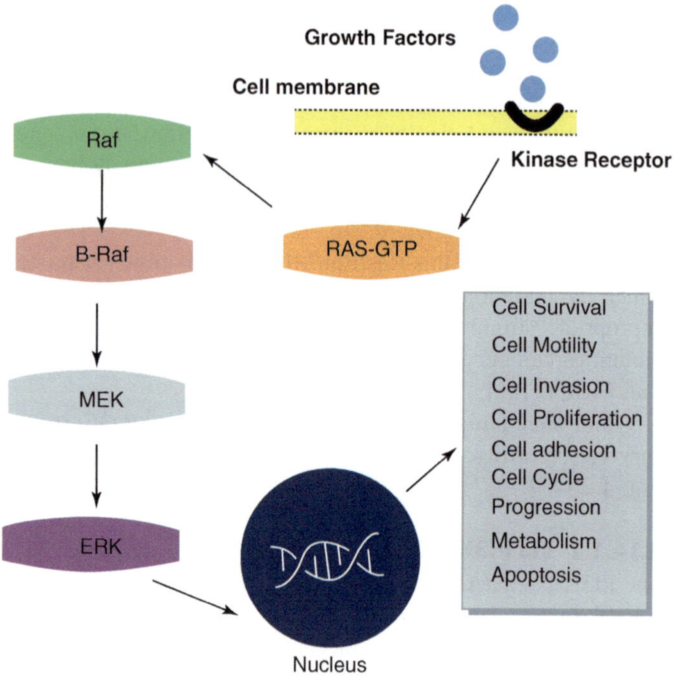


**Fig. 4.2** Ras/Raf/MEK/ERK signaling pathway – Growth factors and growth factor receptors activate Ras gene phosphorylation which will trigger the activation of other B-Raf/MEK/ERK genes, resulting in activities in the cell nucleus that will result in the maintenance of cell survival, motility, invasion, and proliferation

The Ras/Raf/MEK/ERK and PI3K/PTEN/Akt/mTOR cascades are often activated by genetic alterations in signaling molecules such as receptor tyrosine kinases (RTKs). The integral components of these pathways, Ras, B-Raf, PI3K, and PTEN, are also activated/inactivated by mutations. These pathways have profound effects on proliferative, apoptotic, and differentiation pathways. Dysregulation of these pathways may contribute to resistance to chemotherapy drugs, cancer-initiating cell proliferation, and premature aging. These pathways play important roles in

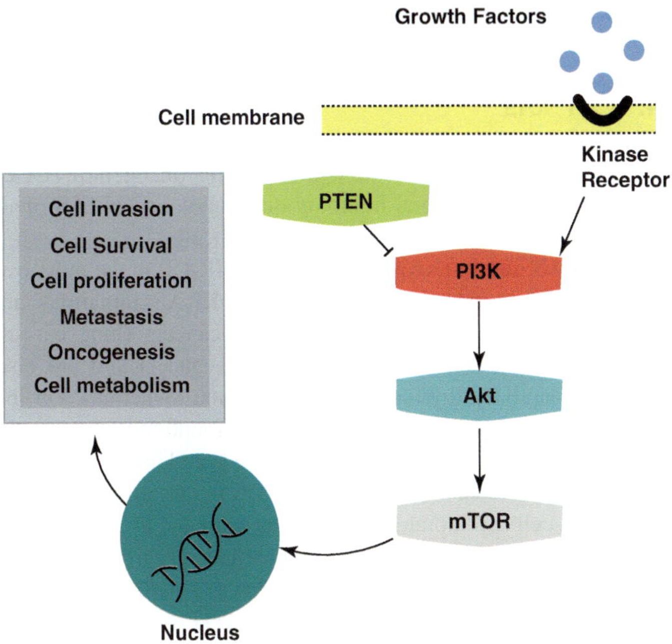


**Fig. 4.3** PI3K/PTEN/Akt/mTOR signaling pathway – Growth factors and growth factor receptors activate the PI3K protein that will trigger the activation of the other AKT and mTOR genes, resulting in activities in the cell nucleus that will result in an activation of oncogenesis, maintenance of survival and increase in cell metabolism, proliferation, invasion, and metastasis. PTEN inhibits the activation of PI3K; therefore it inhibits the activation of this signaling pathway

regulating the growth of normal and malignant cells. Inhibitors that target these pathways have many potential uses in suppressing cancer, proliferative diseases, as well as aging [45, 46].

There are several effective inhibitors specific to many of the major components of Ras/Raf/MEK/ERK and PI3K/PTEN/Akt/mTOR. These specific inhibitors have been developed and are currently used in clinical practice around the world in anticancer therapies [46].

## 4.14.2 Description of the Main PTKs Involved in the Signaling Pathways

### 4.14.2.1 RAS

The RAS (rat sarcoma) gene family consists of three members: KRAS (Kirsten rat sarcoma viral homolog oncogene), HRAS (Harvey rat sarcoma viral homolog oncogene), and NRAS (neuroblastoma RAS viral oncogene homolog) [50].

The RAS family (KRAS, NRAS, and HRAS) is the most frequent mutated gene family in cancers. KRAS mutations are known causes of three of the deadliest cancers (lung cancer, colorectal cancer (CRC), and pancreatic cancer) and are also found in papillary thyroid cancers and some leukemias. On the other hand, mutations in NRAS genes are found more frequently in cases of melanoma, but they can also be found in anaplastic and follicular thyroid cancers, whereas HRAS mutations are found in squamous cell carcinomas (SCC) of the head and neck, urothelial carcinoma of the bladder, and rarely in renal cell carcinomas [50].

In normal cells, RAS is activated through growth factor receptors on cell membranes, and when in its GTP-bound state, RAS interacts by activating various effector pathways, for example, mitogen-activated protein kinase (MAPK) and phosphatidylinositol 3-kinase (PI3K) pathway. RAS mutations keep the RAS in its active state, bound to GTP, activating the signaling pathways that result in tumor cell growth [50].

RAS proteins are activated through extracellular stimuli in the plasma membrane surface receptors, e.g., receptor tyrosine kinases (RTKs). These signals replace the inactive RAS bound to GDP with GTP, and this binding of RAS to GTP makes it active by stimulating intracellular signaling from various pathways, causing changes, for example, in mechanisms that lead to cell transformation, invasion, and metastasis. The most widely studied effectors for RAS signaling are the Raf serine/threonine kinases (c-Raf-1, A-Raf, B-Raf). The recent identification of mutated B-Raf in several types of human cancers provides validation of the importance of this effector pathway in oncogenesis. RAS promotes the association of Raf with the plasma membrane, where other events facilitate Raf activation. Raf then phosphorylates and activates the dual specificity kinases MEK1 and MEK2 which are mitogen-activated protein kinases ERK1 and ERK 2 (MAPKs) [51].

#### 4.14.2.2 RAF

RAF proteins are essential components of the RAS/RAF/MEK/ERK signaling cascade, and there are three isoforms: CRAF, BRAF, and ARAF. CRAF (also called Raf −1) is the first RAF protein identified, followed by ARAF and BRAF [47, 52].

Although they have similar molecular structures, RAF proteins perform quite different activities. BRAF is one of the main targets of genetic mutations in oncogenesis; it has the highest activity among three isoforms. [47, 52]

For RAF research, the first attentions were on the CRAF and after, were transferred to the BRAF after the discovery in 2002 that BRAF mutations (especially BRAF V600E) had a substitution of V600E (valine for glutamate) that occurs adjacent to a phosphorylation site, which occurs in a large percentage of certain types of cancer, especially melanoma [47, 52].

*BRAF Inhibitors:* Dabrafenib, Encorafenib, Vemurafenib, Sorafenib [4].

#### 4.14.2.3 MEK (Methyl Ethyl Ketone)

MEK was independently identified by various groups as an RAF substrate in 1992. Recent studies have provided detailed mechanisms of RAF phosphorylation and MEK activation. As substrate, MEK needs to be recruited by RAF prior to activation. In quiescent cells, BRAF and MEK form a heterodimer in the cytosol. In contrast to RAS and RAF mutations, MEK mutations are much less common in cancer genomes [52].

MAPK (MEK) is a RAS pathway kinase also known as MAPKs found in two different forms MEK1 and MEK2. These kinases, when phosphorylated, later activate to ERKs (ERK1 and ERK2). They are the only known catalytic substrates for RAF kinase. When RAS binds to RAF, it activates MAP-ERK kinases that are responsible for cell growth, proliferation, survival, translation, lipid metabolism, transcription, and protein acetylation [53].

Selective MEK inhibitors represent a new therapeutic option, having been shown to inhibit growth and induce cell death in melanoma cells with BRAF and NRAS mutations [52].

MEK1 and MEK2 inhibitors in combination with BRAF, KRAS, and PI3K inhibitors have shown promising results in mutated metastatic melanoma, colorectal adenocarcinoma with KRAS mutation, metastatic pancreatic adenocarcinoma, GIST, solid tumor, recurrent or refractory multiple myeloma, and recurrent melanoma [53].

*MEK Inhibitors:* Binimetinib, Cobimetinib, Trametinib [4].

#### 4.14.2.4 ERK

ERK1 and ERK2 are serine/threonine protein kinases that participate in the RAS-Raf-MEK-ERK signal transduction cascade. While the RAF kinases and MEK families have narrow substrate specificity, ERK1 AND ERK2 catalyze the phosphorylation of hundreds of cytoplasmic and nuclear substrates, including regulatory molecules and transcription factors [54].

ERK cascades are involved in physiological responses as [4]well as in maladaptive processes leading to diseases, for example, oncogenes have been identified within the ERK 1/2 signaling pathway in tumor cells [5].

Of several MAPKs, signal transduction via extracellular signal-regulated kinase (ERK) 1/2 is crucial for neurotrophin and growth factor-mediated neuronal responses. The RAS protein recruits RAF kinase to the membrane, where it is phosphorylated and activated by Ser /Thr /Tyr kinases. This leads to activation of ERK kinase (known as MEK). MEK then phosphorylates and activates ERK1/2 at Ser /Thr residues. After activation, ERK1 and ERK2 can phosphorylate regulatory targets in the cytosol or translocate to the nucleus and phosphorylate common substrates, including extracellular proteins, effectors, and transcription factors, resulting in a variety of responses such as cell proliferation, differentiation, expression gene, and the cell cycle response of neurons to neural activity [55].

#### 4.14.2.5 PI3K

Phosphatidylinositol-3-kinases (PI3Ks) are a family of intracellular heterodimeric lipid kinases that respond to nutrition, growth factor, and play a critical role in the regulation of many biological functions, including cell growth, proliferation, survival, differentiation, metabolism, motility, genomic stability, protein synthesis, and angiogenesis [56].

PI3Ks are divided into three classes (I–III) based on structural and biochemical properties. Class I PI3Ks are the main family of PI3K, and the enzymes are known to boost oncogenesis. Class IA PI3Ks are given activation through tyrosine kinase receptor signals (including HER, FGFR, and IGF-1) and G-protein-coupled receptors [56].

When PI3K is activated, it catalyzes the phosphorylation of PIP2 and PIP3 which will activate kinases involved in cellular mechanisms of activation of cell proliferation and multiplication [49].

Mutations in PI3K are often seen in the case of breast cancer, resulting in an uncontrolled, drug-resistant cell growth tumor [56].

Inhibition of PI3K can result in decreased cell proliferation and increased cell death [49].

*PI3K Inhibitors:* Alpelisib, Copanlisib, Duvelisib, Idelalisib [4].

#### 4.14.2.6 AKT

AKT kinases are molecules that signal cell growth and differentiation. AKT is a well-characterized effector of PI3K in the PI3K / Akt / mTOR signaling pathway and its dysregulation plays an important role in the development of many human cancers. Increased AKT kinase activity has been reported in breast cancer, epithelial ovarian, prostate, and gastric cancers. Many oncoproteins and tumor suppressors cross in the AKT pathway that results in cell proliferation, differentiation, and inhibition of apoptosis. The AKT pathway acts as an effective mediator by transmitting signals from a wide range of regulatory proteins, such as PTEN, PI3K, and receptor tyrosine kinases [57].

AKT kinase activity is induced by various growth factors, such as fibroblast growth factor (FGF), vascular endothelial growth factor (VEGF), nerve growth factor, epidermal growth factor (EGF), and growth factor similar to insulin (IGF), among others [57].

#### 4.14.2.7 mTOR

The mTOR kinase is called the rapamycin mechanistic target or rapamycin target in mammals. Numerous studies in non-neuronal cells from different species suggest mTOR as a main signal of the PI3K/AKT pathway in regulating the cell growth process. It has the remarkable ability to detect and integrate signals for cellular nutrients and energy to control protein synthesis and cell growth. The activity of this kinase is stimulated by insulin, mitogens, growth factors, and inhibited by low nutrient levels, growth factor deprivation, and cellular stress [59].

The regulation of mTOR activity by growth factors is mediated by the PI3K / AKT signaling pathway. Activation of AKT will result in other activities that will develop in the activation of mTOR. Activation of mTOR often results in cell growth and cell size increase [59].

MTOR inhibitors have been and are still intensively tested in oncological indications; their use in genetically defined syndromes and mTOR-related pathologies are promising pathways for pharmacological interventions [58].

*mTOR Inhibitors:* Everolimus, Temsirolimus [4].

#### 4.14.2.8 PTEN

The phosphatase and tensin homolog (PTEN) regulates the dephosphorylation of PIP2 and PIP3, preventing the activation of kinases. Therefore it is a tumor suppressor and negative regulator of PI3K function catalyzing the reverse reaction. The PTEN mutation and loss of its function are signaling activators and activation of PI3K in many tumors [58].

### 4.14.3 Description of Top RTKs

#### 4.14.3.1 VEGFR/VEGF

Members of the vascular endothelial growth factor (VEGF) family act by activating tyrosine kinase-like receptors. VEGF receptors (VEGFR, vascular endothelial growth factor receptor) are predominantly expressed on vascular endothelial cells. There are three VEGF receptors, and the selective activation of each one of them results in different biological responses. Activation of the Flt-1 receptor (or VEGFR-1) induces organizational effects on the vascular structure; activation of the KDR receptor (or VEGFR-2) induces vascular endothelial cell mitosis; and activation of the Flt-4 receptor (or VEGFR-3, predominantly expressed in lymphatic vessels) induces lymphoangiogenesis [60].

*VEGF Inhibitors:* Axitinib, Lenvatinib, Selpercatinib, Vandetanib, Sunitinib, Pazopanib, Sorafenib, Regorafenib, Sorafenib [4].

#### 4.14.3.2 EGFR/EGF

The epithelial growth factor receptor (EGFR) is a plasma membrane glycoprotein composed of an extracellular binding domain, a lipophilic transmembrane segment, and an intracellular tyrosine kinase domain. EGFR is a member of the human epidermal growth factor (HER) receptor family, which includes HER-1, HER-2, HER-3, and HER-4, important mediators of cell growth, differentiation, and survival. EGFR is activated by homodimerization with another EGFR or heterodimerization with another member of the HER family, e.g., HER-2. The EGFR family comprises four growth factor tyrosine kinase receptors: EGFR itself (ErbB1), (EGFR/HER1), ErbB2 (HER2/neu), ErbB3 (HER3), and ErbB4 (HER4) [60].

*EGFR Inhibitors:* Gefitinib, Erlotinib, Dacomitinib, Afatinib, Lapatinib, Neratinib, Osimertinib, Vandetanib, Cabozantinib [4].

#### 4.14.3.3 HER

Among the RTKs, the human epidermal growth receptor (HER) family plays an important role in the development and progression of human cancer. Family members are extensively regulated, mutated, and overactivated in human cancer, and they regulate various characteristics of cancer and serve as a prototype for targeting cell surface RTKs in cancer therapy [61].

The human EGF receptor (HER) family consists of four members that belong to the ErbB proteins (ErbB1–4). The epidermal growth factor receptor gene family includes (i) EGFR /ERBB1/ HER1, (ii) ERBB2/HER2/NEU, (iii) ERBB3 / HER3, and (iv)

ERBB4/HER4. Although similar, the HER is the most commonly used nomenclature in articles and clinical reports, while the ErbB nomenclature is associated with biological sciences [62].

Members of the HER family – EGFR, HER2, HER3, and HER4 – exhibit distinct and also shared structural characteristics, which allow these receptors to recognize growth factors in a differential way, using various mechanisms of activation of these receptors [61].

Since the discovery of the founding member of the HER family, the EGFR, the HER field has made progress in all three areas of HER research: basic, translational, and clinical. The central role of HERs in cancer biology has become more apparent, and this understanding has fueled some of the greatest advances in cancer therapy. Understanding the biology of HER3 initially took time because some of the paradigms applied to EGFR, HER2, and RTK are not applied to HER3, which is a pseudokinase receptor. These advances have led to the acceptance of the HER family as the preferred therapeutic target in a large number of types of epithelial tumors [61].

*HER Inhibitors:* Lapatinib inhibits HER-2, neratinib inhibits HER-2 and HER-4, and tucatinib inhibits HER-2 [4].

#### 4.14.3.4 FGFR

Fibroblast growth factor receptors (FGFRs) are a family of RTKs encoded by four different genes, namely, FGFR1, FGFR2, FGFR3, and FGFR4. These receptors are involved in signaling axes that result in cell proliferation, differentiation, and angiogenesis. Furthermore, they influence MAPK activation, inhibition of apoptosis, and promotion of cell survival through the PI3K/AKT pathway and are involved in cell migration through the activation of phosphokinase C (PKC), in addition to triggering the Janus kinase (JAK)-signal transducer and activator of transcription (STAT) pathway [63].

More than 4000 solid tumors have been evaluated and molecularly sequenced, and the analysis of results indicates that approximately 7% of cancers are characterized by FGFR gene mutations, the majority by gene amplification, others by gene mutations and a minority by genetic rearrangements [63].

FGFR1 has been identified in types of non-small cell lung cancer and small cell lung cancer, hormone positive breast tumors, bladder cancer, glioblastoma, and Ewing's sarcoma. FGFR2 amplification was found in small percentages of triple negative breast cancer, endometrial, gastric tumors, urothelial tumors, and lung cancer. They are present in adenocarcinomas and squamous cell carcinomas of the lung, thyroid, prostate, and cholangiocarcinomas. FGFR3 amplification is found in autothelial, breast, thyroid, gallbladder, and adenoid cancers. Somatic FGFR3 mutations are reported more frequently in non-muscle invasive bladder cancer than in invasive bladder tumors. Also found in cervical cancer, multiple myeloma, and seminomas. The FGRF4 mutation is rarely found in human neoplasms; however, it has been reported to induce the activation of rhabdomyosarcoma in childhood [63].

*FGFR Inhibitors:* Erdafitinib, Pemigatinib [4].

#### 4.14.3.5 c-KIT

c-KIT, a type III receptor tyrosine kinase (RTK), plays a crucial role in cancer occurrence. Currently, c-KIT is mainly considered a stem cell factor (SCF), which participate in vital functions of the human body, such as fertility, homeostasis, and melanogenesis; however, early studies of c-KIT introduced it as an oncogene [64].

Dysregulation of c-KIT, including overexpression and gain of function mutations, has been detected in several human cancers. Leukemia is the first cancer linked to c-Kit mutation. Subsequent studies reported that the c-KIT activating mutation is found in almost all cases of systemic mastocytosis and other hematopoietic tumor diseases. These findings support the hypothesis that the c-KIT target is possibly located in the stem cell compartment. It has been reported that c-KIT is primarily related to gastrointestinal stromal tumor (GIST), with 80% of all GIST cases. Therefore, the use of KIT inhibitors has provided new discoveries for the treatment of cancer. In addition, KIT mutations have been detected in cancers such as leukemia, unilateral ovarian dysgerminoma, and melanoma, among others [64].

Studies reveal that targeting c-KIT as an oncogene using kinase inhibitor drugs is a promising approach to cancer treatment. However, a number of issues have been raised in relation to this approach. For example, resistance to imatinib, a famous c-KIT inhibitor drug, has been observed in several cases and is attributed to alterations in c-KIT mutations; in addition, c-KIT is expressed in normal tissues such as breast epithelial, vascular endothelial, sweat glands, and retinal astrocytes. In this regard, c-KIT mutations cannot be considered a risk factor for the occurrence of cancer. Therefore, targeting c-KIT for cancer treatment is only feasible in cases where c-KIT is the "conductor" of cancer [64].

*KIT Inhibitors:* Nilotinib, Ripretinib, Sorafenib, Cabozantinib (Cabometyx), Pazopanib [41].

In Table 4.1, we have listed the main protein kinases and their main inhibitors currently used in clinical practice in oncology [4], as it follows:

## 4.15 Immunomodulators

The first compound of this class was thalidomide, developed in 1954 with sedative hypnotic purpose, and later scandalized due to its teratogenicity (pregnant women who used thalidomide had babies with developmental disabilities, such as phocomelia) [65].

However, a few years later, therapeutic properties and advantages were discovered for thalidomide, such as the treatment of leprous erythema nodosum, autoimmune diseases, and multiple myeloma. Once again in market, it was approved for other uses. It is one of the most successful cases of drug repositioning. In countries like the USA, Japan, and Brazil, it is controlled by specific and rigorous systems of access and dispensing [65].

With properties such as reduced production of tumor necrosis factor, antiangiogenic, antiproliferative effects and down-regulation of crucial cytokines, thalidomide has gained some analogs: lenalidomide and pomalidomide (INN; marketed as Pomalyst in the USA and Imnovid in the European Union and Russia) [65, 66].

The three drugs mentioned are administered orally.

Thalidomide (first generation drug) has significant toxicity in elderly patients. As it has a sedative effect, it is recommended to be administered at night. Do not ingest with food. One of the

**Table 4.1** Protein kinases and drugs whose mechanism of action is through their inhibition

| *Protein kinase* | *TRK/NTRK* | *BCR-ABL* | *ALK* | *ROS1* | *RET* | *MET* | *JAK* |
|---|---|---|---|---|---|---|---|
| *Protein kinase inhibitors* | Entrectinib<br>Larotrectinib | Dasatinib<br>Imatinib<br>Nilotinib<br>Ponatinib<br>Bosutinib | Alectinib<br>Brigatinib<br>Ceritinib<br>Crizotinib<br>Lorlatinib | Cabozantinib<br>Crizotinib | Pralsetinib<br>Selpercatinib<br>Cabozantinib<br>Regorafenib<br>Cabozantinib | Capmatinib<br>Cabozantinib | Ruxolitinib |
| *Protein kinase* | *BTK* | *CDK* | *PARP* | *BCL-2* | *FLT3* | *CSF1R* | *CLK* |
| *Protein kinase inhibitors* | Acalabrutinib<br>Ibrutinib<br>Zanubrutinib | Palbociclib<br>Ribociclib<br>Abemaciclib | Enasidenib<br>Talazoparib<br>Niraparib<br>Olaparib<br>Rucaparib | Talazoparib<br>Venetoclax | Gilteritinib<br>Sunitinib<br>Midostaurin<br>Sorafenib<br>Cabozantinib | Pexidartinib | In clinical trials |

most common reactions, and delicate management is peripheral neuropathy. It can also cause fatigue, edema, and muscle weakness [4, 67].

Lenalidomide (second generation drug) is more potent, has fewer adverse effects, is used in newly diagnosed multiple myeloma, relapsed refractory myeloma, and as maintenance therapy after autologous stem cell transplantation (ASCT). It inhibits hematopoietic tumor cell profiling, increases mediated immunity to T cells and NK cells, and increases the number of NKT cells; inhibits angiogenesis by blocking migration and adhesion of endothelial cells and the formation of microvessels; increases fetal hemoglobin synthesis by CD34+ hematopoietic stem cells and inhibits the production of proinflammatory cytokines (e.g., TNF-α and IL-6) by monocytes. It can be taken with or without food. It may cause reactions such as myelosuppression, diarrhea, nausea, and peripheral edema [4, 5, 67]..

Pomalidomide (a third-generation drug), on the other hand, is 10 times more potent than lenalidomide and has shown excellent results in patients with relapsing multiple myeloma and in those refractory to lenalidomide and bortezomib. Smoking reduces its plasma concentration curve due to CYP1A2 induction. It can cause reactions such as fatigue, neutropenia, hypercalcemia, and muscle spasms [5, 67].

During therapy using these drugs, the patient is at an increased risk of suffering thrombotic events, such as deep vein thrombosis and pulmonary embolism. It is recommended that the need for concomitant use of prophylactic anticoagulant (such as acetylsalicylic acid/aspirin) be evaluated [5].

## 4.16 Radiopharmaceuticals

It is known as radiopharmaceutical therapy (RPT); the use of radioactive atoms seeking targets associated with tumors is an emerging treatment modality with several advantages over existing treatments [68]. Some of the drugs used in this modality are:

- Radium chloride (223 RA): It emits alpha particles and mimics calcium, presenting an antineoplastic effect on bone metastases due to DNA breakage in adjacent cells [4].
- Iobenguane I 131: It is a Iobenguane labeled with Iodine-131. It accumulates in innervated adrenergic tissues such as the heart, lungs, adrenal medulla, salivary glands, liver, and spleen; as well as in tumors originating from the neural crest that express high levels of the NE transporter on their cell surfaces. It promotes cell death and tumor necrosis [4].
- Lutetium-Dotatate (177Lu-Dota): radiolabeled somatostatin analogue; it is used for malignant tumors that express somatostatin receptors. It provokes cell damage, through the formation of free radicals, also reaching neighboring cells [4].

## 4.17 Other Drugs

- Arsenic Trioxide: Indicated for acute promyelocytic syndrome, usually with associated tretinoin. This drug is for intravenous use, and does not have a fully elucidated action mechanism. In vitro, it causes morphological changes and DNA fragmentation in human promyelocytic leukemia NB4 cells, generating apoptosis. It also damages and degrades the PML/RARα fusion protein. It can cause reactions such as differentiation syndrome, abnormalities in cardiac conduction, and encephalopathy [4, 5].
- Bexarotene: It is a retinoid, which induces tumor regression by activating the retinoid receptor X, regulating genes that control cell differentiation. It has hepatic metabolism and renal excretion. It can suppress TSH levels, causing hypothyroidism, so it's important to monitor. Other possible reactions can be pancreatitis, photosensitivity, and lipid abnormality [5].
- Tretinoin: It is a retinoid that induces differentiation and inhibition of cell proliferation in transformed hematopoietic cell lines. It is used for acute promyelocytic leukemia, but its mechanism of action on this disease is not fully known yet. It

has hepatic metabolism and renal and fecal excretion. Administered orally, it is recommended to be ingested with or after a meal. Some of its reactions are cardiotoxicity, fever, and otalgia [4].

## References


1. Dickens E, Ahmed S. Principles of cancer treatment by chemotherapy. Surgery (Oxford). 2018;36(3):134–8.
2. Singh RK, Kumar S, Prasad DN, Bhardwaj TR. Therapeutic journey of nitrogen mustard as alkylating anticancer agents: historic to future perspectives. Eur J Med Chem. 2018;151:401–33.
3. American Cancer Society [Internet]. How chemotherapy drugs work. Available in https://www.cancer.org/treatment/treatments-and-side-effects/treatment-types/chemotherapy/how-chemotherapy-drugs-work.html. Access on 14 July 2021.
4. MOC. Clinical Oncology Manual [Internet]. Extract from the Cancer agents. 2021. Available in https://mocbrasil.com/moc-drogas/agentes-oncologicos/. Access on 19 July 2021.
5. Medscape [Internet]. Drugs & Diseases. Available in https://reference.medscape.com/. Access on 10 July 2021.
6. Albert Einstein Hospital. Guide to protocols and drugs for treatment in Oncology and hematology. São Paulo. 2013.
7. Teles KA, Medeiros-Souza P, Lima FAC, de Araújo BG, Lima RAC. Rotina de administração de ciclofosfamida em doenças autoimunes reumáticas: uma revisão. Rev Bras Reumatol. 2017;57(6):596–604.
8. Mori T, Aisa Y, Yamazaki R, et al. Cryotherapy for the prevention of high-dose melphalan-induced oral mucositis. Bone Marrow Transplant. 2006;38:637–8. https://www.nature.com/articles/1705494#citeas
9. Lilleby, K., Garcia, P., Gooley, T., McDonnnell, P., Taber, R., Holmberg, L., . . . Bensinger, W. A prospective, randomized study of cryotherapy during administration of high-dose melphalan to decrease the severity and duration of oral mucositis in patients with multiple myeloma undergoing autologous peripheral blood stem cell transplantation. Bone Marrow Transplant 2006; 37, 1031–1035. https://doi.org/10.1038/sj.bmt.1705384
10. UP TO DATE [Internet]. Drugs Information. Available in https://www.uptodate.com/contents/search. Access on 3 July 2021.
11. de Almeida VL, et al. Cancer and cell-cycle-specific and non-cellular-cycle-specific antineoplastic agents that interact with DNA: an introduction. New Chem [online] 2005;28(1):118–29. Available in: https://doi.org/10.1590/S0100-40422005000100021.

12. Hassan SA, et al. Chemotherapeutic agents and the risk of ischemia and arterial thrombosis. Curr Atheroscler Rep. 2018;20:10.
13. Herrmann J, et al. Vascular toxicities of cancer therapies: the old and the new—an evolving avenue. Circulation. 2016;133(13):1272–89. https://doi.org/10.1161/CIRCULATIONAHA.115.018347.
14. Saif MW, Shah MM, Shah AR. Fluoropyrimidine-associated cardiotoxicity: revisited. Expert Opin Drug Saf. 2009;8(2):191–202. https://doi.org/10.1517/14740330902733961.
15. Sudhoff T, et al. 5-fluorouracil induces arterial vasocontractions. Ann Oncol. 2004;15(4):661–4.
16. Bispo Junior W, et al. Capecitabine-induced hand-foot syndrome: a case report. Cogitare Enferm. 2017;22(1):01–4. https://doi.org/10.5380/ce.v22i1.45824.
17. Lass JH, Lazarus HM, Reed MD, Herzig RH. Topical corticosteroid therapy for corneal toxicity from systemically administered cytarabine. Am J Ophthalmol. 1982;94(5):617–21. https://doi.org/10.1016/0002-9394(82)90006-x.
18. Mayer RJ, Van Cutsem E, Falcone A, et al. Ensaio randomizado de TAS-102 para câncer colorretal metastático refratário. N Engl J Med. 2015;372(20):1909–19. [PubMed 25970050 ]
19. Lord S, Ghersi D, Gattellari M, Wortley S, Wilcken N, Thornton CE, Simes J. Antitumour antibiotic containing regimens for metastatic breast cancer. Cochrane Database Syst Rev 2004;2004:CD003367. https://doi.org/10.1002/14651858.cd003367.pub2.
20. Perry MC, editor. The chemotherapy source book. 2nd ed. Williams and Wilkins; 1997. [ISBN 0-683-06868-7].
21. McGowan JV, Chung R, Maulik A, Piotrowska I, Walker JM, Yellon DM. Anthracycline chemotherapy and cardiotoxicity. Cardiovasc Drugs Ther. 2017;31(1):63–75. https://doi.org/10.1007/s10557-016-6711-0.
22. Pommier Y. Topoisomerase I inhibitors: camptothecins and beyond. Nat Rev Cancer. 2006;6:789–802. https://doi.org/10.1038/nrc1977.
23. Sinha BK. Topoisomerase Inhibitors. Drugs. 1995;49:11–9. https://doi.org/10.2165/00003495-199549010-00002.
24. Branco A, et al. Rubrofusarin, a natural polyketide as new human topoisomerase II-D inhibitor. Brazilian J Pharmacognosy 2008;18(Supl):703–8.
25. Tsao AS, Papadimitrakopoulou V. Mitotic inhibitors. J Thorac Oncol. 2011;6(11):S1789–90.
26. Garon EB, Dubinett SM. Mitotic inhibitors. J Thorac Oncol. 2011;6(11):S1791–2.
27. Olziersky A-M, Labidi-Galy SI. Clinical development of anti-mitotic drugs in cancer. Cell Div Mach Dis. 2017:125–52.
28. McCabe MT, Mohammad HP, Barbash O, Kruger RG. Targeting histone methylation in cancer. Cancer J. 2017;23(5):292–301.
29. Fricker LD. Proteasome inhibitor drugs. Annu Rev Pharmacol Toxicol 2020;60:15.1–15.20.

30. Quaglio D, Infante P, Di Marcotullio L, Botta B, Mori M. Hedgehog signaling pathway inhibitors: an updated patent review (2015–present). Expert Opin Ther Pat. 2020;1354–3776:(Print) 1744–7674 (Online).
31. Batool T, Makky EA, Jalal M, Yusoff MM. A comprehensive review on L-Asparaginase and its applications. Appl Biochem Biotechnol. 2016;178:900–23.
32. Heo YA, Syed YY, Keam SJ. Pegaspargase: A Review in Acute Lymphoblastic Leukaemia. Drugs Springer Nature Switzerland. 2019;79:767–77. https://doi.org/10.1007/s40265-019-01120-1.
33. Longui CA. Corticoterapia: minimizing side effects. J Pediatr Rio de Janeiro 2007;83(5 suppl).
34. Student S, Hejmo T, Poterała-Hejmo A, Leśniak A, Bułdak R. Anti-androgen hormonal therapy for cancer and other diseases. Eur J Pharmacol. 2019;172783.
35. Gamat M, McNeel DG. Androgen deprivation and immunotherapy for the treatment of prostate cancer. Endocr Relat Cancer. 2017;24:T297–310.
36. Ritch C, Cookson M. Recent trends in the management of advanced prostate cancer. F1000 Res. 2018;7:F1000. Faculty Rev-1513.
37. Guedes JBR, et al. Factors associated with adherence and persistence in hormone therapy in women with breast cancer. Rev Bras Epidemiol. 2017;20(04):636.
38. Shagufta IA. Tamoxifen a pioneering drug: an update on the therapeutic potential of tamoxifen derivatives. Eur J Med Chem. 2018;143:515–31.
39. Pruskowski JA. Another strike against Megestrol acetate therapy? Am J Geriatr Psychiatry. 2020;28(6):644–5.
40. Kharb R, et al. Aromatase inhibitors: Role in postmenopausal breast câncer. Arch Pharm. 2020;1–20.
41. Murphy E, Prommer EE, Mihalyo M, Wilcock A. Octreotide. J Pain Symptom Manage. 2010;40:140–8.
42. Leite CAVG, Costa JVG, Callado RB, Torres JNL, Lima Júnior RCP, Ribeiro RA. Receptor tyrosine kinases: therapeutic implications in cancer. Brazilian J Clin Oncol. 2012;8:29.
43. Avila CM, Romeiro NC. Protein tyrosine kinases: challenges in the development of drugs aimed at cancer therapy. Rev Virtual Quim. 2010;2(1):59–82.
44. Engh RA, Bossemeyer D. The protein kinase activity modulation sites: mechanisms for cellular regulation. Adv Enzyme Regul. 2001;41:121.
45. McCubrey JA, et al. Roles of the RAF/MEK/ERK and PI3K/PTEN/AKT pathways in malignant transformation and drug resistance. Adv Enzyme Regul. 2006;46:249–79.
46. McCubrey JA, Steelman LS, Chappell WH, Abrams SL, Franklin RA, Montalto G, Martelli AM. (2012). Ras/Raf/MEK/ERK and PI3K/PTEN/Akt/mTOR Cascade inhibitors: how mutations can result in therapy resistance and how to overcome resistance. Oncotarget. 2012;3(10):1068–111.

47. Babbitt GA, Lynch ML, McCoy M, Fokoue EP, Hudson AO. Function and evolution of B-Raf loop dynamics relevant to cancer recurrence under drug inhibition. J Biomol Struct Dyn. 2020;1–16.
48. Aoki M, Fujishita T. Oncogenic roles of the PI3K/AKT/mTOR Axis. Curr Top Microbiol Immunol. 2017;407:153–89.
49. Yang J, Nie J, Ma X, Wei Y, Peng Y, Wei X. Targeting PI3K in cancer: mechanisms and advances in clinical trials. Mol Cancer. 2019;18(1):26.
50. Moore AR, Rosenberg SC, McCormick F, Malek S. RAS-targeted therapies: is the undruggable drugged? Nat Rev Drug Discov. 2020;19(8):533–52.
51. Griffin JE, Ojeda SR. Texbook of endocrine physiology. New York: Oxford University Press; 1992. p. 66–7, 149.
52. Degirmenci W, Hu J. Targeting aberrant RAS/RAF/MEK/ERK signaling for cancer therapy. Cell. 2020;9(1):198.
53. Mahapatra DK, Asati V, Bharti SK. MEK inhibitors in oncology: a patent review (2015-present). Expert Opin Ther Pat. 2017;27(8):887–906.
54. Roskoski R. ERK1/2 MAP kinases: structure, function, and regulation. Pharmacol Res. 2012;66(2):105–43.
55. Dwivedi Y, Rizavi HS, Zhang H, Roberts RC, Conley RR, Pandey GN. Aberrant extracellular signal-regulated kinase (ERK)1/2 signalling in suicide brain: role of ERK kinase 1 (MEK1). Int J Neuropsychopharmacol. 2009;12(10):1337.
56. Ellis H, Cynthia XM. Curr Oncol Rep. 2019;21:110.
57. Revathidevi S, Munirajan AK. Akt in cancer: Mediator and more. Semin Cancer Biol. 2019;59:80–91. https://doi.org/10.1016/j.semcancer.2019.06.002. Epub 2019 Jun 4. PMID: 31173856.
58. Hillmann P, Fabbro D. PI3K/mTOR pathway inhibition: opportunities in oncology and rare genetic diseases. Int J Mol Sci. 2019;20(22):5792.
59. Park KK, Liu K, Hu Y, Kanter JL, He Z. PTEN/mTOR and axon regeneration. Exp Neurol. 2010;223(1):45–50.
60. Karkkainen M, Petrova T. Vascular endothelial growth factor receptors in the regulation of angiogenesis and lymphangiogenesis. Oncogene. 2000;19:5598–5605. https://doi.org/10.1038/sj.onc.1203855.
61. Kumar R, George B, Campbell MR, Verma N, Paul AM, Melo-Alvim C, et al. HER family in cancer progression: From discovery to 2020 and beyond. Adv Cancer Res. 2020;147:109–60.
62. Roskoski R. Small molecule inhibitors targeting the EGFR/ErbB family of protein-tyrosine kinases in human cancers. Pharmacol Res. 2018.
63. Ghedini GC, Ronca R, Presta M, Giacomini A. Future applications of FGF/FGFR inhibitors in cancer. Expert Rev Anticancer Ther. 2018;18(9):861–72.
64. Abbaspour Babaei M, Kamalidehghan B, Saleem M, Zaman Huri H, Ahmadipour F. Receptor tyrosine kinase (c-Kit) inhibitors: a potential therapeutic target in cancer cells. Drug Des Devel Ther. 2016;10:2443–59.

65. Ito T, Handa H. Molecular mechanisms of thalidomide and its derivatives. Proc Jpn Acad Ser B Phys Biol Sci. 2020;96(6):189–203. https://doi.org/10.2183/pjab.96.016. https://www.ncbi.nlm.nih.gov/pmc/articles/PMC7298168/#.
66. Quach H, Ritchie D, Stewart AK, Neeson P, Harrison S, Smyth MJ, Prince HM. Mechanism of action of immunomodulatory drugs (IMiDS) in multiple myeloma. Leukemia. 2010;24(1):22–32. 10.1038/leu.2009.236. Epub 2009 Nov 12. PMID: 19907437; PMCID: PMC3922408. https://www.ncbi.nlm.nih.gov/pmc/articles/PMC3922408/.
67. Raza S, Safyan RA, Lentzsch S. Immunomodulatory drugs (IMiDs) in multiple myeloma. Curr Cancer Drug Targets. 2017;17(9) https://doi.org/10.2174/1568009617666170214104426.
68. Sgouros G, Bodei L, McDevitt MR, et al. Radiopharmaceutical therapy in cancer: clinical advances and challenges. Nat Rev Drug Discov. 2020;19:589–608. https://doi.org/10.1038/s41573-020-0073-9.

**Samanta Oliveira da Silva** graduated from UnG – Guarulhos University. Specialist in Clinical Pharmacology and Pharmacotherapy from SENAC University Center. Specialist in Oncology Pharmacy and Pharmaceutical Care in Oncology by Instituto Racine. She has been working in clinical pharmacy since 2016 and has solid experience in Oncohematology and Hematopoietic Stem Cell Transplantation (HSCT). Samanta has also worked in ICU, CIM, and Pharmacovigilance. She lectures at symposiums and events, in addition to occasionally giving classes in undergraduate and graduate courses. Participated in the publication of the first BMT Manual for Pharmacists (SOBRAFO), and is a member of the HSCT Committee of the Brazilian Society of Pharmacists in Oncology in the 2020–2022 administration.

**Ellen Mayara Corrêa** graduated in Pharmacy from the University of Amaro. Master's student in the professional program "Patient Centered Cancer Care" by Hospital A. C. Camargo Cancer Center. Specialist in Hospital Pharmacy from Oswaldo Cruz University. Capacity in Clinical Research at Center Paulista of Clinical Investigation. More than 8 years of experience in Oncology Pharmacy at Hospital Beneficence from São Paulo and at the Prevent Senior Health Operator.

Currently Pharmacist responsible for Clinical Research in Oncology at Hospital A. C. Camargo Cancer Center.

# Protocols 5

Kaléu Mormino Otoni,
Karla Bruna Nogueira Torres Mormino,
Sandna Larissa Freitas dos Santos,
and Maria Liliane Luciano Pereira

## 5.1 Introduction

According to the World Health Organization (WHO), there are more than 20 million new cases of cancer in the world by 2025, which makes cancer a public health problem, especially among still developing countries, where the impact is expected to be corresponding to 80% of new cases forecast for 2025 [9].

There are also an estimated 5210 new cases of non-Hodgkin's lymphoma (NHL) in men and 5030 in women in 2016. These values correspond to an estimate of 5.27 new cases for every 100,000 men and 4.88 for every 100,000 women. Regarding the cases of

K. M. Otoni (✉)
Jesus Maria José Maternity Hospital, Quixadá, Ceará, Brazil

Postgraduate Program in Integrated and Multidisciplinary Care for Women's and Children's Health, Federal University of Ceará, University Campus – Rectory, PICI, Fortaleza, CE, Brazil

K. B. N. T. Mormino
Catholic University Center of Quixadá, Unicatólica, Quixadá, Ceará, Brazil
e-mail: Karlabruna@unicatolicaquixada.edu.br

S. L. F. dos Santos · M. L. L. Pereira
Graduate Program in Pharmaceutical Sciences, Federal University of Ceará, Fortaleza, CE, Brazil



C. W. P. Schmidt, K. M. Otoni (eds.), *The Golden Guide to Oncologic Pharmacy*, https://doi.org/10.1007/978-3-030-98596-7_5

leukemia, there were a total of 5540 new cases in men and 4530 in women, with values of 5.63 new cases per 100,000 men and 4.38 per 100,000 women. More current data show that, in the 2018–2019 biennium, there were more than 600,000 new cases of cancer per year, of which 10,800 were leukemic, 10,180 NHL, and 2530 LH [10].

The basic treatment for onco-hematologic diseases is chemotherapy. Such methodology uses chemical compounds, called chemotherapeutics, in the treatment of diseases caused by biological agents. When applied to cancer, it is called anticancer chemotherapy. Chemotherapy drugs do not act exclusively on tumor cells, affecting both tumor and normal cells as well. Therefore, some structures such as bone marrow, hair, and digestive tube mucosa can be affected by their action, mainly due to the degree of renewal of these tissues [13].

Neutropenia is one of the most common complications resulting from chemotherapy, causing a decrease in the number of neutrophils, a decrease in protective barriers, and changes in the microbiota, predisposing a high potential for infection, being considered a case of medical emergency, as it can evolve quickly and can lead to death of individuals [17].

## 5.2 Oncohematological Cancers

### 5.2.1 Leukemias

Leukemia is one of the main diseases afflicted by the population, has an unknown origin most of the time, and mainly affects the leukocyte-type defense cells, with the main characteristic of the accumulation of young abnormal cells in the bone marrow, which end up replacing the normal cells of the body [8].

Leukemias can be grouped and classified in different ways, and one of them is the evolution time, which can be chronic or acute. In acute leukemia, leukemic cells grow exorbitantly and very quickly in a short period of time. In chronic leukemia, the disease slowly worsens as the number of white blood cells increases. In addition, there is another classification for leukemia, which can be classified according to the type of cell that is affected by the disease, that is, those that affect lymphoid cells are called lymphoid, lymphocytic, or lymphoblastic cells; those that affect myeloid cells are called myeloid or myeloblastic [15].

Therefore, the most common leukemic cancers are chronic lymphoid leukemia (CLL), acute lymphoid leukemia (ALL), chronic myeloid leukemia (CML), and acute myeloid leukemia (AML) [7].

#### 5.2.1.1 Acute Lymphoid Leukemia (ALL)

ALL is a disease derived from undifferentiated lymphoid cells that are present in different organs of our body, such as bone marrow, thymus, and lymph nodes. There is an accumulation of these cells at different stages of the maturation process, having the ability to multiply a lot, but not for mature and normal cells, but for young and immature cells. ALL can occur at any age, but its recurrence is greater among children aged 2–5 years, white and male [5].

The most commonly used treatment schemes in pediatric and adult ALL are, in general, the same drugs in different combinations and schemes. Superiority of one scheme over another is not established. Many of the schemes, particularly pediatric ones, included cranial caudal radiotherapy (RT) as CNS prophylaxis. However, with a higher rate of medium- and long-term complications with RT in the pediatric population, studies and analyses were conducted to assess the impact of omission of RT in treatment protocols that included CNS penetrating drugs and intrathecal applications. A prospective study with 501 patients treated with a scheme without RT showed CNS recurrence rates similar to protocols with RT [39].

Pediatric schemes incorporate asparaginase which in adults can present significant toxicity, especially in those aged >40–45 years. The function of this agent is to deplete the serum levels of asparagine, a fundamental amino acid for lymphoblasts to maintain their viability. Asparaginase formulations come from *Escherichia coli* (*E. coli*) or *Erwinia chrysanthemi*. Thus, allergic and infusional reactions can occur with the administration of these agents (stimulated by the bacterial protein). The allergic reaction may be associated with the production of anti-asparaginase antibodies with greater clearance of this medication and subsequent lower efficacy. Serum asparaginase levels >0.1 IU/mL in the nadir are associated with more effective asparagine depletion and greater antitumor activity. Serum levels below this value may compromise the antileukemic activity of this agent. Therefore, it is important to measure the serum level of asparaginase in patients who present allergic reactions to the drug. If there is documentation of inadequate serum levels, it is necessary to switch to an alternative formulation (*Erwinia*). In fact, serum asparaginase levels have been correlated with antileukemic activity and survival in pediatric studies [40].

| Initial default scheme | |
|---|---|
| Induction (4 weeks) | Vincristine, 1.5 mg/m$^2$/week IV, for 4 weeks on D0, D7, D14, and D21; daunorubicin, 25 mg/m$^2$/week IV, for 4 weeks on D0, D7, D14, and D21; prednisone, 60 mg/m$^2$/day VO, for 28 days, on D0, D7, D14, and D21; asparaginase, 6000 IU/m$^2$ IM, 3×/week, for 9 doses (start in the first week); cytarabine, 100 mg intrathecal on D0; and methotrexate, 12 mg intrathecal on D14 |
| Consolidation (5 weeks) | Prednisone, 7.5 mg/m$^2$ VO, in D0, 3.75 mg/m$^2$ VO, in D1 and D2; cyclophosphamide, 1000 mg/m$^2$ EV, in D0 and D14; 6-mercaptopurine, 60 mg/m$^2$/day VO, from D0 to D27; vincristine, 1.5 mg/m$^2$ EV, on D14, D21, D42, and D49; cytarabine, 75 mg/m$^2$/day EV, from D1 to D4, from D8 to D11, from D15 to D18, and from D22 to D25; methotrexate, 12 mg intrathecal, in D1, D8, D15, and D22; cranial RT, 1800 cGy in 10 fractions if CNS not involved in the initial presentation, 2400 cGy cranial in 12 fractions, and 600 cGy in the axial spine in 3 fractions if involvement of the CNS in the initial presentation |
| Maintenance (8 weeks) | 6-mercaptopurine, 60 mg/m$^2$/day PO, from D0 to D41; methotrexate, 15 mg/m$^2$ PO, in D0, D7, D14, D21, D28, and D35 |

| Initial default scheme | |
|---|---|
| Late intensification (7 weeks) | Reinduction phase (4 weeks): dexamethasone, 10 mg/m²/day orally, from D0 to D20, with gradual decrease for 7 days; vincristine, 1.5 mg/m² IV in D0, D14, and D21; doxorubicin, 25 mg /m² EV, in D0, D7, and D14. Reconsolidation phase (3 weeks): asparaginase, 6000 IU/m² IM, on D3, D5, D7, D10, D12, and D14; vincristine, 1.5 mg/m² EV, on D42 and D49; cyclophosphamide, 1000 mg/m² IV, on D28; thioguanine, 60 mg/m²/day orally, from D28 to D41; cytarabine, 75 mg/m²/day IV or SC, from D29 to D32 and from D36 to D39; methotrexate, 12 mg intrathecal, in D29 and D36 |
| Extended maintenance (12 weeks) | Vincristine, 1.5 mg/m² IV, on D0, D28, and D56; prednisone, 40 mg/m²/day VO, from D0 to D4, from D28 to D32, and from D56 to D60; 6-mercaptopurine, 75 mg/m²/day PO, from D0 to D83; methotrexate, 20 mg/m² PO, on D7, D14, D21, D28, D35, D42, D49, D56, D63, D70, and D77; methotrexate, 12 mg intrathecal, on D0 |
| Dose reduction | Suspension of asparaginase if there is liver, pancreatic, or allergic disorder. Reduce vincristine to 1 mg if bilirubin is >2 mg/dL; doxorubicin by 25% if bilirubin is 2–3 mg/dL; in 50% if it is 3–4 mg/dL and in 75% if >4 mg/dL; prednisone by 30% if there is hypertension or diabetes. Use it in the prevention of hemorrhagic cystitis by cyclophosphamide (dosing from 80 to 100% of the dose of cyclophosphamide, 40% IV immediately before, 20% during and 20% after 4 and 8 h) |

*Source*: Williams et al. [39]

With all schemes, long-term consequences can occur, particularly when affecting younger individuals. Among the complications are melanoma, sarcoma, breast cancer, colorectal cancer, hormonal changes, sexual dysfunction, lung and heart diseases, as well as cognitive changes. Less exposure to chemotherapy and radiotherapy treatment has contributed to the reduction of these late complications [41].

#### 5.2.1.2 Acute Myeloid Leukemia (AML)

AML is a neoplasm derived from hematopoietic precursors or myeloid stem cells, which causes anemia, neutropenia, and thrombocytopenia precisely because of the accumulation of blast cells in the marrow. It accounts for about 90% of leukemias in adult life, affecting mainly young people and adults with more advanced ages (Table 5.1). The diagnosis became more specific due to monoclonal cells and through the laboratory test called flow cytometry [21].

**Table 5.1** Chemotherapy protocols according to adopted criteria

| Criteria | Recommendations |
|---|---|
| Patients <60–70 years old eligible for intensive chemotherapy | Induction: the standard treatment, known as 7 + 3, consists of daunorubicin, 60–90 mg/m$^2$ EV, in D1, D2, and D3 or idarubicin, 12 mg/m$^2$ EV, in D1, D2, and D3 and cytarabine, 100 at 200 mg/m$^2$ IV, by continuous infusion, for 24 h, from D1 to D7, for a maximum of 2 cycles. One can also consider as an alternative: (a) daunorubicin, 60–90 mg/m$^2$ IV, in D1, D2, and D3 or idarubicin, 12 mg/m$^2$ IV, in D1, D2, and D3; cytarabine, 100–200 mg/ m$^2$ IV, by continuous infusion, for 24 h, from D1 to D7; cladribine, 5 mg/m$^2$ IV, in 3 h, from D1 to D5, for a maximum of 2 cycles; (b) FLAG-Ida with or without gentuzumab mainly in young patients with favorable cytogenetic risk: fludarabine, 30 mg/m$^2$ IV, from D2 to D6; cytarabine, 2 g/m$^2$ IV, in 4 h, starting 4 h after fludarabine D2 to D6; filgrastim, 300–480 mcg SC, from D1 to D7 and idarubicin, 8 mg/m$^2$ IV, from D4 to D6. When used, the dose of gentuzumab ozogamycin is 3 mg/m$^2$ IV in 2 h on D1 of cycle 1 only. Repeat FLAG-Ida for a maximum of 2 cycles, with gentuzumab being used only in the first cycle |
| Patients under 60–70 years of age eligible for intensive care – consolidation | Consolidation: patients at favorable or intermediate risk receive 3 or 4 cycles of high doses of cytarabine, 1.5–3.0 g/m$^2$ (HiDAC), for 3 h, every 12 h on alternate days, on D1, D3, and D5 – total of 6 doses or 1–2 cycles of HiDAC followed by autologous bone marrow HSCT. Individuals at intermediate cytogenetic risk may be considered for allogeneic HSCT as a consolidation regimen. Unfavorable risk patients should be referred for allogeneic HSCT in first remission if they have a related histocompatible donor |

**Table 5.1** (continued)

| Criteria | Recommendations |
|---|---|
| Patients aged 60–75 years old | Patients over 60 years old, with good performance index and without comorbidities should be considered for the "7 + 3" regimen (idarubicin, 12 mg/m$^2$ IV, or daunorubicin, 45–90 mg/m$^2$) IV, in D1, D2, and D3 and cytarabine, 100–200 mg/m$^2$ IV, by continuous infusion, for 24 h, from D1 to D7. Consolidation: individuals who achieve CR after induction should be considered for reduced intensity allogeneic HSCT. At least one cycle of consolidation with HiDAC should be considered with doses adjusted according to age – 2 g/m$^2$ (patients over 60 years old) or 1.5 g/m$^2$ (patients over 70 years old) for 3 h, every 12 h on alternate days, on D1, D3, and D5 – total of 6 doses – potentially followed by HSCT |
| Patients not eligible for intensive chemotherapy | (a) Azacitidine, 75 mg/m$^2$, from D1 to D7, IV or subcutaneously or decitabine, 20 mg/m$^2$, from D1 to D5 IV + venetoclax, 400 mg daily (dose is rapidly escalated with 100 mg in the D1, 200 mg in D2 and 400 mg in D3); (b) cytarabine, 20 mg/m$^2$ subcutaneous, from D1 to D10 + venetoclax, 600 mg daily (dose is rapidly escalated with 100 mg on D1, 200 mg on D2, 400 mg on D3, and 600 mg on D4 |
| Patients with relapsed acute myeloid leukemia who have gene mutations | Patients with relapsed and/or refractory AML who have an HDI1 mutation should be treated, if available, with ivosidenib, 500 mg VO, 1×/day, continuously, from D1 to D28. Patients with relapsed and/or refractory AML who have an IDH2 mutation should be treated, if available, with enasidenib, 100 mg VO, 1×/day, continuously, from D1 to D28. Alternatives for treating these AML subtypes in the absence of these drugs include the chemotherapy schemes abovementioned and venetoclax as a single agent |

#### 5.2.1.3 Chronic Lymphoid Leukemia (LLC)

CLL accounts for about one third of all leukemias, affecting mainly older people, rarely seen in patients under 30–40 years of age and quite rare in children. It is characterized by the accumulation of monoclonal lymphocytes [4].

The following is the description of the recommendation for fit patients with mutated IGHV: (a) FCR (fludarabine, 25 mg/m$^2$/day

IV, from D1 to D3; cyclophosphamide, 250 mg/m²/day IV, from D1 to D3; rituximab, 375 mg/m²/day IV, on D1 of cycle 1 and 500 mg/m²/day IV, on D1 of cycles 2–6), every 28 days, for 6 cycles. Recommended anti-infective prophylaxis, continuous and maintained up to 6–12 months after the end of treatment: sulfamethoxazole/trimethoprim, 160–800 mg orally, 3×/week and valaciclovir, 500 mg orally, daily (or acyclovir, 200 mg orally, 2 ×/day). Growth factors (G-CSF) should be used as there is an 85% chance of grade 3–4 neutropenia; (b) acalabrutinib, 100 mg (1 caps.) PO, 12/12 h, in cycles of 28 days, continuous, from cycle 1 to progression, toxicity or doctor/patient decision, associated or not with obinutuzumab (G), starting only from cycle 2, in this cycle: 100 mg on D1, 900 mg on D2, 1000 mg on D8 and D15; from cycles 3 to 7: 1000 mg on D1, for a total of 6 cycles of 28 days. The same prophylactic guidelines for ibrutinib should be followed, reinforcing the use of antivirals due to the anti-CD20 antibody; (c) ibrutinib, 420 mg (3 caps. of 140 mg) VO continuous until progression, toxicity, or decision of the doctor/patient [42].

#### 5.2.1.4 Chronic Myeloid Leukemia (CML)

CML is a myeloproliferative disorder, in which there is a lot of release of granulocytic cells as a result of the clonal expansion process (Table 5.2). Signs of the disease are leukocytosis, myeloid hyperplasia, basophilia, and neutrophilia. It is characterized by an acquired mutation that affects hematopoietic stem cells, differing from other leukemias in that approximately 90% of patients have a marker karyotype, the Philadelphia chromosome (Ph), resulting from a translocation involving chromosomes 9 and 22, allowing us to relate this change and/or mutation to CML [20].

### 5.2.2 Lymphoma

Lymphomas (LF) start from the transformation of a lymphocyte into the lymphatic system. The prefix "lymph" indicates its origin from the transformation of a lymphocyte, and the suffix "oma" is

**Table 5.2** Initial recommendations for CML

| **Treatment of the Chronic Phase in First Line** | |
|---|---|
| First generation tyrosine kinase inhibitor | First line treatment: imatinib, 400–800 mg orally, 1×/day |
| Second generation tyrosine kinase inhibitor | First line treatment: dasatinib, 100 mg orally, 1×/day, or nilotinib, 300 mg orally, 2×/day. Patients with an intermediate or high ETLS score should preferably be treated with second generation TKIs |
| **Treatment of advanced phases** | |
| Accelerated and blastic | Mutation analysis before starting therapy. FA: Patients who have not previously received imatinib, imatinib, 600 mg/day PO, or second-generation TKI, dasatinib, 140 mg, 1×/day PO or nilotinib, 400 mg, 2×/day PO or bosutinib, 500 mg, 1 ×/day VO. Ponatinib, 45 mg, 1×/day orally, in case of T315I mutation. Patients who progress to advanced stages during imatinib: Second- or third-generation TKI. Omacetaxin, 1.25 mg/m$^2$ SC, 2×/day, from D1 to D14, every 28 days until hematological response or 6 cycles, followed by maintenance of 7 days of treatment at the same dose every 28 days can be considered in patients who progress to AF after treatment with TKI |

*Source*: Castagnetti et al.[43]

derived from the Greek word meaning “tumor.” They are the result of damage to the DNA of a lymphocyte that occurs after birth and therefore represents an acquired disease rather than an inherited disease. This alteration or mutation in the lymphocyte DNA generates a malignant transformation: it results in the uncontrolled and excessive growth of the lymphocyte, providing a competitive advantage to the malignant lymphocytes and the cells formed from their multiplication. The accumulation of these dividing cells results in tumor masses in lymph nodes and other locations [27].

Lymphomas usually start in lymph nodes or in clumps of lymph tissue present in organs such as the stomach and intestines. In some cases, lymphomas can involve the bone marrow and blood: they may spread to other locations. Lymphocytic leukemias originate and occur mainly in the bone marrow and then pass into the blood. They can spread to the lymph nodes [23].

Non-Hodgkin lymphomas (NHL) account for about 2.5% of all malignant tumors diagnosed in Brazil, excluding non-melanotic skin cancer. The symptoms of general weakness with fever, weight loss, and pallor usually intensify with the evolution of the untreated disease. Bleeding is not a frequent symptom, but it can be present and very serious when the tumor infiltrates the bone marrow, progressing to the stage of blood dissemination (leukemized lymphoma or leukosarcoma) [22].

Hodgkin's lymphoma is a lymphoproliferative neoplasm defined by the clonal multiplication of cells with a peculiar morphological and immunophenotypic pattern, known as Reed-Sternberg cells, derived from the malignant transformation of B lymphocytes from the germinal center. Although lymphoma is usually disseminated at the time of diagnosis and indolent in its clinical course, it has been recognized that clinical aggressiveness and the risk of transformation to diffuse large B-cell lymphoma (LDGC-B) increase proportionally with the number of centroblasts ("large cells") and the fraction of proliferating cells. Thus, lymphoma is classified, for purposes of therapeutic planning and prognosis, based on the number of centroblasts present in the pathological specimen: LF grade 1–2, up to 15 centroblasts per field of highest magnification; grade 3A, above 15 centroblasts, centrocytes present; and grade 3B, above 15 centroblasts, absence of centrocytes (11). Grade 3B LF has a genetic profile, immunophenotypic and clinical behavior that can be considered as a follicular variant of LDGC-B [23, 27].

Clinical staging is performed according to the Ann Arbor criteria (adopted by the TNM/UICC Classification – International Union Against Cancer), modified at the Cotswolds conference, in Stage I: disease restricted to a single lymph node chain (I) or to a single organ or extralymphatic location (IE); » Stage II: disease affects two or more lymph node chains on the same side of the diaphragm (II) or involvement located in a single organ or extralymphatic location and its regional lymph node(s), with or without involvement of other chains lymph nodes on the same side of the diaphragm (IIE); » Stage III: disease affects lymph node chains on both sides of the diaphragm (III), which may also be accompanied by localized involvement in an organ or related extralymphatic location (IIIE), or involvement of the spleen (IIIS), or both (IIIE+S); » Stage IV: disease affects one or multiple extralymphatic sites, with or without associated lymph node involvement, or affects the extranodal area with non-regional lymph node involvement; » Descriptor X: presence of tumor mass greater than 10 centimeters; » Descriptor E: extranodal involvement by contiguity or single isolated site of extranodal disease; » Descriptor A or B: absence (A) or presence (B) of symptoms "B" – unexplained weight loss greater than 10%, unexplained fever, and night sweats [24].

LF is radiosensitive and nodal irradiation is standard treatment in the early stages, i.e., I and II. Symptomatic advanced stage (stage III or IV) LF patients are treated with the expectation that the disease will evolve in a relapsing and remitting form, which may require several lines of treatment during the course [25].

For many years, the standard of first line care was based on alkylating agents, often in combinations with vinca alkaloid and corticosteroid. Attempts to increase the intensity of chemotherapy by adding an anthracycline have failed to demonstrate a survival advantage. Any improvement in the response rate to anthracycline polychemotherapy must be weighed against the inevitable increase in toxicity and the exclusion of anthracycline as a therapeutic agent in the case of subsequent transformation to high-grade lymphoma [25].

Fludarabine is a drug with LF activity, whether used as a single agent or in combination. No studies have identified a survival advantage of fludarabine-based treatments compared to the use of alkylants. The comparison between fludarabine and the combination of cyclophosphamide, vincristine, and prednisolone (CVP) in 381 patients with previously untreated LF showed higher response rates in the fludarabine group, without resulting in improvement in time to progression parameters. The use of fludarabine in first line therapy may, however, have a detrimental effect on the mobilization of hematopoietic stem cells for autologous transplantation, leads to an increased risk of opportunistic infections, and may be associated with an increased risk of secondary myelodysplasia and leukemia [26].

### 5.2.3 Myeloma

Multiple myeloma (MM) is a malignant yet incurable neoplasm characterized by clonal proliferation of plasma cells in the bone marrow that secrete monoclonal protein in the blood and/or urine (97%) and may be associated with organ dysfunction. It represents 1% of malignant tumors and 10–15% of hematological neoplasms. It is preceded by at least 8–10 years by monoclonal gammopathy of undetermined significance (GMSI), which has a fixed risk of 1% per year of progression to MM/another related disorder. Every patient with active (symptomatic) MM should be treated. With the new treatments – immunomodulators (IMiDs) and proteasome inhibitors (PIs) – the relative 5-year survival has improved from 30% (1990) to 50% (2013) [29, 30].

The goals of initial therapy are rapid disease control and reversal of complications, minimizing toxicity and early mortality, and allowing collection of hematopoietic stem cells (HCTH) in eligible patients. In these, melphalan-based induction therapy should be avoided, as it compromises the collection. However, many of the induction regimens that incorporate newer drugs do not significantly affect collection, and in these cases, the need to classify patients based on TCTHA eligibility has diminished over time (Table 5.3). The main objective is to obtain complete response (CR) after induction followed by TCTHA, a strong predictor of long-term prognosis [29].

Treatment is based on a combination of immunomodulatory drugs (IMiDs) (thalidomide, lenalidomide, pomalidomide), proteasome inhibitors (PIs) (bortezomib, carfilzomib, ixazomib), traditional chemotherapy (QT) (cyclophosphamide, doxorubicin, liposomal doxorubicin), and more recently antibodies monoclonals (daratumumab and elotuzumab) [28].

**Table 5.3** Myeloma recommendations

| Sequencing | Recommendation |
|---|---|
| Induction | (a) RVD (bortezomib, 1.3 mg/m$^2$ SC, in D1, D4, D8, and D11; lenalidomide, 25 mg PO, from D1 to D14; dexamethasone, 20 mg PO, in D1, D2, D4, D5, D8, D9, D11, and D12) every 21 days for 4 cycles; or (b) VTD (bortezomib, 1.3 mg/m$^2$ SC, in D1, D4, D8, and D11; dexamethasone, 40 mg VO, in D1, D2, D4, D5, D8, D9, D11, and D12; thalidomide, 200 mg PO, from D1 to D21) for 4 cycles of 21 days; or (c) dara-VTD (bortezomib, 1.3 mg/m$^2$ SC, on D1, D4, D8, and D11, oral thalidomide, 100 mg per day in all cycles, and oral or IV dexamethasone, 40 mg on D1, D2, D8, D9, D15, D16, D22, and D23 of induction cycles 1 and 2 and in D1 and D2 of induction cycles 3 and 4, and 20 mg in D8, D9, D15, and D16 of induction cycles 3 and 4 and in D1, D2, D8, D9, D15, and D16 of the two consolidation cycles). Daratumumab was administered IV at a dose of 16 mg/kg body weight once weekly in induction cycles 1 and 2 and once every 2 weeks during induction cycles 3 and 4 and consolidation; (d) CyBorD (or VCD) – cyclophosphamide, 300 mg/m$^2$ PO, bortezomib, 1.5 mg/m$^2$ SC and dexamethasone, 40 mg PO, on D1, D8, D15, and D22, every 28 days for 4 cycles. When a faster response is desired, cyclophosphamide, 300 mg/m$^2$ VO, in D1, D8, D15, and D22 can be considered; bortezomib, 1.3 mg/m$^2$ IV or SC, on D1, D4, D8, and D11; dexamethasone, 40 mg VO, from D1 to D4, from D9 to D12, and from D17 to D20, every 28 days, in cycles 1 and 2 |
| Consolidation | Autologous transplantation (melphalan, 200 mg/m $^2$) |
| Maintenance | Lenalidomide, 10–15 mg orally continuously (or from D1 to D21 every 28 days in case of cytopenia). Addition of bortezomib, 1.3 mg/m$^2$ SC every 2 weeks as part of maintenance, may also be considered in high-risk individuals. All patients should receive zoledronic acid, 4 mg IV, in 15 min or denosumab, 120 mg SC, every 4 or 12 weeks, for at least 2 years |

*Source*: Ravi et al. [44]

## 5.3 Pediatric Cancer

Tumors in juvenile patients can be subdivided into two large groups: hematological tumors such as leukemia and lymphoma and solid tumors such as those in the central nervous system/ brain, abdominal tumors (neuroblastomas, hepatoblastomas, nephroblastomas), bone tumors, and soft tissue tumors (rhabdomyosarcomas, synovial sarcomas, fibrosarcomas), among others. The prognosis of cancer in children and adolescents is positively influenced by early diagnosis strategies and continuity of care through appropriate treatment at the right time [32].

Pediatric cancer is not a preventable disease. Although several studies point to the existence of potential risk factors for the child's intrauterine exposure, there is no scientific evidence that clearly shows the association between the disease and environmental factors. Therefore, the prevention of childhood cancer is still a challenge for the future, and the current emphasis on the approach to this cancer must be given to early diagnosis and timely referral for timely and quality treatment, which enables higher cure rates [31].

Diagnosis of the disease, treatment, and implications have an important impact on children and family members. In Brazil, cancer accounted for eighth place among the causes of death among children aged zero to 4 years, but it is the leading cause of death in the age group from 5 to 19 years in 2014, according to the Mortality Information System (Table 5.4). While in adults, the main risk factors for cancer are environmental, related to exposure to carcinogens, and inadequate lifestyle habits, in the first two decades of life, the development of cancer is strongly linked to inherited genetic factors or acquired mutations of the uncertain cause [33].

Cancer in children and adolescents has characteristics that make it different from cancer in adults. It predominantly originates from embryonic cells, has a short latency period and, in general, rapid growth, being very important to obtain better results, prompt diagnostic suspicion and prompt referral to start treatment [37].

**Table 5.4** Main childhood cancers

| Type of cancer | Main symptoms |
|---|---|
| Acute leukemias | The clinical manifestations of acute leukemia are secondary to the excessive proliferation of immature (blastic) cells in the bone marrow, which infiltrate the body's tissues, such as tonsils, lymph nodes (buttocks), skin, spleen, kidneys, central nervous system (CNS), and others |
| Tumors of the central nervous system | Signs and symptoms are multiple and progressive, such as vomiting and headache, mood change, behavior change, gait and coordination change, seizures, nonspecific signs and symptoms of intracranial hypertension (ICH), strabismus, macrocephaly, cranial nerve palsy, lethargy, abnormal eye movements (nystagmus), hemiplegia, weight loss, and focal motor deficit |
| Lymphomas | Adenomegaly is considered suspicious when, after ruling out an infectious cause, it presents together with the following characteristics: fever without a determined cause, weight loss, and night sweats; alterations in two or more series of the blood count (anemia and/or leukopenia/leukocytosis and/or thrombocytopenia); hepatosplenomegaly, negative serology (toxoplasmosis, rubella, HIV, cytomegalovirus, infectious mononucleosis, syphilis); persistence of lymph node infarction greater than 3 cm after 6 weeks of evolution, even after appropriate specific treatment |
| Retinoblastoma | Patients who have more common warning signs such as the "cat's eye reflex" – a yellowish white reflex in the eye due to alteration of light refraction in the retina |
| Osteosarcomas | Signs and symptoms suggestive of bone neoplasm permeate the request and evaluation of imaging tests, such as radiography, computed tomography, and magnetic resonance imaging of the affected region. Other changes that prompt referral: signs of rarefaction and bone lysis; osteolytic lesions; periosteal reaction – thickening or rupture of the periosteum line and Codman's triangle |

(continued)

**Table 5.4** (continued)

| Type of cancer | Main symptoms |
|---|---|
| Rhabdomyosarcoma | The signs and symptoms of rhabdomyosarcoma depend mainly on the location of the tumor: tumor located in the trunk, limbs, or groin (including the testes). The first sign is usually a mass or swelling. Most of the time, it doesn't cause any pain or other problems. Tumors around the eyes may cause swelling or the child may look cross-eyed. Tumors in the ear or sinuses can cause earache, headache, or nasal congestion |

*Source*: Brasil [33]

In pediatrics, there is an extended off-label use of chemotherapy agents such as carboplatin, which is indicated for ovarian carcinoma, small cell lung carcinoma, head and neck squamous cell carcinomas, and uterine cervix carcinomas. Other uses, such as in the treatment of brain tumors, are off-label. Contraindications: hypersensitivity to the drug or other constituents of the formula or to cisplatin; severe renal failure, severe myelosuppression, and/or in the presence of massive bleeding [37].

Cisplatin is approved by the National Health Surveillance Agency (ANVISA) for adult and pediatric use, for metastatic testicular tumors, metastatic ovarian tumors, advanced bladder cancer, head and neck squamous cell carcinomas. Other uses, such as in the treatment of brain tumors, are off-label. Contraindications: hypersensitivity to the drug or formula components, myelosuppression, severe kidney failure, hearing disorders, generalized infections [38].

There is no standard treatment for children under 3 years of age with malignant brain tumors. Patients with incomplete resection have an unsatisfactory prognosis and reduced prolonged progression-free survival.

### 5.3.1 Wilms' Tumor

Wilms' tumor (or nephroblastoma) is the most common primary renal malignancy in childhood. It is an embryonic tumor that develops from immature renal remnants (nephrogenic remains or nephroblastomatosis). In most cases they are unicentric, but they can be multifocal in one or both kidneys. The occurrence of Wilms' tumor is often associated with the development of various syndromes, such as sporadic aniridia syndrome, WAGR syndrome (Wilms, aniridia, genitourinary anomalies, and mental retardation), Denys-Drash syndrome (Wilms, intersex disorders, and nephropathy), and others [36].

Wilms' tumor treatment is an example of success resulting from the association of the efforts of integrated multidisciplinary teams with cooperative groups in the United States and Europe. The National Wilms Tumor Study (NWTS) was founded in 1969 and currently records more than 80% of estimated cases in the United States. Studies by the Société Internationaled'OncologieP édiatrique or International Society of Pediatric Oncology (ISPO) began in 1971, with the collaboration of several European countries [35].

The ISPO-2001 protocol is based on international collaboration with collection of relevant data that allow answering questions of clinical interest that are important to patients. Its main objectives are to maintain risk stratification according to preoperative response, minimize acute and late toxicity, and establish a tumor bank for research on molecular prognostic factors (Table 5.5) [36].

As with most solid tumors that appear in the pediatric age group, surgery is essential in the treatment of nephroblastoma. Nephrectomy should be performed on the affected side via the abdominal route. For bilateral tumors, conservative surgery with partial nephrectomies or even enucleations is indicated, in order to preserve renal function. Lung metastases that do not disappear completely after chemotherapy must be resected. Pulmonary radiotherapy is indicated to complete disease control [35].

**Table 5.5** Therapeutic recommendations of the ISPO-2001 protocol

| Phase | Low risk | Intermediate risk | High risk |
|---|---|---|---|
| I | – | Actinomycin<br>+<br>Vincristine | Actinomycin<br>+<br>Vincristine<br>+<br>Adriamycin |
| II | Actinomycin<br>+<br>Vincristine | Actinomycin<br>+<br>Vincristine<br>+–<br>Adriamycin | 5<br>Medicines<br>+<br>Radiotherapy |
| III | Actinomycin<br>+<br>Vincristine | Actinomycin<br>+<br>Vincristine<br>+–<br>Adriamycin | 5<br>Medicines<br>+<br>Radiotherapy |

*Source*: Weirich et al. [34]

## 5.4 Solid Tumors: Breast Carcinoma

### 5.4.1 Classification

With two histopathological types (ductal infiltrating carcinoma (DIC) and lobular infiltrating carcinoma (LIC)), breast cancer will be staged by locoregional extension and distance, which will guide the treatment. The IUAC (International Union Against Cancer) Classification of Malignant Tumors is the most accepted staging system that uses the categories T (tumor), N (lymph node involvement), M (distant metastasis), and Tis (ICIS – introlobular carcinoma **in situ**) for this clinical process [2, 3].

Discussing the molecular classification, this may have the luminal A, luminal B, hybrid luminal, human epidermal growth factor receptor 2 (HER-2), and basal-like subtypes. In the case of immunohistochemistry (IHC), this will address the positivity of estrogen (ER) and progesterone (PR) receptors with percentage of involvement, and in clinical practice, for the treatment to be defined, the status of hormone receptors and the assessment of

HER-2 status play a crucial role, and therefore, the IHC will quantify the positivity of HER-2 receptors in 0/3 crosses, 1/3 crosses, 2/3 crosses, or 3/3 crosses [2, 3, 16].

Regarding the classification T (tumor), it is important to note that in the case of Tis (Paget), the classification will occur according to the size and characteristics of the parenchymal neoplasm, which can be classified as T1 (tumor with 2 cm or less in its largest dimension) and T1mic (when there is microinvasion: there is a tumor measuring up to 0.1 cm in its largest dimension). Thus, the status of these receptors, the assessment of the status of HER-2 together with the clinicopathological criteria, the TNM classification and the breast cancer risk classification will guide the therapeutic decision [2, 3].

### 5.4.2 Chemotherapeutic Protocols

As mentioned, the therapeutic approach (surgery of the primary tumor, assessment of axillary involvement, radiotherapy, and systemic drug treatment) will be defined by the criteria previously scored. With an emphasis on systemic drug therapy, it may have an adjuvant (prophylactic), prior (neoadjuvant/cytoreductive), and palliative character [1–3].

As one of the main therapeutic protocols, chemotherapy affects normal and neoplastic cells, and, in the case of adjuvant therapy, the analysis of the characteristics of the patient and the tumor is taken into account, in which patients with intermediate or high risk are elective for this type of therapy (Table 5.6). As for previous therapy, it is indicated when the patient presents an advanced stage of the pathology or through some other points to be analyzed; however, for these therapies, there is an assessment of the degree of risk and therapeutic regimens according to this degree [2, 3, 16].

With regard to palliative therapy, there is no consensus on the conduct to be adopted, as well as there are no guidelines that provide specific treatment and, thus, the selection of medications used occurs according to numerous factors related to the patient and the tumor. Currently, hormonal manipulations for advanced

**Table 5.6** Suggested chemotherapy regimens of treatment according to risk

| Risk/hormonal status | Pre menopause | Post menopause |
|---|---|---|
| Low risk | Tamoxifen – if RH positive – for 5 years. Individual cases: AC for 4 cycles, TC for 4 cycles, or CMF for 6 cycles | Tamoxifen or upfront aromatase inhibitor, or switch – if RH positive |
| Intermediate risk | Tamoxifen if RH positive – for 5 years. AC or FAC or FEC or TC or AC for 4 cycles followed by 4 cycles of docetaxel 100 mg/m$^2$ every 21 days | Tamoxifen or upfront aromatase inhibitor or switch – if RH positive. AC or FAC or FEC or TC or AC for 4 cycles followed by 4 cycles of docetaxel 100 mg/m$^2$ every 21 days |
| High risk | FAC or FEC for 6 cycles or AC for 4 cycles followed by 4 cycles of docetaxel 100 mg/m$^2$ every 21 days or paclitaxel 80 mg/m$^2$ weekly for 12 cycles | FAC or FEC for 6 cycles or AC for 4 cycles followed by 4 cycles of docetaxel 100 mg/m$^2$ every 21 days |

*Source*: Brasil [3], [2]

breast cancer are widely used; among them are the drugs tamoxifen, aromatase inhibitors (exemestane, anastrozole or letrozole), LHRH analogues, and fulvestrant [2, 3].

### 5.4.3 Main Effects Caused by Drugs Used in Breast Cancer Therapeutic Schemes

Kameo et al. [11] argue that, according to the amount of medication administered, there is an increase in the occurrence of adverse reactions arising from drug interactions. And, in this context, Amaral [1] emphasizes that the effectiveness of breast cancer therapy is related to the combination of two or more drugs and, in this combination, are the groups of anthracyclines (doxorubicin, daunorubicin, epirubicin, mitoxantrone, and idarubicin) or taxanes (paclitaxel and docetaxel), in addition to fluorouracil, cyclophosphamide, and carboplatin.

The group of anthracyclines are the most used chemotherapeutics in the treatment of breast cancer, and, among the effects caused by these drugs, cardiotoxicity is cited. In addition, cardiac conduction disturbance, myocarditis, pericarditis, and arrhythmias are present [1].

In the group of taxanes, the elimination of these drugs is complex and, as side effects, cutaneous reactions stand out, and the patient may manifest erythema, phlebitis, desquamation, pain, and others. In addition to these, paclitaxel stands out, which, regardless of the dose administered, can lead to the onset of alopecia, myelosuppression, and peripheral neuropathy. Fluorouracil may cause vomiting, pain, oral mucositis, taste changes, and nausea. Cyclophosphamide can cause alopecia, cystitis, infection, and gastrointestinal problems. Carboplatin, on the other hand, is related to dry cough, muscle spasms, sweating, and tachycardia, among others [1, 18, 19].

By blocking the action of the aromatase enzyme, aromatase inhibitors (aminoglutethimide, fedrazole and formestane, anastrozole, letrozole, and exemestane) have more favorable side effects, with less frequency of cardiovascular, thromboembolic, and gynecological events (Table 5.7). However, there are side effects, with musculoskeletal effects being the most reported, in which exemestane has a higher incidence of diarrhea and arthralgia [12, 14].

In the case of the use of monoclonal antibodies, trastuzumab stands out, considered the standard treatment for patients with HER2+ breast cancer. In addition to this, pertuzumab, lapatinib, and neratinib also act on the HER2 protein. Pertuzumab can cause heart problems that can be aggravated by concomitant use of chemotherapy with doxorubicin or epirubicin; on the other hand, trastuzumab is associated with the possibility of developing reversible heart failure (type II) by some patients [6, 16].

**Table 5.7** Pharmacodynamic profile of AI (aromatase inhibitors)

| Aromatase inhibitors | Action mechanism | Effects |
|---|---|---|
| Aminoglutetimide | Inhibits aromatase, which is essential for the generation of estrogens from androstenedione and testosterone | Respiratory depression, hypoventilation, hypotension, hypovolemic shock due to dehydration, drowsiness, lethargy, coma, ataxia, dizziness, fatigue, nausea, and vomiting |
| Formstan | Inhibits aromatase, which is essential for the generation of estrogens from androstenedione and testosterone | Itching, rash, lethargy, drowsiness, headache, leg swelling, vaginal or leakage bleeding |
| Anastrozole | Inhibits aromatase; inhibits the conversion of androgens to estrogens | Hot flashes, asthenia, arthralgia, headache, nausea, and reddening skin lesions |
| Exemestane | Inhibits aromatase; inhibits the conversion of androgens to estrogens | Convulsion |
| Letrozole | Inhibits aromatase; inhibits the conversion of androgens to estrogens | Headache, nausea, bloating, tiredness, hot flashes, hair thinning, skin allergies, vomiting, indigestion, weight gain, muscle aches, increased or loss of appetite, vaginal bleeding, vaginal discharge, constipation, dizziness, and enlargement of sweating |

*Source*: ESCÓRCIO et al. [48]

## 5.5 Cancers of the Head and Neck

### 5.5.1 Nasopharynx Carcinoma

In nasopharyngeal tumors, unlike what occurs in other sites in the head and neck region, surgery as an initial treatment is not routinely performed due to the difficulty of obtaining free surgical margins, in addition to the complexity of the access, aesthetic and functional morbidities, and high cure rates achieved with external RT. The key role of early stage RT was demonstrated in a retrospective analysis with 702 stage I patients treated with conventional RT or IMRT and a median follow-up of 105 months, which demonstrated a 5-year overall survival (OS) rate of 99.3% [47].

| | |
|---|---|
| Stages I and II | In stage I patients, we favor isolated radiotherapy (RT), preferably with modulated intensity (IMRT), at a dose of 7000 cGy in daily fractions directed to the primary site. In stage II patients, we favor concomitant treatment of RT and chemotherapy (QT) with cisplatin, 30 mg/m$^2$/week IV. Targeted doses and extension of the RT field to bilateral cervical regions vary according to the presence or absence of lymph node involvement, i.e., lymph node negative, 5000 cGy in the upper cervical region (up to level III); positive lymph node, 6500–7000 cGy in total cervical region |
| Stages III to IVA | Induction systemic QT, followed by concomitant radiochemotherapy with cisplatin, 40 mg/m$^2$ IV, in 2 h, weekly or, alternatively, cisplatin, 100 mg/m$^2$ IV, in 2 h, in D1, D22, and D43, combined with IMRT in dose of 7000 cGy in daily fractions from 180 to 200 cGy. Preferred induction systemic QT options include gemcitabine, 1000 mg/m$^2$ IV, on D1 and D8, and cisplatin, 80 mg/m$^2$ IV, on D1, repeated every 3 weeks for 3 cycles; cisplatin, 75 mg/m$^2$ IV and docetaxel, 75 mg/m$^2$ IV, both on D1 and repeated every 3 weeks for 3 cycles. Less favored systemic QT induction options include cisplatin, 60 mg/m$^2$ IV, on D1, docetaxel, 60 mg/m$^2$ IV, on D1 and 5-FU, 600 mg/m$^2$/day IV in continuous infusion from D1 to D5, with G-CSF support, repeated every 21 days for 3 cycles; or cisplatin, 80 mg/m$^2$ IV, on D1 and 5-FU, 800 mg/m$^2$/day IV in continuous infusion, from D1 to D5, repeated every 21 days for 2 cycles |
| Follow-up after initial treatment of stage I disease to IVA | Perform nasofibroscopy and imaging tests, preferably MRI of the face and neck. PET-CT can be considered 3 months after completion of RT. repeat nasofibroscopy periodically and check TSH to monitor thyroid function. After 2 years of follow-up, we favor semiannual follow-up until the fifth year and annually thereafter |

*Source*: Sun et al. [46]

### 5.5.2 Salivary Gland

The 10-year survival achieved with stage I and II surgery is 90% and 65%, respectively. Apparently, there is no difference according to the place of origin of the primary tumor (parotid gland, submandibular gland, and minor salivary glands), and overall survival rates (OS) are correlated with tumor grade.

| Staging | Recommendations |
|---|---|
| Stages I and II | Tumor resection with free margins and lymph node dissection in T2 tumors, with lymphovascular invasion, minor salivary glands, and high histological grade, and surgery should address chains I–III. Consider postoperative radiotherapy (RT) to the primary site in early high-risk tumors (intermediate or high grade, positive margins, perineural or intraneural invasion, lymphovascular invasion, and adenoid cystic carcinoma) |
| Stages III and IV (resectable) | Surgery considering primary tumor resection and prophylactic lymph node dissection for chains I–III, in case of clinically negative lymph nodes, and therapeutic lymph node dissection for chains I–V, in case of clinically positive lymph nodes, followed by postoperative RT. If available, consider using RT with the IMRT technique |
| Stage IVM0 (unresectable) | RT in doses of 6000–6500 cGy, given in daily fractions over 6–7 weeks. In patients with good clinical condition and without comorbidities, we favor the concomitant use of QT containing platinum |

| Staging | Recommendations |
|---|---|
| Stage IVM1 | There is no standard guideline regarding the most effective combination due to the lack of studies with a representative number of individuals. Systemic treatment must be defined considering the histological subtype. For patients with adenoid cystic carcinoma, we only recommend systemic treatment for symptomatic individuals or those with rapidly progressive disease, in which case we suggest lenvatinib, 24 mg VO, 1×/day (preferably) or axitinib, 5 mg VO, 2×/day. If not available, consider cisplatin, 80 mg/m$^2$ IV, in 120 min, on D1 and vinorelbine, 25 mg/m$^2$ IV, on D1 and D8, repeated every 3 weeks or CAP regimen (cyclophosphamide combination, 500 mg/m$^2$ IV, doxorubicin, 50 mg/m$^2$ IV and cisplatin, 50 mg/m$^2$ IV, on D1), repeated every 3 weeks. For patients with HER-2 positive ductal carcinoma, we recommend preferably ado-trastuzumab emtansine, 3.6 mg/kg IV, every 3 weeks. If not available, we recommend a combination of carboplatin, AUC 6 IV, on D1, docetaxel, 75 mg/m$^2$ IV, on D1 and trastuzumab, on D1 (8 mg/kg IV as a loading dose followed by 6 mg/kg IV), every 3 weeks, followed, if response after 4–6 cycles, of maintenance with trastuzumab, 6 mg/kg IV, every 3 weeks or the combination of docetaxel, 70 mg/m$^2$, IV in D1 and trastuzumab in D1 (8 mg/kg IV as a loading dose followed by 6 mg/kg IV) every 3 weeks, for 6 cycles, and then followed by trastuzumab, 6 mg/kg IV, every 3 weeks. For carriers of secretory carcinoma with TRK fusion, we recommend larotrectinib, 100 mg orally, 2×/day or entrectinib, 600 mg orally, 1×/day. For the other histological subtypes, we recommend cisplatin and vinorelbine, CAP or carboplatin, AUC 5 EV and paclitaxel, 175 mg/m$^2$ EV, in 3 h, both on D1, every 3 weeks |

*Source*: Ning et al. [45]

## References


1. Amaral LBMX. Cuidado de enfermagem nos efeitos adversos na quimioterapia para câncer de mama: revisão narrativa da literatura. Monografia (Graduação em Enfermagem) – Universidade Federal do Tocantins. Palmas; 2019. p. 50.
2. Brasil. Ministério da Saúde. Secretaria de Atenção à Saúde. Secretaria de Ciência, Tecnologia e Insumos Estratégicos. Portaria conjunta n° 5: aprova as diretrizes Diagnósticas e Terapêuticas do Carcinoma de Mama. Brasília-DF. 2019.
3. Brasil. Ministério da Saúde. Instituto Nacional de Câncer José Alencar Gomes da Silva. Estimativa 2020: incidência de Câncer no Brasil. Rio de Janeiro: INCA; 2019.
4. Chisesi T. State of the art in the treatment of CLL. Rev Bras Hematol Hemoter. 2009;31(2):51–6.
5. Farias MG, Castro SM. Diagnóstico laboratorial das leucemiaslinfóides agudas. J Bras Patol Med Lab. 2004;40(2):91–8.
6. Galvan ADC, Porath H. Perfil epidemiológico de pacientes que desenvolveram insuficiência cardíaca em tratamento com trastuzumabe para câncer de mama HER-2 positivo em centro de oncologia de hospital universitário. Monografia (Graduação em Medicina) – Faculdade Evangélica Mackenzie do Paraná. Curitiba; 2020. p. 58.
7. Howlader N, et al., editors. SEER cancer statistics review, 1975–2014. National Cancer Institute: Bethesda; 2017.
8. Instituto Nacional de Câncer José Alencar Gomes da Silva (INCA). Coordenação de Prevenção e Vigilância. Estimativa 2018: incidência de câncer no Brasil. Rio de Janeiro: INCA; 2017.
9. Instituto Nacional de Câncer José Alencar Gomes da Silva (INCA). Coordenação de Prevenção e Vigilância. Estimativas 2016: incidência de câncer no Brasil [Internet]. Rio de Janeiro, INCA; 2015. Available from: http://www.inca.gov.br/estimativa/2016/estimativa-2016-v11.pdf.
10. Instituto Nacional de Câncer José Alencar Gomes da Silva (INCA). ABC do câncer: abordagens básicas para o controle do câncer [Internet]. Rio de Janeiro: INCA; 2017. Available from: http://www1.inca.gov.br/inca/Arquivos/comunicacao/livro_abc_3ed_8a_prova_final.pdf.
11. Kameo SY, Silva GM, Sawada NO, Santana ME. Neutropenia febril de recorrência pós-quimioterapia em paciente com câncer de mama. Rev Enferm UFPI. 2015;4(2):111–8.
12. Lucarelli AP, Martins MM, Forattini A. Inibidores da aromatase no tratamento de pacientes com câncer de mama. Arq Med HospFacCienc Med Santa Casa São Paulo. 2013;58:88–91.
13. Lopes FC. Neutropenia febril no pacienteoncológico [Internet]. 2011.
14. Martinez AS, Queiroz FJG, Cangiani EE. Estudo das características terapêuticas dos antineoplásicos orais. Revista Eletrônica de Ciências da

Saúde. Centro Universitário Planalto do Distrito Federal – UNIPLAN. Águas Claras/DF. 2019;1(1):20–24.
15. Mesa MJ, Restrepo DM, Ramírez-Pulgarín S, Martínez-Sánchez LM, Gázquez MA, Forero JP. Perfil clínico y microbiológico de niños Con neutropenia febril posterior a tratamientos antineoplásicos tratados en una institución hospitalaria de Medellín (Colombia), 2009-2010: estudio de serie de casos. Arch med. 2015;15(1):25–32.
16. Nascimento AS, Mello EVSL, Schneider LCL, Almeida FLA. Principais tratamentos utilizados no combate ao câncer de mama: uma revisão de literatura. Arquivos do MUDI. 2019;23(3):201–19.
17. Nascimento TG, Andrade M, Oliveira RA, Almeida AM, Gozzo TO. Neutropenia: ocorrência e manejo em mulheres com câncer de mama em quimioterapia. Rev latinoamenferm [Internet]. 2014.
18. Piranda DN, Freitas-Alves DR, Vianna-Jorge R. Farmacogenética e Implicações Terapêuticas no Câncer de Mama. Revista Brasileira de Cancerologia. 2013;59(3):449–52.
19. Sidney KMM, Romeu GA, Pinheiro CG. Estudo de reações adversas ao paclitaxel em pacientes com câncer de mama em um hospital de referência. Rev Bras Farm Hosp Serv Saúde São Paulo. 2017;8(1):37–42.
20. Silva, Colet da F, Araðjo, da Silva L, Frizzo, Nunes M. Neoplasias Hematológicas No Idoso: Uma Revisão. Rev Sau Int, Rio Grande do Sul. 2016;8(15):1–13.
21. Vasconcelos RC. Avaliação dos marcadores celulares por citometria de fluxo em pacientes com leucemia mieloide aguda. Rev Bras Hematol Hemoter. 2010;32(3):275–6.
22. Sander CA, Flaig MJ, Jaffe ES. Cutaneous manifestations of lymphoma: a clinical guide based on the WHO classification. World Health Organization. Clin Lymphoma. 2001;2(2):86–100.; ; discussion 101–2. https://doi.org/10.3816/clm.2001.n.014.
23. Judith AF. Scientific advances and the evolution of diagnosis, subclassification and treatment of lymphoma. Arch Med Res. 2020;51(8):749–64. https://doi.org/10.1016/j.arcmed.2020.05.022. Epub 2020 Jun 14
24. Eich HT, Heimann M, Stutzer H, Kriz J, Reiser M, Muller RP. Long-term outcome and prognostic factors in early-stage nodal low-grade non-hodgkin's lymphomas treated with radiation therapy. Strahlenther Onkol. 2009;185(5):288–95.
25. Hagenbeek A, Eghbali H, Monfardini S, Vitolo U, Hoskin PJ, Wolf-Peeters C, et al. Phase III intergroup study of fludarabine phosphate compared with cyclophosphamide, vincristine, and prednisone chemotherapy in newly diagnosed patients with stage III and IV low-grade malignant non-Hodgkin's lymphoma. J Clin Oncol. 2006;24(10):1590–6.
26. Waterman J, Rybicki L, Bolwell B, Copelan E, Pohlman B, Sweetenham J, et al. Fludarabine as a risk fator for poor stem cell harvest, treatment-related MDS and AML in follicular lymphoma patients after autologous hematopoeetic cell transplantation. Bone Marrow Transplant. 2012;47(4):488–93.

27. Jiang M, Bennani NN, Feldman AL. Lymphoma classification update: T-cell lymphomas, Hodgkin lymphomas, and histiocytic/dendritic cell neoplasms. Expert Rev Hematol. 2017;10(3):239–49. https://doi.org/10.1080/17474086.2017.1281122. Epub 2017 Jan 29
28. Rajkumar SV. Multiple myeloma: 2016 update on diagnosis, risk-stratification, and management. Am J Hematol. 2016;91(7):719–34.
29. Swerdlow SHA. WHO classification of tumours of haematopoietic and lymphoid tissues. 4th ed. Lyon: International Agency for Research on Cancer; 2008.
30. Rajkumar SV. International myeloma working group updated criteria for the diagnosis of multiple myeloma. Lancet Oncol. 2014 Nov;15(12):e538–48.
31. Pasqualini C, Rialland F, Valteau-Couanet D, Michon J, Minard-Colin V. Nouvelles perspectives dans l'immunothérapie des cancer pédiatriques. Bull Cancer. 2018;105(Suplemento 1):S68–79. https://doi.org/10.1016/S0007-4551(18)30392-8.
32. Snaman J, Kaye EC, Baker JN, Wolfe J. Pediatric palliative oncology: the state of the science and art of caring for children with cancer. Curr Opin Pediatr. 2018;30(1):40–8. https://doi.org/10.1097/MOP.0000000000000573.
33. Brasil. Ministério da Saúde. Secretaria de Atenção à Saúde. Departamento de AtençãoEspecializada e Temáticas. Protocolo de diagnóstico precoce do câncer pediátrico [recursoeletrônico]/Ministério da Saúde, Secretaria de Atenção à Saúde, Departamento de AtençãoEspecializada e Temáticas. Brasília: Ministério da Saúde; 2017.
34. Weirich A, Leuschner I, Harms D, Vujanic GM, Troger J, Abel U, et al. Clinical impact of histologic subtypes in localized non-anaplastic nephroblastoma treated according to the trial and study SIOP-9/GPOH. Ann Oncol. 2001;12:311–9.
35. Charlton J, Irtan S, Bergeron C, Pritchard-Jones K. Bilateral Wilms tumour: a review of clinical and molecular features. Expert Rev Mol Med. 2017;18(19):e8. https://doi.org/10.1017/erm.2017.8.
36. Treger TD, Chowdhury T, Pritchard-Jones K, Behjati S. The genetic changes of Wilms tumour. Nat Rev Nephrol. 2019;15(4):240–51. https://doi.org/10.1038/s41581-019-0112-0.
37. Filbin M, Monje M. Developmental origins and emerging therapeutic opportunities for childhood. Cancer Nat Med. 2019 Mar;25(3):367–76. https://doi.org/10.1038/s41591-019-0383-9.
38. Landier W, Armenian S, Bhatia S. Late effects of childhood cancer and its treatment. Pediatr Clin N Am. 2015 Feb;62(1):275–300. https://doi.org/10.1016/j.pcl.2014.09.017.
39. Williams MTS, Yousafzai YM, Elder A, Rehe K, Bomken S, LironFrishman-Levy ST, Sinclair P, Dormon K, Masic D, Perry T, Weston VJ, Kearns P, Blair H, Russell LJ, Heidenreich O, Irving JAE, Izraeli S, Vormoor J, Graham GJ, Halsey C. The ability to cross the

blood–cerebrospinal fluid barrier is a generic property of acute lymphoblastic leukemia blasts Crossmark: check for updates. Blood. 2016;127(16):1998–2006.
40. Levinsen M, Marquart HV, Groth-Pedersen L, Abrahamsson J, Albertsen BK, Andersen MK, Frandsen TL, Harila-Saari A, Pronk C, Ulvmoen A, Vaitkevičienė G, Lähteenmäki PM, Niinimäki R, MerviTaskinen MJ, Schmiegelow K. Leukemic blasts are present at low levels in spinal fluid in one-third of childhood acute lymphoblastic leukemia cases. Pediatr Blood Cancer. 2016;63(11):1935–42. https://doi.org/10.1002/pbc.26128. Epub 2016 Jul 22.
41. Vora A, Andreano A, Pui C-H, Hunger SP, Schrappe M, Moericke A, Biondi A, Escherich G, Silverman LB, Goulden N, Taskinen M, Pieters R, KeizoHoribe MD, Locatelli F, Valsecchi MG. Influence of cranial radiotherapy on outcome in children with acute lymphoblastic leukemia treated with contemporary therapy. J Clin Oncol. 2016;34(9):12–17.
42. Messina M, Del Giudice I, Khiabanian H, Rossi D, Chiaretti S, Rasi S, Spina V, Holmes AB, Marinelli M, Fabbri G, Piciocchi A, Mauro FR, Guarini A, Gaidano G, Dalla-Favera R, Pasqualucci L, Rabadan R, Foà R. Genetic lesions associated with chronic lymphocytic leukemia chemo-refractoriness. Crossmark: Check for Updates. Blood. 2014;123(15):2378–88.
43. Castagnetti F, Gugliotta G, Breccia M, Stagno F, Iurlo A, Albano F, Abruzzese E, Martino B, Levato L, Intermesoli T, Pregno P, Rossi G, Gherlinzoni F, Leoni P, Cavazzini F, Venturi C, Soverini S, Testoni N, Alimena G, Cavo M, Martinelli G, Pane F, Saglio G, Rosti G, M Baccarani on behalf of the GIMEMA CML Working Party. Long-term outcome of chronic myeloid leukemia patients treated frontline with imatinib. Leukemia. 2015;29:1823–31. © 2015 Macmillan Publishers Limited
44. Vij R, Kumar S, Zhang M-J, Zhong X, Huang J, Dispenzieri A, Abidi MH, Bird JM, Freytes CO, Gale RP, Kindwall-Keller TL, Kyle RA, Landsburg DJ, Lazarus HM, Munker R, Roy V, Sharma M, Vogl DT, BaldeepWirk PN, editors. Hari impact of pretransplant therapy and depth of disease response before autologous transplantation for multiple myeloma. Biol Blood Marrow Transplant. 2015;21:335e341.
45. Ning C, Zhao T, Wang Z, Li D, Kou Y, Huang S. Cervical lymph node metastases in salivary gland adenoid cystic carcinoma: a systematic review and meta-analysis. Cancer Manag Res. 2018;10:10–14.
46. Sun X, ShengfaSu CC, Han F, Zhao C, Xiao W, Deng X, Huang S, Lin C, Lu T. Long-term outcomes of intensity-modulated radiotherapy for 868 patients with nasopharyngeal carcinoma: an analysis of survival and treatment toxicities. Radiother Oncol. 2014;110(3):398–403. https://doi.org/10.1016/j.radonc.2013.10.020. Epub 2013 Nov 11
47. Tang L-Q, Lu T-Y, Yang L, Guo S-Y, Zhong Q-Y, Zou M-S, Chen B-L, Tang Q-N, Chen W-H, Guo S-S, Liu L-T, Chen Q-Y, Guo L, Mo H-Y, Dong RS. Patterns of failure and survival trends of 720 patients with stage

I nasopharyngeal carcinoma diagnosed from 1990-2012: a large-scale retrospective cohort study. J Cancer. 2018;9:7–13.
48. ESCÓRCIO et al. Study pharmacokinect and pharmacodynamic profile of the substances used in breast cancer treatment. Revista Saúde em Foco, Teresina. v. 4, n. 1, art. 6, p. 67–93, jan./jul.2017.

# Handling Chemotherapy 6

Sandro Luis Ribeiro Ness
and Laura Alegria Martins

S. L. R. Ness (✉)
Hospital de Clínicas de Porto Alegre – HCPA,
Porto Alegre, Brazil

College of Medicine – Universidade Federal do Rio Grande do Sul – UFRGS, Porto Alegre, Brazil

Hospital Pharmacy and Clinical Oncology – IBRAS, Ponta Grossa, PR, Brazil

Oncology Pharmacy – Centro Universitário São Camilo, São Paulo, Brazil

SOBRAFO (Sociedade Brasileira de Farmacêuticos em Oncologia), São Paulo, Brazil

Clinical Pharmacy by SBRAFH (Sociedade Brasileira de Farmácia Hospitalar e Serviços de Saúde), São Paulo, Brazil

L. A. Martins
Hospital de Clínicas de Porto Alegre – HCPA,
Porto Alegre, Brazil

SOBRAFO (Sociedade Brasileira de Farmacêuticos em Oncologia), São Paulo, Brazil

College of Pharmacy – Universidade Federal do Rio Grande do Sul – UFRGS, Porto Alegre, Brazil

Institute of Education and Research Hospital Moinhos de Vento, Porto Alegre, Brazil

Oncology Pharmacy – Institute of Education and Research Hospital Moinhos de Vento - IEP/HMV,
Porto Alegre, Brazil





C. W. P. Schmidt, K. M. Otoni (eds.), *The Golden Guide to Oncologic Pharmacy*, https://doi.org/10.1007/978-3-030-98596-7_6

## 6.1 Occupational Exposure to Antineoplastic Drugs

Antineoplastic drugs present risks of occupational exposure to professionals responsible for handling them, as they have carcinogenic, mutagenic, teratogenic, and/or genotoxic characteristics and can produce toxic effects at low doses when administered to humans or animals. Several international agencies, which develop guidelines for good practices and care in the handling and administration of these drugs, consider any agent that presents at least one of these effects as a dangerous substance [1–5].

The fact that they do not have a selective action on cancer cells and may also cause effects on healthy cells largely explains the risk to these professionals [3, 5, 6].

The risks to professionals responsible for handling cytotoxic drugs are the result of the combination of the characteristic of toxicity and the extent to which workers are exposed daily in the course of their work activities through inhalation, absorption, and ingestion of these agents. Thus, it is essential to describe work practice guidelines to limit exposure and what equipment is needed to carry out safe and appropriate practices [6].

In 2004, the National Institute for Occupational Safety and Health (NIOSH) published a warning on the prevention of occupational exposure to antineoplastic drugs and other substances considered cytotoxic. In this publication and in subsequent updates, a list of substances that can cause harm to exposed professionals was compiled [2].

Exposure to cytotoxic drugs can cause short- or long-term damage. Short-term damages are headache, dizziness, skin rash, vomiting; long-term damages are infertility, endocrine sequelae, early menopause, musculoskeletal disorders, immune dysfunctions, fetal abnormalities, miscarriages, pregnancy abnormalities, DNA damage, increased micronucleus frequency, increased sister chromatid exchanges, and leukemia or others types of cancer [2, 7, 8]. However, it is difficult to measure the risk, the long-term harm of these agents in the healthy individual, and the magnitude of safe exposure to these drugs [9, 10].

Groups involved in the handling of cytotoxic agents such as patients, pharmaceutical industry workers, pharmacists, nurses, physicians, pharmacy and nursing assistants, cleaning and sanitizing personnel, researchers, family members, and caregivers are potentially exposed [2, 3, 11].

Exposure to contamination may occur at different times: removal of the solution from the vial, reconstitution of drugs, opening of ampoules, removal of air from the syringe containing the drug, adjustment of doses, connection of needles and removal of caps from the syringes, handling of oral antineoplastic drugs, administration to the patient, cleaning and sanitizing of handling and administration areas, and waste disposal [1, 6].

Several studies of environmental and personal contamination have been carried out using different methodologies and workplaces. Environmental contamination can be evidenced through the work surfaces where residues are found on the outside of the laminar flow cabin, walls, floors, shelves, benches, equipment, packaging and medicine bottles, syringes, elastomeric infusers, both in the areas of preparation in the pharmacy how much of the administration drugs in the infirmary. Contact with excreta and bodily fluids or clothing used on patients during the treatment period can also lead to contamination. Although not all samples have detectable drug levels, all studies have shown that surface contamination exists and is common in areas where cytotoxic drugs are stored, prepared, administered, or discarded [2, 3, 12–16].

In the case of antineoplastic drugs, there is no exposure limit allowed for each drug, requiring preventive measures. Thus, it characterizes the importance of environmental monitoring and baseline levels in professionals who handle drugs. The major limitation of these measures is quantification: it is not possible to define the exact individual dose to which the worker was exposed [17]. Thus, it is important to know the amount of compounded drug and the mode of diffusion in the environment, characterize the area of greatest contamination, know the route of absorption of the antineoplastic in question and the proportion between cutaneous and respiratory dose, efficiency of collective and individual protection devices, and the eventual transfer of residual microquantities present in the work environment to contiguous areas [18].

Different studies and methodologies for monitoring the occupational exposure of workers involved in the handling and administration of antineoplastic drugs are being developed: comet assays, micronucleus testing in peripheral blood lymphocytes and salivary fluid, cytogenetic methods of analysis of chromosomal aberrations and chromatid exchange sisters, methods of mutagens and thioesters in urine, and quantification of drugs and their metabolites through chromatography [15].

Ness et al. demonstrated an increase in oxidative stress parameters in pharmacists and nurses who handle and administer antineoplastic drugs, respectively, even with the correct use of individual and collective protective equipment, and no damage to DNA was demonstrated through in comet assays and micronucleus test when compared to a control group of professionals in a hospital in southern Brazil [19]. However, other studies have shown DNA damage through sister chromatid exchange, micronucleus enlargement, and comet assay [20–22], and several review and meta-analysis studies analyze different studies and methodologies [23–27].

## 6.2 Individual and Collective Protection Equipment

Drugs considered cytotoxic and that present risks of contamination must be handled, taking into account strict safe handling techniques and use of individual (PPE) and collective (CPE) protection equipment, ensuring personal protection of the team and the environment [2, 3, 28].

## 6.3 Collective Protection Equipment (CPE)

### 6.3.1 Biological Safety Cabinet (BSC)

All handling must take place in a biological safety cabinet (BSC), class II, type B2, or class III, indicated for handling sterile and highly toxic products. It features a high-efficiency particulate air (HEPA) filter that removes particles and microorganisms from the air, producing sterile work areas. Class II B2 has 100% external exhaust, with the air passing through a HEPA filter, ensuring per-

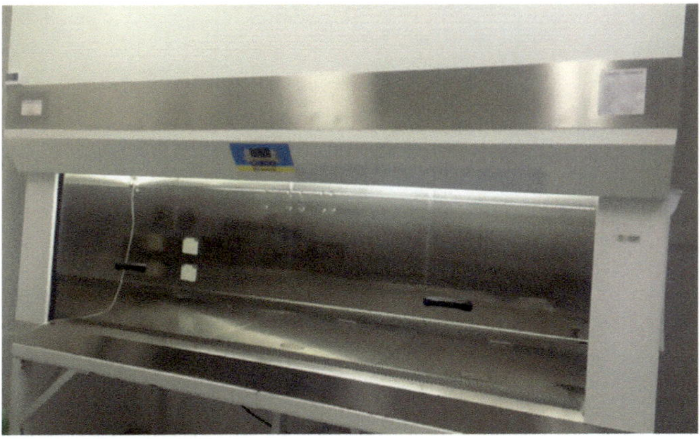

**Fig. 6.1** Biological safety cabinet (BSC), class II, type B2

sonal and environmental protection (Fig. 6.1). This flow works under negative pressure, preventing the contaminated air inside from expanding outward, contaminating the handling room. In this way, its air movement technology protects the operator, the handled product, and the external environment.

As per the 2006 ASHP guidelines, professionals must understand that BSC Class II does not prevent contamination inside the cabinet and that effectiveness in containing contamination by antineoplastic drugs depends on the use of proper techniques by the operators [29].

The BSC Class III (Fig. 6.2) is a fully enclosed vented, gas-tight enclosure. Operations are conducted using gloves that are attached and observed through a viewing window that does not open. This BSC is kept under negative pressure, and air is drawn into the cabinet through HEPA filters. The exhaust air is treated by double filtration of HEPA filters. The passage of material in and out of the cabin is usually accomplished through a double-door passage hatch.

The Class III of biological safety cabinets (BSCs) have the advantage that there is a physical barrier between the products and the handler [30].

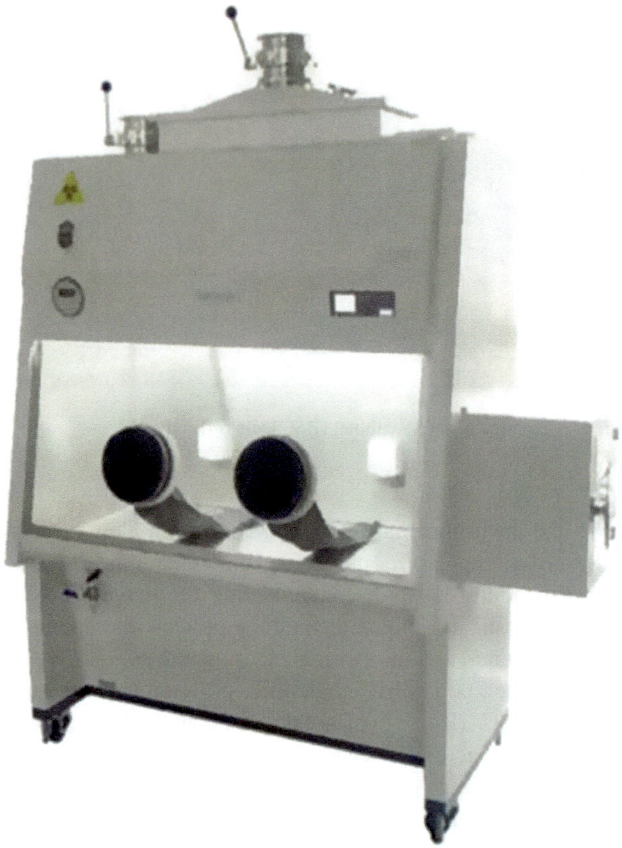

**Fig. 6.2** Biological safety cabinet (BSC), class III

ASHP recommends that BSCs be certified by qualified technicians every six months or whenever the cab is moved or needs repair [29]. Technicians who maintain these cabinets or change HEPA filters must be aware of the risks and must use the same PPE recommended for large spills. Any interruption in its operation implies the immediate stoppage of preparation activities [2, 6].

**Table 6.1** Types of biological safety cabinets

| |
|---|
| *Class II* |
| Down air and HEPA filter |
| *A* – It recirculates 70% of the internal air and 30% discharged into the preparation area. |
| *B* – Extracted air is expelled to the outside. |
| *B1* – It recycles 30% and expels 70% of the air. |
| *B2* – It expels 100% of the air. |
| *B3* – It recycles 70% and expels 30% of the air. |
| *Class III* |
| Closed cabinets, handling with rubber gloves attached. The pressure must be negative and does not require a clean area. |

Most biological safety cabinets have built-in ultraviolet (UV) light. Ultraviolet light is intended to destroy microorganisms in the air or on exposed surfaces when the BSC blower is turned off. When the cabinet runs continuously, this light is not needed.

Horizontal type cabinets should not be used for the preparation of cytotoxic drugs, as they represent a risk to the handler.

Table 6.1 refers to the types of biological safety cabinets

### 6.3.2 Biological Safety Cabinet Certification

All equipment and processes used in the preparation of parenteral cytotoxics that affect sterility or product attributes must be validated and/or certified.

The biological safety cabinet must be certified by a qualified person and must meet the requirements of biosafety standards such as design, construction, performance, and field certification. Documentation for this purpose must be approved, maintained, revised, and signed by a designated pharmacist, and the cabinet must be recertified every six months when the cabinet is changed or repaired or the HEPA filter is changed [31, 32].

Tests include the following:

- HEPA filter integrity test
- Airflow
- Particle count
- Pressure and sterilization
- Fume test

### 6.3.3 Shower and Eye-Wash

The shower and eye-wash are equipment used in places of storage or handling of chemically hazardous products to be used in case of accidents. Their function is to immediately clean the eyes, face, hands, and any other part of the body that has been contaminated. The equipment has a controlled water flow with low speed, allowing for efficient decontamination (Fig. 6.3).

They must be in the room before the handling room and be checked weekly for functionality [32, 33].

#### 6.3.3.1 Personal Protective Equipment (PPE)

Personal protective equipment is defined by OSHA as equipment used to minimize exposure to hazards that cause serious injury

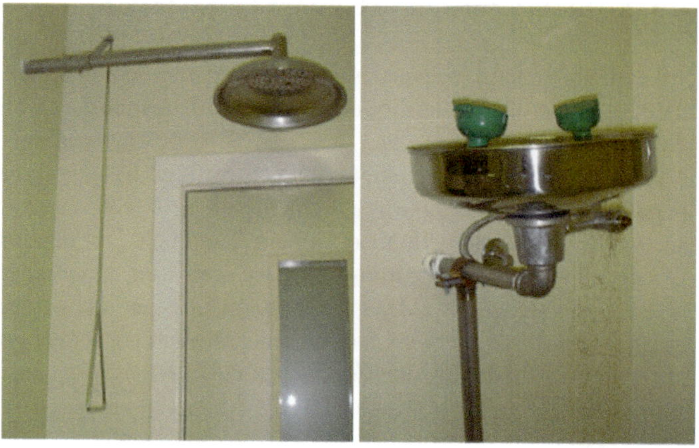

**Fig. 6.3** Shower and eye-wash

and illness in the workplace. They must be designed and built safely and must be kept clean and reliably [1].

The correct selection and use of PPE are essential both to guarantee the sterility of the final product and to protect the operator. PPE should be used to protect the professional during the reconstitution of cytotoxics and during all other activities in which they may come into contact with these medications.

Activities may include packaging opening, handling, transportation, administration, spill control, labeling, disposal of drug residues, and handling of patient excreta and bodily secretions [28].

Thus, personal protective equipment must be provided by the employer and used by all professionals involved in the handling of cytotoxic drugs, both in preparation and administration.

USP specifies that the composition garment (Fig. 6.4) for sterile doses must include the following [34]:

- Powder-free sterile gloves
- Clothing closed at the back and neck, with sleeves that fit comfortably on the wrists
- N95/PFF2 respirator
- Protective goggles
- Exclusive shoes or shoe covers
- Caps/protectors for beard and hair

#### Waterproof Overalls or Apron

Appropriate clothing protects the handler from spills and splashes of waste materials, providing a physical barrier to particles generated during the handling process. Overalls and/or gowns must not have seams or zips that could allow the passage of medicines.

Even though there is no specific standard for clothing, disposable gowns made of materials coated with polyethylene, polypropylene, or other waterproof laminated materials offer protection for all activities that may result in direct exposure of the worker and should not be used in other areas to avoid spreading contamination and exposing other health professionals [29, 34, 36].

The overalls or long aprons are for use restricted to the handling area, with low release of particles, low permeability, and

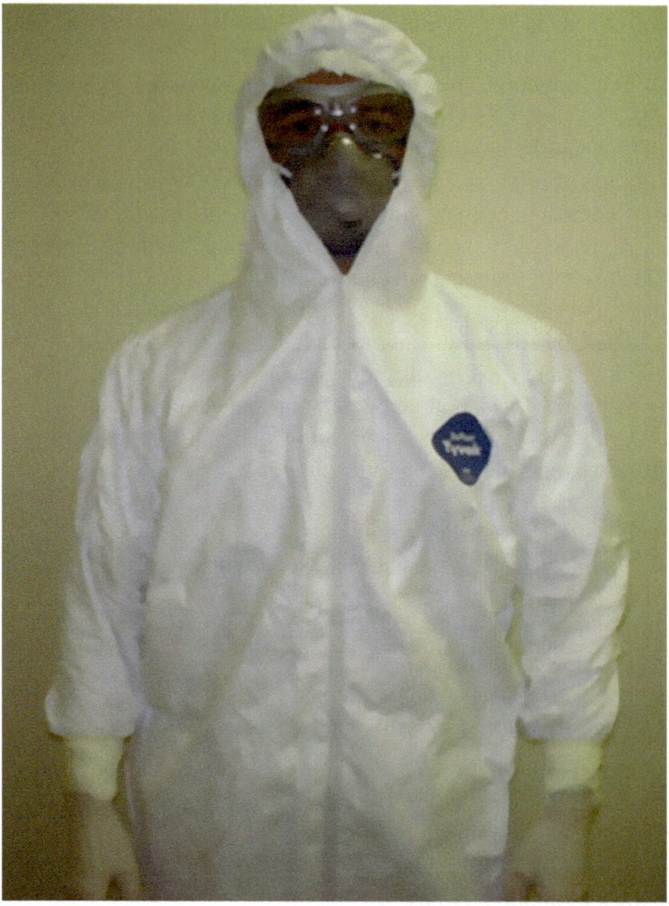

**Fig. 6.4** Attire in the handling of antineoplastic drugs [35]

closed front with long sleeves and a tight cuff. It must be used by all professionals directly involved in the handling of cytotoxic drugs, activities that present the possibility of splashes or spills. After use, it must be disposed of in toxic waste containers. Reuse increases the probability of exposure [3].

### Surgical Glove

Gloves are essential for handling cytotoxics and must be worn at all times, including receipt, storage, and in contact with cytotoxic drug packages, boxes, and vials.

NIOSH and ASHP recommend the use of two pairs of gloves when preparing, administering, and disposing of potentially hazardous drugs, both to reduce penetration of antineoplastic agents and to improve work practices, because the use and removal of a single glove allows the skin to be exposed to a number of contaminated surfaces [29, 36].

Gloves must not contain dust, considering the possibility of causing contamination, absorption, and retention of antineoplastics in the work area. Gloves must be changed regularly. Recommendations range from 30 to 60 minutes or whenever they are damaged or contaminated [34].

### Respiratory Protection

Respiratory protection should always be used when there is exposure to aerosols from cytotoxic drugs. In activities that require respiratory protection, the respirator type PFF2/N95 is sufficient and must be perfectly adjusted to the operator's face, adequately covering the nose and mouth. The disposable or semifacial use model with a double filter periodically changed can be used.

The N95 disposable respirator is a type of particulate respirator that only protects against inhaling particulates – not gases or vapors.

NIOSH-approved chemical cartridge respirators protect from airborne exposure to vapors or gases and are most suitable for preparation, cleaning of hazardous drug spills, decontamination, or cleaning of BSC with the viewing window raised [37, 38].

The use of a disposable respirator is also recommended when administering medication.

Surgical masks are not recommended as they do not offer adequate protection because they do not have aerosol retention power [28, 39].

#### Eye Protection

Eye protection is necessary in view of the possibility of splashing in the eyes from antineoplastic drugs, which, when absorbed, can be irritating to the eyes and mucous membranes. Thus, it is recommended in all activities that present a risk of splashing cytotoxic drugs, as well as having side barrier protection [28].

#### Beanie or Disposable Head Cover

Disposable head covers (and beard protectors, if necessary) are used to minimize the release of hair and skin particles into the clean area. Disposable head covers must completely cover the hair and ears and the beard protector (if necessary to cover the facials) must be placed on the dirty side of the demarcation line in the anteroom, and they are for single use and must not be kept for reuse [28].

#### Is There a Difference Between Shoe Covers and Protective Foot Covers?

Shoe covers and protective foot covers help minimize the spread of particle contamination from worn shoes in the clean area. A pair of shoe covers should be put on by all caregivers who pass from the dirty side of the demarcation line in the anteroom to the clean side. These shoe covers must be disposed of in hazardous waste containers and must not be kept for reuse. They must be worn over closed shoes or nonslip boots [28].

### 6.3.3.2 Closed-System Drug-Transfer Device (CSTD)

The use of closed-system transfer devices (CSTDs) (Fig. 6.5) in the handling and administration of cytotoxic drugs has increased considerably over the years. The system is intended to prevent the release of the drug into the environment through the formation of aerosols or spillage and the occurrence of a puncture accident during the handling process. The devices are connected to syringes, vials, and sets (Luer-lock connection), eliminating the use of needles [40, 41].

NIOSH recommends its use and defines CSTD as "a drug transfer device that mechanically prohibits the transfer of envi-

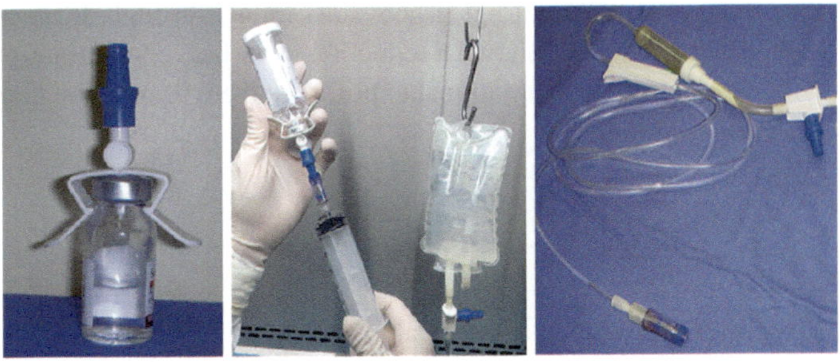

**Fig. 6.5** Closed-system drug-transfer device (CSTD)

ronmental contaminants into the system and the escape of hazardous drug or vapor concentrations out of the system" [2]. Several international societies and bodies recommend its use in the handling and administration of dangerous drugs [1–3, 28, 42, 43].

However, it is not certain that all available CSTDs perform fully adequate and equally protective. To date, there is no standardized test protocol to assess the performance of available CSTDs. Therefore, they should be carefully evaluated, based on independent peer-reviewed studies, with demonstrated reduction in contamination [43]. NIOSH is developing an independent vapor containment performance protocol for CSTDs in healthcare environments [44].

CSTDs should not be used as a substitute for other protective equipment listed and are therefore not the only means of worker protection. They should be used as part of a hazardous drug safety program and used in conjunction with PPE, CPE, and engineering controls [2, 43]. They should also not be used with physically or chemically incompatible drugs.

Handling a used syringe and needle usually results in contamination. Drops, leakage from the butyl rubber stopper after multiple punctures, and aerosol generation resulting from increased pressure within drug vials have also been observed [28].

There is no short-term or long-term data to inform whether specific CSTDs impact health outcomes [44].

Studies have been carried out to demonstrate the impact and efficiency of these devices when compared to the use of needles to dilute and reconstitute drugs. The results found, through different techniques used, have shown a reduction in surface contamination with a reduction in occupational exposure and environmental contamination [13, 18, 24, 40, 45].

### 6.3.4 Medical Surveillance

Medical surveillance is a medical examination program that aims to detect and monitor potential health effects on workers exposed to hazardous chemical or physical substances in the workplace. Thus, the objective is to minimize and allow early treatment of adverse health effects for everyone involved in the handling of dangerous drugs that are at risk from daily exposure.

When a damage is identified, it can be corrected early, and the employer can limit worker exposure and prevent everyone's health through protective actions on other workers. NIOSH recommends conducting medical surveillance but points out that it is a second line of defense, increasing the protection already provided by engineering, administrative, work practices, individual and collective protective equipment, and education and training on the risk of exposure to these agents [1, 2].

The following surveillance data must be performed preplacement of the worker and repeated annually, according to medical criteria and implemented surveillance program:

- *Medical history* including reproductive status, smoking, work history, and occupational exposure, through a questionnaire
- *Complete physical examination* including skin, mucous membranes, and lymphatic system
- *Laboratory tests* such as full blood count with differential, reticulocytes, liver function tests, urea nitrogen, creatinine, and urine monitoring (damage to the bladder or dipstick for blood in urine)
- *Biological monitoring*, which does not become clear as there is no reliably published data of a standard or best practice. Not used as routine exams.

The employer must provide a safe workplace, quality protective equipment and proper use training, and good safety practices [1].

- Identify risk situations and activities and exposed staff.
- Preserve and maintain each employee's medical and exposure records.
- Make all records available to employees.
- Provide any and all informational material about.

Workers should be counseled and encouraged to report any occupational health problem to employee health services.

When handling cytotoxic drugs, the reproductive status of employees and the risk of toxicity in handling such drugs must be considered, diverting from this activity, professionals who want to become pregnant, pregnant and who are breastfeeding.

In the case of accidents and occupational exposure to antineoplastic drugs, the type and size of exposure should be evaluated: splashes, needle prick containing cytotoxic drugs, skin shedding (analysis of skin and mucous membranes), and inhalation of aerosols (evaluation of the pulmonary system). In addition to the exams mentioned above, an accident notification report must be generated.

### 6.3.5 Physical Area

All projects in the physical area of health facilities must be prepared in accordance with the provisions of regulatory standards (within their territory of operation) on the minimum requirements for infrastructure and quality of care provided to the health of the population.

Antineoplastic treatment includes preparation, administration, storage, transport, disposal, and management of health waste. Thus, antineoplastic and cytotoxic drugs must be handled under conditions that promote patient safety, worker safety, and environmental protection.

Several studies demonstrate that vials of antineoplastic drugs are contaminated upon receipt [13, 46]. Therefore, both pharmacists, pharmacy technicians, and other health professionals involved in the process of caring for cancer patients may be exposed when handling or touching contaminated surfaces.

International guidelines recommend that the preparation of antineoplastic drugs be carried out in a restricted area and preferably centralized [37, 47, 48]. Specific demarcations with signs through pictograms or texts should be evidenced before entering the production and storage areas of potentially dangerous drugs. Access to areas must be restricted to authorized personnel in order to protect individuals not directly involved in the manipulation process [30].

All handling of cytotoxic (hazardous) drugs must be carried out in a Class II Type B2 biological safety cabinet.

Bedrooms, rest areas, and circulation areas for employees, patients, visitors, and employees should be located away from areas of potential contamination in order to reduce unnecessary exposure to these agents. Chapter 800 USP determines that specific areas are designated for defined tasks, including receipt and storage of sterile and nonsterile drugs. The requirement that areas surrounding the handling area be under negative pressure to contain and minimize the risk of exposure is also evidenced [34, 47].

Antineoplastics and all cytotoxic and potentially dangerous drugs must be stored in a way to avoid spillage from falling and breaking vials. Sterile and nonsterile products can be stored simultaneously, but sterile handling must be carried out in a separate place.

There must be a storage area for refrigerated antineoplastics with a dedicated refrigerator in a negative pressure area. Engineering controls are required to protect preparations from cross and microbiological contamination (if the preparation is sterile) during all phases of the handling process.

To avoid microbiological contamination and to ensure the comfort of professionals working in the area, the temperature of the preparation rooms must be controlled. The temperature in the range of 18–22 °C is acceptable. Humidity must be controlled to prevent corrosion and condensation on work surfaces and also to provide operator comfort. The human comfort zone is generally in the range of 30–70% relative humidity [30].

The locker room of the chemotherapy dilution rooms must have an eyewash, in addition to the washbasin and the dressing area.

### 6.3.6 Area Classification

The International Standards Organization (ISO), in view of the need for classification and international standards for clean rooms, establishes a set of classification standards for particles in ambient air that are evaluated according to the number of particles per cubic meter in a size of specified particle (Table 6.2).

For sterile medications, room classification must take into account particulate and microbiological contamination. The room should be designed to facilitate asepsis in the handling and preparation of cytotoxic drugs and should also be designed to provide containment of cytotoxic drugs, particularly in the case of failure of the biosafety cabinet.

The preparation of sterile cytotoxic drugs can be defined as aseptic preparation and must therefore be carried out in a Grade A environment that corresponds approximately to ISO Class 5 [44].

**Table 6.2** Classification of particulate matter in ambient air [34]

| ISO classification of particulate matter in ambient air (limits are on particles 0.5 μm and larger per cubic meters [current ISO] and cubic feet [former Federal Standard No. 209E, FS 209E]) | | | |
|---|---|---|---|
| Class name | | Particle count | |
| ISSO classification | US FS 209E | ISO, $m^3$ | FS 209E, $ft^3$ |
| 3 | Class 1 | 35.2 | 1 |
| 4 | Class 10 | 352 | 10 |
| 5 | Class 100 | 3520 | 100 |
| 6 | Class 1000 | 35,200 | 1000 |
| 7 | Class 10,000 | 352,000 | 10,000 |
| 8 | Class 100,000 | 3520,000 | 100,000 |

Positive and negative pressure differentials with the surrounding environment must be established for cytotoxic preparation rooms with the dual purpose of protecting operators and maintaining the sterility of the parenteral finished products.

"Pass-through hatches" are essential to avoid direct access between the cytotoxic cleanroom and the external environment. There are two possibilities for locating such equipment: they can be between the clean room and the anteroom or between the clean room and the external environment. If the last option is selected, interlocking ports must be used, and the unit must be HEPA filtered.

Hatch doors should preferably be equipped with an audible or visual alarm to prevent the doors from being opened simultaneously.

When the air pressure is positive in the handling room and the air pressure is negative in the anterooms and "through hatches," the negative air pressure in the hatches and in the staging room, in this case, acts as a trap to isolate the potentially contaminated air.

When the air pressure is negative in the handling room and the air pressure is positive in the "passage hatches" and in the anterooms, the positive air pressure of the hatches, in this case, acts as a protective barrier.

### 6.3.7 Manipulation Area

It must consist of at least two separate controlled rooms, a clean room and an anteroom, closed off and physically separated by a wall. The anteroom can be subdivided into a dressing room and a storage room for medicines and finished products. The activities carried out in the manipulation area are directly related to the preparation of parenteral drugs.

The antineoplastic drug and cytotoxic drug preparation area is designed to minimize entry, generation, retention of particles, and microbial contamination. Preparation rooms must meet specific International Standards Organization (ISO) classification standards.

Access to the hazardous area must be limited to authorized and trained personnel. Each and every professional who accesses the classified area must follow proper hand hygiene and clothing procedures as the first major step in preventing microbial contamination of sterile preparations.

The clean room containing the biological safety cabinet is used for the preparation of drugs considered potentially dangerous and must have at least 5 $m^2$ per BSC. The cleanroom must maintain an ISO Class 7 environment and have negative pressure to the anteroom with air filtered by HEPA (high-efficiency particulate arrestance) filters. A HEPA filter is a high-efficiency particulate air filter that retains approximately 99.9% of the 0.3-micron particulate material to provide ultra-clean air.

Anterooms help maintain the ISO rating and pressure differential in the cleanroom and can be used for the storage of supplies and medication as long as these activities do not interfere with maintaining the ISO rating. It must maintain an ISO Class 7 environment and be positive pressure for both the clean room and the rest of the pharmacy.

The anteroom should be divided into a "clean" side (closer to the clean room) and a "dirty" side (closer to the other areas), which can be demarcated with a visible line on the floor.

## 6.4 Technique of Handling Antineoplastic Drugs

### 6.4.1 Decontamination of the Biological Safety Cabinet

The decontamination of a biological safety cabinet must take place under the following conditions:

- After a manipulation has been completed and removed from the BSC
- Before pausing use for a long period of time
- When returning to use after a long period of time
- After a small spill involving the work surface

For the biological safety cabinet decontamination procedure, disinfectant solution, sterile water, wet wipes with 70% alcoholic solution, sterile gauze or clean, lint-free towels, and disposable or reusable containers (for example, sterile stainless steel bowl) are required.

Before decontaminating the biological safety cabinet (BSC), it must be purged for at least five minutes after the last dangerous drug preparation (HD).

For this procedure, complete personal protective equipment (PPE) is required, including N95 respirator, overalls, and safety glasses. Ultraviolet light must be off, and cab must be in operational mode with indoor/outdoor fans on. Disinfectant solution, sterile water, wet wipes, 70% alcoholic solution, and sterile gauze or towels (enough to use at least one towel per surface) must be arranged on a cart next to the BSC.

The internal surfaces – roof grid, rear wall, fittings, sidewalls, and work surface – must be sanitized vertically from top to bottom and horizontally from back to front (in the direction of airflow, from the cleanest area to the most contaminated area). To perform the same cleaning process on the bottom surface of the work tray, it is necessary to raise or support the tray to allow access below the work surface and perform decontamination of the top and bottom parts of the front entrance grill and shelves that hold the work tray.

After cleaning with disinfectant solution, rinse the site with sterile water to remove any residue of the cleaning agent. After cleaning, purge the BSC for at least 30 minutes before any aseptic procedure takes place inside the cab. Place all disposable PPE and contaminated waste into the proper chemical waste disposal after completion of the procedure [37].

## 6.5 Dressing Technique

Handling dangerous drugs requires attention and care to ensure that sterility is not compromised by the contamination of nonsterile substances and that no drug residues will contaminate the environment and the handler.

Before performing the attire, all adornments, including bracelets, rings, and watches, must be removed in order to prevent contaminants from becoming attached to their surfaces [29].

The step-by-step procedure for placing the PPEs includes the following:

- Access the anteroom on the dirty side of the demarcation line.
- Wearing disposable head cover or beanie (including beard cover, where applicable), making sure all hair and ears are covered by the head cover.
- Placing a shoe cover and stepping with that foot over the demarcation line to the clean side of the anteroom.
- Placement of the second shoe cover and enter to the clean side of the anteroom.
- Handwashing technique must precede the attire of personal protective equipment (PPE).
- Washing hands and wrists with soap and water for at least 30 seconds.
- Hand hygiene must be performed by all professionals before entering the clean room to minimize microbiological contamination of sterile products.
- Hand hygiene agents must be designed to remove visible dirt and dangerous drug contamination.
- The common soap has limited antimicrobial activity; therefore, soaps containing detergent and an antimicrobial agent (for example, chlorhexidine) are indicated for these cases, associated with alcohol-based hand products.
- Alcohol-based products used to disinfect hands prior to handling antineoplastics must have a minimum alcohol concentration of 70% and be used in conjunction with regular soap or antimicrobial.
- Drying hands and wrists with paper towels (using the towel to close the faucets, if the faucet does not have foot pedal operation).
- Placement of the first pair of gloves examining integrity, holes, tears, or other defects.
- Placement of clothing consisting of a sterile apron or jumpsuit (in waterproof material, with long sleeves, adjustable elastic collar and cuffs, with low particle emission, without front opening), examining the integrity of the surface to ensure total closure of the PPI.

- Placement of the jumpsuit cuffs over the cuffs of the first pair of gloves.
- Use an N95 or chemical cartridge-type respirator and safety glasses with side shields.
- To ensure that the respirator is placed correctly, perform a seal check of the respirator through the internal and external pressure difference.
- DO NOT wear a surgical mask under a respirator.
- Wearing the second pair of sterile gloves, placed over the apron cuffs until the wrists are fully covered.

## 6.6 Biological Safety Cabinet Use

The manipulation must be carried out at least 15 centimeters from the front opening of the cabinet. Contaminated air must be expelled through the rear grill and not through the front opening [49].

It is important to avoid overloading the BSC and avoid filling the workspace completely in order that the airflow paths remain free, with no vial or materials imposing cab circulation. In addition, for operator protection, rapid movements in or near the front opening or insertion movements in and out of the front opening (activities that interrupt or block the airflow inside the BSC should be avoided).

Before starting the handling process, the medication vials must be disinfected and wrapped with pre-moistened gauze with 70% alcohol, placing them directly on the work surface of the BSC.

Sterile materials (syringes, covers, equipment, safety devices, etc.) must be placed directly on the work surface inside the BSC, avoiding placing them on the front grill. The outer packaging (protective wrap) of sterile supplies must be opened immediately prior to use.

Select syringes that will not have more than three-quarters capacity when containing the partial or full dose of the drug.

Select appropriate gauge and length needles for the vial and final container.

If the syringe is the final application device, select a locking cap for the syringe. If the dose is placed in another container, such as an intravenous diluent bag or vial, select and prepare the container for injection of the antineoplastic or cytotoxic drug, removing any external wrapping and equipping it with the appropriate device.

Wipe the sealing rubber of the vials with a gauze soaked in alcohol, and let it dry. The use of drug transfer devices by a closed system can prevent the dispersion of aerosols during handling.

Unperforated vials can have positive or negative pressure in relation to the work area. When making the first perforation, always anticipate the positive pressure to prevent leakage of the vial contents by droplets or aerosol.

### 6.6.1 Technique of Filling Secondary Equipment with Diluent

- Before adding dangerous drugs to the intravenous (IV) solution bag: make sure the correct solution/secondary administration set and the IV solution bag for the drug to be administered have been selected according to what has been validated in the medical prescription.
- Squeeze the diluent solution pouch to check for leaks. Close the secondary administration set roller clam.
- Remove the protective cap from the administration port of the diluent pouch and remove the protective cap from the spike in the solution and from the secondary administration set (equipment).
- Place the secondary administration set inserter firmly into the administration port of the diluent pouch. Hold the solution pouch upright or lift the pouch using a hook to allow the solution to flow freely from the pouch into the tube. Squeeze the secondary administration set drip chamber to fill the chamber halfway with the diluent solution.
- Remove the protective cap from the distal end of the secondary administration set tube and keep it for later use, or dispose of it in waste inside the BSC if connecting a safety device to the distal end of the tube.

- Slowly open the secondary administration set roller clamp to allow the solution to completely fill the tube and close the roller clamp when the solution reaches the distal end of the tube.
- Examine the tubing for air bubbles and remove when hitting the sides of the tubing, allowing them to move through the tubing to either end.
- Place the diluent solution pouch on the work surface of the BSC. Do not hang the diluent solution bag on the BSC bar while injecting the drug, as the solution may run through the needle out of the injection port, resulting in spillage.

### 6.6.2 Aseptic Technique for Handling Dangerous Drugs (Powder Reconstitution)

- Make sure the correct drug vial has been selected for preparation.
- To reconstitute powdered medicine in a vial, calculate the amount of diluent needed to reach the desired concentration.
- Remove the exact amount of diluent in a syringe in such a way that it is enough not to be more than three-quarters full when containing the entire dose, with the needle attached.
- With the vial on the work surface, position the syringe and needle so that the bevel of the needle is facing up away from the manipulator. Insert the needle at a 45-degree angle into the vial sealing rubber until the bezel is half covered. Make sure the needle is in the vial and that no part of this location was exposed during reconstitution.
- Pull the syringe plunger and draw air from the vial into the syringe, creating negative pressure in the vial. Allow the syringe's diluent to enter the vial (to correct negative pressure) without pushing the plunger. If it is necessary to push the plunger, push it slowly and carefully, exchanging small amounts of liquid and air.
- Repeat these steps until all the diluent is in the vial and air is in the syringe. With the needle fully in the vial, hold the syringe

and vial firmly by rotating the medicine vial to ensure all the medicine powder is in the solution.

- Gently shake the vial (if appropriate or for medications that specifically do not blister) and inspect the solution for undissolved medication and particles.
- Thereafter, write reconstitution date and time, or date in use (stability) and time directly on the bottle, for future use.
- Move the needle to the top of the vial into the air space above the drug solution. Hold the syringe and plunger firmly in one hand and the medicine vial in the other and carefully separate the syringe and needle from the medicine vial.
- Once the correct dose is contained in the syringe, hold the syringe and plunger firmly and place the empty vial vertically on the work surface.
- Maintain traction on the plunger and rotate the syringe to bring all air bubbles to its surface.
- The syringe should not be more than three-quarters full with the desired contents of the vial, and no air bubbles should be in the solution. This will ensure greater precision in the syringe.
- Repeat this process, if necessary, to make sure all air bubbles are out of the syringe.
- Do not draw additional air into the drug solution as this will require removing the air bubble from the syringe.
- Check that the correct volume of medication for the dose is contained in the syringe. Hold the injection port perpendicular to the airflow so that the first air can flow, clearing the point where the needle will enter.
- To remove air from the syringe while the syringe is still filled with medicine, make sure the needle is capped.
- Hold the syringe in an upright position so that the tip of the covered syringe is pointing up and pull the syringe plunger down slightly at first to remove any solution from the needle or syringe tip.
- Tap the syringe barrel with fingers together or tweezers just below any air bubbles to bring them to the top of the syringe or tilt and rotate the syringe causing larger air bubbles to move through the solution, collecting smaller air bubbles at the top of the syringe.

- Remove the needle cover by placing it beside the work surface. Clean the sealing rubber of the container with a 70% alcoholic solution.
- Place the needle tip in the center of the injection port by pressing the needle tip straight through the membrane into the pouch with the needle shaft parallel to the port walls.
- Inject the drug into the diluent container.
- Clean the needle by pulling air from the IV bag/vial into the syringe before removing the needle and syringe from the final container.
- Remove the injection port needle from the diluent solution and securely replace the needle cap.
- Discard needle in a sharps container.
- Clean the sealing rubber of the medicine bottle with gauze soaked in 70% alcohol to remove any chemotherapeutic residue.
- Clean the outside of the container to remove any residue generated during handling that may have contaminated the container or gloves used during the process and before labeling the final container.
- To remove a dose of already reconstituted medicine from the vial, it is ideal to use a needle of a smaller gauge than the original puncture, if possible, to avoid increasing the perforation of the vial and causing leakage.
- Draw a volume of air into the syringe a little less than the volume of solution you will draw.
- Examine the vial closure to identify the previous puncture. Make sure the closure has been sealed around the existing hole and repeat the previous steps to remove the drug.
- To recap the needle, place the cap on a flat surface such as a table or counter with something firm to "push" the cap against the needle.
- Hold the syringe in one hand and slide the needle into the cap without using the other hand.
- Push the capped needle against a firm object to "seat" the cap firmly on the needle.
- Immediately place a Luer lock or non-Luer lock (sliding) tip cap on the tip of the syringe.

- Do not remove the needle and place the syringe with the syringe tip exposed on the work surface of the BSC if the syringe was used to withdraw dangerous drugs.

### 6.6.3 Aseptic Technique for Handling Dangerous Drugs (Ready-to-Use Liquid Medicines)

- To use a vial containing ready-to-use liquid medications, consider that the unperforated vial may be at positive, negative, or neutral pressure in relation to the workplace.
- Given this uncertainty, it is prudent to draw a volume of air into the syringe that is slightly less than the volume of solution you will draw.
- Create and maintain negative pressure in the bottle as described above. Once you have mastered these manipulation techniques, any combination of them can be used to produce a partial dose from one vial, multiple doses from one vial, multiple doses from multiple vials, and so on.
- If it is necessary to use negative pressure, care must be taken. Accumulation of positive pressure within the vial will cause a splash of solution and spillage from the needle bevel when the needle is removed.
- The ampoules must be handled with care to avoid any form of contamination and to avoid cuts or scratches resulting from the sharp edges of the open ampoule.
- Make sure all liquid is removed from the neck of the ampoule. If not, gently tap the work surface to clean the neck.
- Position the ampoule away from open spaces or other professionals. Holding the ampoule at a small angle, grasp the top of the ampoule and break it with a quick snapping motion, pulling it up and away from the ampoule.
- A gauze must contain the top of the ampoule and any droplets that come off during opening.
- Contain and discard the top of the ampoule in an appropriate sharps waste container.

### 6.6.4 Removal of the Finished Product From the Interior of the Biological Safety Cabinet (BSC)

- Before removing the final product from the interior of the BSC, gently invert the IV solution bag to check the final product for leaks and inspect the solution for the presence of suspended particles.
- Dispose of contaminated waste inside the BSC using gauze moistened with a 70% alcohol solution.
- Remove the final product from the interior of the BSC and place it on a clean or disposable surface and affix the patient's specific label and all auxiliary labels to the final product.
- Once it has been removed from the interior of the BSC and labeled, place the final product in a bag and seal.
- Clean and disinfect the work surface using an aqueous antibacterial agent (e.g., chlorhexidine) followed by gauze moistened with 70% alcohol between each preparation.

### 6.6.5 Aseptic Technique for Handling Dangerous Drugs in Elastomeric Infusers

- Make sure the correct dangerous medicine bottle has been selected.
- Make sure the correct infuser model and size have been selected.
- Make sure the proper type and size have been selected.
- Select an appropriately sized syringe and withdraw the calculated total volume of diluent.
- Make sure that the elastomeric reservoir (balloon) is not twisted, preventing breakage during filling.
- Make sure the Luer cap is secured to the distal end of the infuser delivery tubing. Remove the fill compartment cover on top of the infuser.
- Attach a syringe filled with the appropriate diluent and volume for preparation to the filling compartment.

- Inject the diluent into the infuser. Do not use a needle to inject the solution into the filling compartment as this may damage the infuser.
- In an upright position on the work surface of the BSC, remove the syringe from the infuser supply compartment before adding any medication solution.
- Remove the Luer cap from the distal end of the infuser by resting it on alcohol-soaked gauze to visually confirm that the contents of the infuser are flowing through the infuser line.
- Allow three drops of thinner to fall onto alcohol-soaked gauze.
- Replace the Luer cap on the distal end of the infuser delivery tubing and clamp the line.
- Add drug to the infuser through the filling port of the infuser. Once all diluent and drugs have been added to the infuser, replace the cap on the infuser supply compartment.
- Check the infuser for leaks and inspect the solution for the presence of particles.
- When adding the diluent or drug to the infuser, invert it with the syringe attached, placing it on a flat work surface.
- Hold the syringe barrel with one hand, and use slow, steady downward pressure to inflate the balloon while stabilizing the infuser with the other hand.
- Do not inject the solvent and drug with too much force creating turbulence in the solution as this can create too many bubbles in the elastomer.
- A small amount of bubbles is allowed as they will not cause problems as they will gradually dissipate as the air in the tube moves through the filter.

## 6.7 Spill of Dangerous Drugs

To minimize the exposure of staff and patients to dangerous drugs, spills must be properly managed in accordance with established institutional policies and procedures.

All employees working in areas where spills could potentially occur must participate in on-the-job training.

Spill kits must be located in all areas where exposures may occur, including areas of preparation, distribution, storage, and receipt of hazardous drugs, and must be carefully reviewed to ensure that they contain all necessary supplies with adequate validity and integrity.

Kits must contain the following PPEs:

- Disposable and waterproof apron, with long sleeves, elastic cuffs, and back closure
- Two pairs of procedure gloves
- Disposable safety glasses or face shields
- Shoe cover and head cover
- N95/PFF2 respirator
- Sharps shovel and container
- Gauze pads or absorbent towels
- Two high-density garbage bags for chemical waste disposal
- Decontamination agent (detergent and water or equivalent solution)
- Chemical waste container
- Documents for recording the accident

### 6.7.1 Procedure in the Case of Spillage into the Environment

- Stop activities and assess the degree of spillage and personal contamination, if any.
- Open the spill kit.
- Put on respiratory protection first.
- Put on two pairs of procedure gloves, disposable apron, head cover, shoe covers, and glasses.
- Isolate and demarcate the area with paper towels.
- The affected region must be covered with compresses or absorbent paper and, at the limits of the leak, gauze to restrict the advance of the liquid.
- Open the first garbage bag.
- In the case of contamination with dust, use moistened compresses/paper towels.

- In the case of contamination with liquids, use dry swabs/paper towels.
- Place liquid detergent in the affected area.
- If there are any glass fragments, collect them with a disposable shovel and discard them in the plastic garbage bag.
- Clean from the periphery to the center, that is, from the least contaminated area to the most contaminated area.
- Triple wash with detergent and plenty of water.
- Discard all contaminated material (swabs, gauze, absorbent paper, and bottles if present in the garbage bag, followed by the first pair of gloves used).
- Carefully close the plastic bag containing the waste so as not to cause a "sigh."
- Place the bag with the waste inside another plastic garbage bag reserved for this purpose.
- Remove the PPE and discard in the external plastic bag.
- Dispose of in containers identified as toxic waste.
- Record by writing the size of the spill, drugs involved, and people exposed.
- Provide and replace a new spill kit.

## 6.8 Disposal of Hazardous Waste

Hazardous waste must be disposed of separately from general waste in capped chemical waste containers. Waste containers must be leak-proof, have a lid with a safety seal, and must be labeled with an appropriate warning label.

All sharps used for the preparation and administration of dangerous drug mixtures must be placed in a sharps container.

Disposal for sharp piercing objects cannot contain more than three-quarters fill, and the contents must not be pushed down to create more space due to the risk of exposure.

Two pairs of chemotherapy gloves should be worn when handling hazardous waste. Pending removal from the disposal container, waste must be stored in a safe area in properly sealed and labeled containers [1, 9].

## 6.9 Certifications and Quality Assurance

Whenever possible, all equipment and processes used for cytotoxic preparation that affect the sterility or attributes of the product must be qualified or validated.

All certificates issued must be reviewed, approved, and signed by a designated pharmacist and archived for periods that may vary according to local practice and regulations.

Qualification is required for the room and equipment used. This includes the biological safety cabinet, among other equipment.

## References

1. OSHA. Guidance manual for hazardous waste site activities. Occup Saf Heal Guid Man Hazard Waste Site Act; 1985.
2. NIOSH. Preventing occupational exposures to antineoplastic and other hazardous drugs in health care settings; 2004.
3. ASPH. Guidelines on handling hazardous drugs; 2006.
4. McDiarmid MA, Presson A, Fujikawa J. Controlling occupational exposure to hazardous drugs. Occupational Safety and Health Administration. Am J Heal Syst Pharm. 1996.
5. IARC. IARC monographs programme on the evaluation of carcinogenic risks to humans. IARC Monogr Eval Carcinog. Risks to humans; 2004.
6. Yodaiken RE, Bennett D. OSHA - work-practice guidelines for personnel dealing with cytotoxic (antineoplastic) drugs. Am J Heal Pharm. 1986;43:1193–204.
7. de Souza CB, Tovar JR, Antônio LRD, Dourado CDS, Amorim MHC. Antineoplásicos y riesgos laborales para los enfermeros: una revisión integral/Antineoplásicos e os riscos ocupacionais para os enfermeiros: uma revisão integrativa/Antineoplastic and occupational risks for nurses: an integrative review. Enfermería Glob; 2015.
8. Kumari S, Lobo DJ, Sequira L. Potential health risks among oncology staff nurses of selected hospitals due to antineoplastic drug exposure. Indian J Public Heal Res Dev. 2017;8:358–61.
9. Connor TH, McDiarmid MA. Preventing occupational exposures to antineoplastic drugs in health care settings. CA Cancer J Clin. 2009. https://doi.org/10.3322/canjclin.56.6.354.
10. Connor TH, MacKenzie BA, DeBord DG, Trout DB, O'Callaghan JP. NIOSH list of antineoplastic and other hazardous drugs in healthcare settings 2014. Cincinnati, OH: U.S. Department of Health and Human

Services, Centers for Disease Control and Prevention, National Institute for Occupational Safety and Health, DHHS (NIOSH) Publication No. 2014-138 (Supersedes 2012-150).
11. Alcântara AMPP, Venuto LMA, França ALF, Vieira EP, Martins I. Liquid chromatographic method for simultaneous determination of five antineoplastic drugs. Lat Am J Pharm. 2009;28:525–30.
12. Wild CP. International Agency for Research on Cancer. In: Encycl. Toxicol. 3rd ed; 2014. p. 1067–9.
13. Ness SLR, Pilla C, Tubino GV, Corleta HVE, Capp E. Levels of surface contamination with gemcitabine using standard preparation techniques versus closed-system devices. J Chem Pharm Res. 2016;8:686–94.
14. Graeve CU, McGovern PM, Alexander B, Church T, Ryan A, Polovich M. Occupational exposure to antineoplastic agents an analysis of health care workers and their environments. Workplace Health Saf. 2017. https://doi.org/10.1177/2165079916662660.
15. Bernabeu-Martínez MA, Merino MR, Santos Gago JM, Alvarez Sabucedo LM, Wanden-Berghe C, Sanz-Valero J. Guidelines for safe handling of hazardous drugs: a systematic review. PLoS One. 2018;13:e0197172.
16. Redic KA, Fang K, Christen C, Chaffee BW. Surface contamination of hazardous drug pharmacy storage bins and pharmacy distributor shipping containers. J Oncol Pharm Pract. 2018. https://doi.org/10.1177/1078155216679027.
17. Kupczewska-Dobecka M, Pałaszewska-Tkacz A, Czerczak S, Konieczko K. Hygiene and legal aspects of occupational exposure assessment to cytostatics. Med Pr. 2017. https://doi.org/10.13075/mp.5893.00599.
18. Martins I, Rosa HVD. Considerações Toxicológicas da Exposição Ocupacional aos Fármacos Antineoplásicos. Rev Bras Med do Trab. 2004;2:118–25.
19. Ness SLR, Mascarenhas M, Arbo MD, Tonietto BD, Cestonaro LV, dos Santos NG, Garcia SC, Ferreira CF, Capp E. Occupational exposure assessment in professionals who manipulate and administer antineoplastic drugs in a university hospital in Southern Brazil. J Oncol Pharm Pract. 2021;27(5):1205–13.
20. Moretti M, Grollino MG, Pavanello S, et al. Micronuclei and chromosome aberrations in subjects occupationally exposed to antineoplastic drugs: a multicentric approach. Int Arch Occup Environ Health. 2015;88:683–95.
21. Mahmoodi M, Soleyman-Jahi S, Zendehdel K, et al. Chromosomal aberrations, sister chromatid exchanges, and micronuclei in lymphocytes of oncology department personnel handling anti-neoplastic drugs. Drug Chem Toxicol. 2017;40:235–40.
22. Barth A, Brucker N, Moro AM, et al. Association between inflammation processes, DNA damage, and exposure to environmental pollutants. Environ Sci Pollut Res. 2017. https://doi.org/10.1007/s11356-016-7772-0.

23. Zare Sakhvidi MJ, Hajaghazadeh M, Mostaghaci M, Mehrparvar AH, Zare Sakhvidi F, Naghshineh E. Applicability of the comet assay in evaluation of DNA damage in healthcare providers' working with antineoplastic drugs: a systematic review and meta-analysis. Int J Occup Environ Health. 2016. https://doi.org/10.1080/10773525.2015.1123380.
24. Lancharro PM, De Castro-Acuña Iglesias N, González-Barcala FJ, González JDM. Evidence of exposure to cytostatic drugs in healthcare staff: a review of recent literature. Farm Hosp. 2016. https://doi.org/10.7399/fh.2016.40.6.9103.
25. Gianfredi V, Salvatori T, Nucci D, Villarini M, Moretti M. Genotoxic risk in nurses handling antiblastic drugs: systematic review of literature and meta-analysis. Recenti Prog Med. 2017;108(12):511–20.
26. Villarini M, Gianfredi V, Levorato S, Vannini S, Salvatori T, Moretti M. Occupational exposure to cytostatic/antineoplastic drugs and cytogenetic damage measured using the lymphocyte cytokinesis-block micronucleus assay: a systematic review of the literature and meta-analysis. Mutat Res Rev Mutat Res. 2016;770:35–45.
27. Roussel C, Witt KL, Shaw PB, Connor TH. Meta-analysis of chromosomal aberrations as a biomarker of exposure in healthcare workers occupationally exposed to antineoplastic drugs. Mutat Res Rev Mutat Res. 2019;781:207–17.
28. ISOPP. ISOPP standards of practice. Safe handling of cytotoxics. J Oncol Pharm Pract. 2007;13:1–81.
29. Power LA, Coyne JW, Hawkins B. ASHP guidelines on handling hazardous drugs. Am J Heal Pharm. 2018;75:1996–2031.
30. Connor T, McLauchlan R, Vandenbroucke J. Preface. J Oncol Pharm Pract. 2007;13:1–81.
31. BRASIL. RDC nº 50, de 21 de fevereiro de 2002. Ministério da Saúde ANVISA - Agência Nacional de Vigilância Sanitária. 2002. https://doi.org/10.1061/(ASCE)MT.1943-5533.0000298.
32. BRASIL RDC nº 220, de 21 de Setembro de 2004. Ministério da Saúde. ANVISA - Agência Nacional de Vigilância Sanitária; 2004.
33. BRASIL. Portaria MTE nº. 485, de 11 de Novembro de 2005 - NR 32 - Segurança e saúde no trabalho em serviços de saúde. Diário Of da União. 2005;32:1–40.
34. Bulletin R. ⟨ 797 ⟩ Pharmaceutical compounding — STE rile preparations. 2008;5:1–61.
35. Ness SLR. Biossegurança no Manuseio Seguro de Medicamentos Antineoplásicos In: Almeida, José Ricardo Chambum. Farmacêuticos em Oncologia: Uma Nova Realidade, 3º edição. Atheneu, Rio de Janeiro – RJ; 2018.
36. NIOSH, Burroughs G, Connor T, McDiarmid M. NIOSH alert: preventing occupational exposures to antineoplastic and other hazardous drugs in health care settings. Inst Occup. 2004;58.

37. Pan American Health Organization. Safe handling of hazardous chemotherapy drugs in limited-resource settings. 2012:1–53.
38. Andrews R, Fey O'Connor P. NIOSH manual of analytical methods (NMAM). 5th ed; 2020.
39. NIOSH. Personal protective equipment for health care workers who work with hazardous drugs; 2009.
40. Sessink PJM, Connor TH, Jorgenson JA, Tyler TG. Reduction in surface contamination with antineoplastic drugs in 22 hospital pharmacies in the US following implementation of a closed-system drug transfer device. J Oncol Pharm Pract. 2011;17:39–48.
41. Clark BA, Sessink PJ. Use of a closed system drug-transfer device eliminates surface contamination with antineoplastic agents. J Oncol Pharm Pr. 2013;19:99–104.
42. Mekoba BC, Turingan EM, Roberts PA, Mason S, Willoughby I, Taylor C, Stivers A, Valgus J. A pharmacy-led United States Pharmacopeia (USP) chapter 800 compliance collaborative at an academic medical center. Am J Heal Pharm. 2018. https://doi.org/10.2146/ajhp170472.
43. The United States Pharmacopeial Convention. USP General Chapter <800> Hazardous drugs—handling in healthcare settings; 2019.
44. Celano P, Fausel CA, Kennedy EB, Miller TM, Oliver TK, Page R, Ward JC, Zon RT. Safe handling of hazardous drugs: ASCO standards. J Clin Oncol. 2019;37:598–609.
45. Mathias PI, MacKenzie BA, Toennis CA, Connor TH. Survey of guidelines and current practices for safe handling of antineoplastic and other hazardous drugs used in 24 countries. J Oncol Pharm Pract. 2019. https://doi.org/10.1177/1078155217726160.
46. Schreiber C, Radon K, Pethran A, Schierl R, Hauff K, Grimm CH, Boos KS, Nowak D. Uptake of antineoplastic agents in pharmacy personnel. Part II: study of work-related risk factors. Int Arch Occup Environ Health. 2003;76:11–6.
47. Randolph SA. Hazardous drugs: handling in health care settings. Work Heal Saf. 2018;66:264.
48. Fox ER, McLaughlin MM. ASHP guidelines on managing drug product shortages. Am J Heal Pharm. 2018;75:1742–50.
49. BCCA. BCCA pharmacy practice standards for hazardous; 2016.

# Immunotherapy

# 7

Cristiane Souza de Agostinho,
Flávia Mendes Leite,
Marlize Brandão Ribeiro Cardoso,
and Priscila Pinto Costa

## 7.1 Introduction

It is undeniable that the immune system plays a crucial and determining role in the control and development of neoplastic diseases, acting at different stages of the immune window to ensure balance in the cellular functions of the human body.

Immunotherapy has its initial records from 3000 years ago, in ancient Egypt, until the beginning of the nineteenth century, with several reports of how tumors disappeared spontaneously or after an infection with a concomitant high fever. Thus, the following studies were performed [1, 2].

Before the immune system and its functionality were fully understood, the first sparks of inquiry were ignited near the end of the nineteenth century, when a young woman presented with a unique disease state in New York City. Bessie Dashiel's story was featured in Stephen Hall's text, "The Blood Conflict: Life, Death, and the Immune System," published in 1997, chronicling the extraordinary events that precipitated the use of the immune system to fight cancer [3].

In the summer of 1890, Dashiel developed severe pain in his right hand due to an injury sustained while traveling by train. Due

C. S. de Agostinho · F. M. Leite (✉) · M. B. R. Cardoso · P. P. Costa
Salvador, Bahia, Brazil


C. W. P. Schmidt, K. M. Otoni (eds.), *The Golden Guide to Oncologic Pharmacy*, https://doi.org/10.1007/978-3-030-98596-7_7

to the worsening of the infectious condition, she sought out Dr. William Coley, a young surgeon in New York. Coley confirmed the infectious condition and performed a local tissue biopsy, which confirmed round cell sarcoma. At the time, the best therapy available was amputation [2, 3].

On the first appearance, Coley observed that Dashiell's right hand did not have the typical presentation of an infection. On closer examination, which included opening the wound, Coley found a small amount of pus and tissue that seemed "abnormally hard and more of a grayish color than normal." As Dashiell's pain and symptoms increased, Coley reopened the wound to find "grayish granulations" and a bone that appeared normal. It seemed to Coley that this was something other than an infection, and he became increasingly concerned that Dashiell had a sarcoma. In November 1890, two days after the biopsy results, Coley performed an amputation of Dashiell's right arm below the elbow. Following the amputation, however, Dashiell's disease spread rapidly, and tumors appeared throughout her body. Her symptoms were managed with the best supportive care available at that time, but in January 1891, with Coley at her bedside, Dashiell died of her disease at the age of 18 [3].

After Dashiell's death, Coley devoted himself to studies on the basic understanding of sarcoma treatments. He investigated medical records and medical literature accessible to him in the late nineteenth century, including works by his predecessors, uncovering case reports of patients with potentially incurable cancers who underwent spontaneous remission after concomitant treatment with an acute bacterial infection [1].

His determination to prevent the same fate in others led Coley through a scientific journey that began with a retrospective chart review to gain a baseline understanding of sarcoma treatments and outcomes. Coley started a years-old project involving injecting dead bacteria from inactivated heat, called Coley's toxins, into patients with inoperable cancers. It achieved a significant number of regressions and cures in over 1000 patients, many or most with sarcomas, and the method began gaining widespread acceptance and notoriety. However, its toxins gradually disappeared from use because, in addition to not having much knowledge about the immune system at the time, other researchers tried to use Coley's toxins, but all attempts were unsuccessful [3, 4].

He identified and reviewed 90 cases of sarcoma over the previous 15 years. One particular case stood out that involved a man in his thirties with round cell sarcoma. The patient had four tumors on his neck and face and needed multiple surgeries, the last so extensive that it required skin grafts, which ultimately failed. Following his last operation, the patient developed erysipelas, a common infection at the time believed to be caused by *Streptococcus pyogenes*. The patient experienced two occurrences of this infection, but remarkably, his disease disappeared, and his large wound healed [3]. Surprisingly, he found one of these patients alive and well years after his cancer diagnosis. Coley concluded that if an accidental infection could lead to complete regression of this patient's sarcoma, it seemed fair to assume that the same could occur when an infection was artificially produced [3].

Despite the development of radiation therapy and chemotherapy as standard treatments for cancer, scientists remained intrigued by the underlying mechanisms of Coley toxins that led to responses in some patients. In the 1930s and 1940s, animal studies showed that bacteria caused tumor necrosis and that serum from endotoxin-treated tumors could be reintroduced to tumors. The serum caused the tumors to necrose, leading investigators to state that it contained a "tumor necrotizing factor" (TNF) [3].

The discovery of TNF and its relationship with necrosis in sarcomas was associated with the phenomenon of tumor endothelial cell apoptosis, but therapies using TNF brought high systemic toxicity to their patients, with side effects such as fever, headache, hypotension, and edema pulmonary, which made its application for clinical treatments at that time difficult [3, 6].

But William Coley's method increasingly spurred the advance of immunotherapy. In 1976, two Frenchmen, Léon Charles Albert Calmette and Jean-Marie Camille Guérin used the strategy of using bacteria to fight cancer. They applied the Bacillus Calmette-Guérin (BCG), which had been previously discovered, in 1929, by themselves, through the isolation and attenuation of the attenuated strain of the tuberculosis bacillus *Mycobacterium bovis*, found in oxen, bringing a revolution to the treatment of tuberculosis [1, 3].

By injecting a solution containing BCG into the bladder of some patients, an indirect increase in the expression of tumor antigens can be noticed after the tumor cells engulf the bacteria. This promotes an intense, complex coordinated release of multiple cytokines, including those from helper T cells [3, 7].

In 1957, Thomas and Burnet presented the theory that lymphocytes could act as sentinels of the immune system, probably carrying out the identification and elimination of mutated cells, but they still had no knowledge about the specific mechanisms of action of tumor antigens, limiting advances in discoveries. But in 1974, Stutman conducted an experiment showing that mice with immune deficiency developed neoplasms, as well as an increase in killer (NK) cells to support the immune system [1–3].

The innate immune system includes dendritic cells, natural killer (NK) cells, macrophages, neutrophils, eosinophils, basophils, and mast cells. Innate immune cells do not require prior stimulation by antigens and act as a first line of defense against foreign antigens. The adaptive immune system includes B lymphocytes, CD4+ helper T lymphocytes, and CD8+ cytotoxic T lymphocytes (CTLs) and requires formal presentation by antigen-presenting cells (APCs) for its activation. The adaptive immune system generates antigen-specific T and B cell lymphocytes. The immune system is highly variable between individuals but relatively stable over time in a given person [2, 4].

In 1980, new studies brought the identification of antigens linked to melanoma cells, enabling the insertion of targeted immunological therapies, where T cells could be used to attack the tumor, thus identifying the cytotoxic T antigen – lymphocyte 4, which would become the basis for the development of checkpoint inhibitors in the future [3].

Immunotherapies include immunostimulating cytokines, which are small proteins naturally produced and secreted by various cells of the immune system. They are crucial in signaling between immune cells as well as between immune cells and various other types of cells in the body. The first cytokine to be discovered was interferon alpha, also known as type I, described in 1957 by Isaacs and Lindenmann, IL-2, the T-cell growth factor Interleukin 2, was identified in 1976, and this allowed researchers to grow T lymphocytes in vitro for the first time. IL-2 was cloned in 1983 and was immediately used in clinical trials that led to promising results, acting as a synthetic analog of a bacterial cell wall that is capable of activating monocytes and macrophages, including tumor reduction [1, 2, 4].

Gradually, knowledge about the immune system, its actions of immunological surveillance, and protection of the organism enabled decisive advances for improvements in cancer treatments and better quality of survival for cancer patients. Monoclonal antibodies appeared at the beginning of the twentieth century, and they come from B lymphocytes and bind to a specific antigen that will mediate the cytotoxicity reaction induced by this antigen–antibody complex. Paul Ehrlich presented a model for binding a drug to a specific transporter in order to exert its action at the target site, based on the principle of specificity that occurs in the antibody–antigen binding. This model allowed to reduce the unwanted action of the drug in other tissues, as well as to decrease the administered dose, due to the increase in efficacy [2, 3, 5].

The small proteins have since become well established, treating a wide spectrum of diseases, including cancers, acting in various ways, for example, by preventing an antigen from binding to its receptor on the cell surface or by marking an antigen to be antibodies. Monoclonals are generally used, with "mono" inferring that they are a single type of an antibody, targeting a specific antigen, and "clonal" meaning that they are multiplied thousands of times in order to obtain a clinically effective therapeutic dose. The main action of the antibody is to bind to the cell's antigens and mark the cancer cell to be destroyed by specialized immune system cells. Some antibodies act by signaling the immune system and triggering it to continue the attack, while other antibodies can interrupt the signaling that tells cancer cells to grow, divide, and spread [1, 2].

Research into antibody-based therapies flourished over the following decades and eventually led to the development of rituximab, a monoclonal antibody that binds to the CD20 protein present on the surface of immature B cells. In 1997, rituximab became the first approved monoclonal antibody by the FDA for the treatment of cancer, not Hodgkin's lymphoma. The drug targets immature B cells for elimination by NK cells [1, 3, 5].

In order to ensure that an inflammatory immune system response is not constantly activated once a foreign tumor or antigen has stimulated a response, multiple controls or "checkpoints" are in effect or activated. These checkpoints are primarily represented by T cell receptor binding to ligands on cells in the surrounding microenvironment, forming immunological synapses that then regulate T cell functions, which become specialized, or "polarized," to carry out different activities. In order to ensure that an inflammatory immune system response is not constantly activated once a foreign tumor or antigen has stimulated a response, multiple controls or "checkpoints" are in effect or activated. These checkpoints are primarily represented by T cell receptor binding to ligands on cells in the surrounding microenvironment, forming immunological synapses that then regulate T cell functions, which become specialized, or "polarized," to carry out different activities [3–5].

Adoptive cell therapy (ACT) is another type of immunotherapy that primarily involves isolation and in vitro expansion of tumor-specific T cells, followed by infusion back into the cancer patient. These efforts have also extended to the use of natural killer cells, as they exhibit rapid and potent immunity to solid tumor metastases and hematologic cancers. In the early 2000s, genetically modified lymphocytes were introduced. To increase their specificity, T lymphocytes with chimeric antigen receptors (CAR T cells) were developed, which recognize tumor antigens without the need for presentation by APCs. After initial success, chimeric antigen receptors (second generation) were developed, in which costimulatory molecules such as CD28, 4-1BB, or OX40 (molecules of the tumor necrosis factor receptor family) and ICOS (inducible T cell costimulator) were incorporated. Third-generation chimeric antigen receptors incorporate two costimulatory factors. And more recently, shielded chimeric antigen receptors have emerged, where in addition to two co-stimulatory molecules, transgenes for cytokines (IL-2) or ligands are associated (CD40L or 4-1BBL) [2, 3, 5].

Research has shown that lymphocytes present in transplantable tumors are capable of recognizing tumor cells in vitro, where they are clonally expanded and reinfused for treatment, but the technique of clonally isolating and expanding these lymphocytes is very expensive and laborious, which limits their use [4, 5].

Some lead to tumor-associated antigens expressed on the cell surface and therefore become a potential target for new antibody-based therapies. On the other hand, some tumors are known to lose their MHC class I expression, remaining a major challenge for immunotherapy. Furthermore, the entire tumor microenvironment is known to impact cancer growth and development and mediate potential treatment, including the microbiome. Several preliminary trials of fecal microbiota transplants (FMT) have already been conducted with promising results. Identifying relevant biomarkers is a key part of the process [3, 5].

In the early 2000s, genetically modified lymphocytes were introduced. To increase their specificity, T lymphocytes with chimeric antigen receptors (CAR T cells) were developed, which recognize tumor antigens without the need for presentation by adoptive cell therapy. After initial success, chimeric antigen receptors (second generation) were developed, in which costimulatory molecules such as CD28, 4-1BB, or OX40 (molecules of the tumor necrosis factor receptor family) and ICOS (inducible T cell costimulator) were incorporated. Thirdgeneration chimeric antigen receptors incorporate two costimulatory factors. In addition to its high complexity and cost, this treatment modality requires immunosuppression by the patient before its application in order to improve its effectiveness. An alternative source of lymphocytes is peripheral blood; strategies to isolate and expand these rare specific T cells are being developed.

Identifying relevant biomarkers is a key part of the process. For immunological checkpoint inhibitors, the level of expression of CTLA-4, PD-1, or PD-L1 genes is measured before drug administration, although good results are reported with low expression level. It is also well established that tumors with higher overall mutational burden are more responsive to checkpoint inhibitor therapy. In addition, cancers with microsatellite instability as a result of incompatibility repair deficiency are known to exhibit a particularly strong response to PD-1 blockade, regardless of the type of cancer. One of the most important challenges in science is figuring out why some patients respond to immunotherapy so perfectly, while others are not sensitive to this form of treatment. Furthermore, some are believed that patients develop cancer [3–5].

## 7.2 Immune Checkpoint Inhibitors (ICIs)

Immune checkpoint inhibitors are promising immunotherapies with demonstrated sustained antitumor responses in several tumors. Tumor cells exploit multiple complex mechanisms to escape recognition and destruction by the immune system. The ability to induce immune responses against cancer by abrogating an immune-system checkpoint that limits the antitumor activity of preexisting tumor-specific cytotoxic T cells shows the importance of focusing on immune regulatory events for cancer therapy [2, 8].

It was based on immunocytokines such as interleukin-2 and alpha-interferon that were poorly effective and highly toxic. Clinical research trials had tested diverse forms of cancer vaccines that were mostly ineffective, but (Rosenberg) after the first success of ICI and until today, immunotherapy leads the field and immunologists have regained a major influence in cancer research as illustrated by the attribution of the 2018 Nobel Prize in Medicine to the two immunologists who were at the origin of the concept of ICI-based immunotherapy, James Allison and Tasuku Honjo (Ledford).

Immune checkpoints refer to the set of inhibitory pathways that immune cells possess in order to regulate and control the durability of the immune response while maintaining self-tolerance [9]. Among the different immune checkpoint receptors, antibodies blocking two of them can be cited as the first approvals: CTLA-4 (lymphocyte-associated antigen 4) and PD-1 (programmed cell death 1) or its ligand PD-L1.

### 7.2.1 CTLA-4

The CTLA-4 immune checkpoint receptor was first characterized by Brunet et al. [10] in the 1980s. It is expressed by T cells and controls T cell activation during early stages in the lymph nodes. CTLA-4 competes with the co-stimulatory receptor CD28 for the binding to ligands CD80 (B7.1) and CD86 (B7.2), interfering with CD28 interactions, thus preventing costimulation and the priming phase of T-cell activation as demonstrated. By doing so, it prevents and controls further proliferation of the initial T cell response.

### 7.2.2 PD-1

PD-1 was cloned in 1992 [10] with a subsequent characterization of its ligand, PD-L1. It is expressed on activated T cells, B lymphocytes, and natural killer cells and constitutes a main mechanism of tumor immune resistance in peripheral tissues [9].

Interaction of PD-1 with its ligands, PD-L1 and PD-L2, inhibits the effector phase of T-cell activation, thus dampening the immune response [11]. The blockade of PD-1 receptor or its ligand PD-L1 with antibodies enhances preexistent antitumor immune activity, providing patients with major and durable immune responses against the tumor.

For example, we have the following immune checkpoint inhibitors in use nowadays: CTLA-4 inhibitors – ipilimumab; PD-1 inhibitors – nivolumab, pembrolizumab, and cemiplimab; and PD-L1 inhibitors – atezolizumab, durvalumab, and avelumab. The indications are diverse as you can see in Table 7.1:

Although the list of clinical indications is expansive, the clinical response to immune checkpoint inhibitors is variable and differences in clinical response limit their broad applicability. Several factors predict long-term clinical benefit including gene overexpression and the presence of mutations in tumor cells [12]. Often, these novel therapies are not potent enough to be used alone but can potentiate the effects of existing therapy. This synergism may result in an increased incidence and severity of immune-related AEs. New toxicities including "on-target off-tumor" effects have been described, and the effects of these thera-

**Table 7.1** Indication of use of immune checkpoint inhibitors

| Class | Drug | Indication |
|---|---|---|
| Anti-CTLA-4 monoclonal antibody (mAb) | Ipilimumab (Yervoy®) | Unresectable or metastatic melanoma |
| | Tremelimumab | No clinical indication |
| Anti-PD-1 monoclonal antibody (mAb) | Pembrolizumab (Keytruda®) | Hodgkin's lymphoma |
| | | Metastatic nonsquamous NSCLC |
| | | Locally advanced or metastatic urothelial carcinoma |
| | Nivolumab (Opdivo®) | Unresectable or metastatic melanoma |
| | | Nonsquamous and metastatic squamous NSCLC |
| | | Advanced RCC |
| | | Hodgkin's lymphoma |
| | | Locally advanced or metastatic urothelial carcinoma |
| | | Metastatic colorectal cancer |
| | | HCC |
| | | Squamous cell cancer of head and neck |
| Anti-PD-L1 mAb | Atezolizumab (Tecentriq®) | Locally advanced or metastatic urothelial carcinoma, metastatic NSCLC |
| | Avelumab (Bevancio®) | Metastatic Merkel cell carcinoma, locally advanced or metastatic urothelial carcinoma |
| | Durvalumab (Imfinzi®) | Unresectable stage III NSCLC, locally advanced or metastatic urothelial carcinoma |

**Table 7.1** (continued)

| Class | Drug | Indication |
|---|---|---|
| Anti-CTLA-4 mAb + Anti-PD-1 mAb | Ipilimumab + Nivolumab (Yervoy® + Opdivo®) | Unresectable or metastatic melanoma |
| | | RCC |
| | | Metastatic squamous cell carcinoma of the head and neck |
| | | Metastatic NSCLC |

Lewis et al. [45]

pies on healthy tissue remains a concern. Despite these challenges, immune checkpoint inhibitors remain a vital and promising tool in the fight against cancer.

## 7.3 Immunotherapy

### 7.3.1 Atezolizumab

#### 7.3.1.1 Indications

It is indicated for the treatment of urothelial carcinoma, which is locally advanced or metastatic, in adult patients who have undergone previous chemotherapy with platinum or who are not eligible for cisplatin-containing chemotherapy, and whose tumors express PD-L1 $\geq$ 5%. It is also indicated for non-small cell lung cancer (NSCLC) in adults, locally advanced or metastatic after previous chemotherapy. As monotherapy, it is indicated for first-line treatment in adult patients diagnosed with squamous and non-squamous metastatic non-small cell lung cancer, with PD-L1 expression $\geq$50% of tumor cells (TC) or $\geq$10% of tumor-infiltrating (CI) immune cells that do not have mutated EGFR or ALK-positive NSCLC, in addition to locally advanced unresectable or metastatic triple-negative breast cancer with PD-L1 expression $\geq$1% in combination with nab-paclitaxel in adult patients [13, 16].

#### 7.3.1.2 Pharmacokinetics

It is administered by an intravenous infusion (IV) because there are no studies on another form of administration. A population pharmacokinetic analysis performed indicates that the volume of distribution in the central compartment (V1) is 3.28 L and the volume at the state of equilibrium is 6.91 L. There are no direct studies on the metabolism of this drug and its elimination of antibodies mainly by catabolism [14]. The clearance (clearance) of atezolizumab is 0.200 L/day and the half-life of the terminal typical elimination (t1/2) is 27 days [15].

#### 7.3.1.3 Dosage

The recommended dose for first-line diagnosis of metastatic triple-negative breast cancer is 840 mg intravenously followed by 100 mg/m$^2$ of nab-paclitaxel every 28 days, with atezolizumab administered on D1 and D15 and nab-paclitaxel on D1, D8, and D15 [13].

The recommended monotherapy dose for hepatocellular carcinoma is 1200 mg, intravenously every 21 days in combination with bevacizumab, until the disease progression or an unacceptable toxicity. For unresectable or metastatic melanoma, a dose of 840 mg once every 2 weeks (combined with cobimetinib and vemurafenib) is indicated until the disease progression or an unacceptable toxicity. When indicated for small cell lung cancer (extensive stage), as a first-line treatment, a dose of 1200 mg every 3 weeks is recommended [15].

#### 7.3.1.4 Maximum Adult Dose

The maximum dose is 1200 mg IV every three weeks [16].

#### 7.3.1.5 Pediatric Dose

There are no data available on the safety and efficacy of the use of atezolizumab in children and adolescents below 18 years old [14].

#### 7.3.1.6 Maximum Dose in Geriatric Population

It is not necessary for any dose adjustment of atezolizumab in patients ≥65 years old [13].

#### 7.3.1.7 Dose Adjustment

No dose adjustment is necessary in patients with renal insufficiency, as well as in patients with hepatic insufficiency [13, 16].

#### 7.3.1.8 Drug Interactions

Pharmacokinetic drug interaction studies have not been performed with atezolizumab. Existing data shows that atezolizumab is cleared from the circulation via catabolism, which demonstrates that no metabolic drug interactions are expected. However, the use of systemic corticosteroids or immunosuppressants before starting atezolizumab should be avoided due to their potential to interfere with its pharmacodynamic activity and efficacy. However, if necessary, systemic corticosteroids or some immunosuppressants can be used to treat adverse reactions [13, 16].

#### 7.3.1.9 Dilution, Infusion Time, and Stability

Atezolizumab should be diluted in 0.9% SF 250 ml, and it is important to wash the infusion lines and equipment before and after the drug infusion. It must be infused in a time of 30–60 min [13]. It has stability after dilution in a PVC infusion bag for 8 hours at room temperature or 24 hours under refrigeration [16].

#### 7.3.1.10 Main Adverse Reactions

The most common adverse reactions found were fatigue, decreased appetite, nausea, cough, dyspnea, pyrexia, diarrhea, skin rashes, back pain, peripheral edema, vomiting, hypoalbuminia, hypomagnesemia, asthenia, arthralgia, musculoskeletal pain, pruritus, and infection of the urinary tract. It is noteworthy that discontinuation of therapy should only occur for severe reactions (Grade 3) and permanent discontinuation for life-threatening reactions (Grade 4) or recurrent severe reactions [13, 15].

### 7.3.2 Bevacizumab

#### 7.3.2.1 Indications

Bevacizumab is a recombinant monoclonal antibody used in combination with chemotherapeutics for the treatment of metastatic carcinoma of the colon or rectum; metastatic or locally recurrent breast cancer; locally advanced, metastatic, or recurrent non-small cell lung breast cancer; nonsquamous, unresectable, locally advanced, metastatic, or recurrent non-small cell lung cancer; metastatic and/or advanced renal cell cancer [19].

#### 7.3.2.2 Pharmacokinetics

The volume of distribution is 46 mL/kg and has an elimination half-life of 20 days (mean 11–50 days). In addition, it has an excretion rate of 2.75–5 mL/kg/day [16, 17].

#### 7.3.2.3 Dosage

In adult patients, for metastatic colorectal cancer, the recommended dose is 5 mg/kg in the first-line therapy, administered intravenously once every 14 days, or 7.5 mg/kg given once every 21 days per intravenously. For second-line therapy, the recommended dose is 10 mg/kg given once every 14 days or 15 mg/kg given every 21 days intravenously. For metastatic breast cancer, the recommended dose is 10 mg/kg every 14 days or 15 mg/kg given every 21 days intravenously. For advanced, metastatic, or recurrent non-small cell lung cancer, bevacizumab is given in combination with intravenous platinum-based chemotherapy for up to 6 treatment cycles, followed by monotherapy bevacizumab until disease progression is achieved. The recommended dose when combined with carboplatin is 15 mg/kg every 21 days intravenously. For metastatic and/or advanced renal cell cancer, the recommended dose is 10 mg/kg given intravenously every 14 days [19].

#### 7.3.2.4 Pediatric Dose

For refractory solid tumors, the recommended dose is 5–15 mg/kg/dose every 14 days intravenously in a 28-day cycle, or 5–10 mg/kg every 14–21 days. For gliomas and medulloblastoma, the recommended dose is 10 mg/kg/dose every 14 days in combination with irinotecan or 15 mg/kg/dose every 21 days [18].

#### 7.3.2.5 Maximum Adult Dose

The maximum dose an adult can take is 15 mg/kg every 21 days intravenously or 10 mg/kg every 14 days intravenously [16].

#### 7.3.2.6 Maximum Dose in Geriatric Population

There are no special dose recommendations for seniors over the age of 65 years [18, 19].

#### 7.3.2.7 Dose Adjustment

In patients with kidney and liver failure, there are no studies of efficacy and safety [18, 19]. Adjustments are necessary in the presence of reactions. For clinically insignificant mild ones, only decrease the infusion rate, and for those clinically significant reactions, stop the infusion and return to a reduced infusion rate after resolution of symptoms and discontinue the use in the case of severe infusion reactions [17].

#### 7.3.2.8 Drug Interactions

Studies carried out evaluating the drug interaction between bevacizumab and other drugs that make up the therapeutic protocols showed that there were no clinically relevant or statistically significant differences in the clearance of bevacizumab in combination with interferon alfa 2a, erlotinib, or chemotherapeutics, such as irinotecan, leucovorim and fluorouracil, carboplatin, paclitaxel, capecitabine, doxorubicin, or cisplatin, when compared to patients who received monotherapy with bevacizumab. In other words, it does not change the pharmacokinetics of these drugs [16, 19].

#### 7.3.2.9 Dilution, Infusion Time, and Stability

Bevacizumab should be diluted in sodium chloride solution 0.9% in 100 ml; no in-line filter is required in this process. The first infusion must be performed within 90 minutes; if there is no infusion reaction, the second infusion can be performed within 60 minutes. In the absence of infusion reactions, subsequent infusions can be performed within 30 minutes. After dilution of the drug in a pouch, its stability is 48 hours at room temperature [20]. The final concentration must be kept between 1.4 and 16.5 mg/mL [16].

#### 7.3.2.10 Main Adverse Reactions

The most common adverse reactions are febrile neutropenia, leukopenia, thrombocytopenia, anemia, dehydration, hyponatremia, dysgeusia, headache, dysarthria, hypertension, diarrhea, nausea, vomiting, abdominal pain, teeth problems, and others [19].

### 7.3.3 Cetuximab

#### 7.3.3.1 Indication

It is indicated for the treatment of locally advanced head and neck cancer and nonmutated KRAS metastatic colorectal cancer with epidermal growth factor receptor expression associated with irinotecan or FOLFOX4. As monotherapy, it is indicated for patients who have not responded to treatments with irinotecan and/or oxaliplatin [23].

#### 7.3.3.2 Pharmacokinetics

It has an half-life elimination of 112 hours (range 63–230 hours). The volume of distribution ranged from 45 to 62 mL/kg, and plasma concentrations reached stable levels after 21 days of monotherapy. The elimination processes observed in patients with doses equal to or greater than 400 mg/m$^2$ followed zero-order kinetics up to 96 hours after the end of the infusion, with an elimination of 0.4 mL/h/kg [16].

#### 7.3.3.3 Dosage

The recommended initial dose is 400 mg/m$^2$, followed by 250 mg/m$^2$ in subsequent administrations, which should be administered weekly [23].

#### 7.3.3.4 Maximum Adult Dose

The maximum recommended dose is 400 mg/m$^2$ [16].

#### 7.3.3.5 Pediatric Dose

The safety and efficacy of using cetuximab in pediatric patients have not been established [21].

#### 7.3.3.6 Maximum Dose in Geriatric Population

No dose adjustment is necessary in the geriatric population [22].

#### 7.3.3.7 Dose Adjustment

Dose adjustment is not necessary in patients with renal and hepatic impairment, nor is it necessary to add supplemental doses in patients undergoing hemodialysis. For grade 1 or 2 reactions after infusion, the infusion rate should be adjusted by 50%; for reactions of 3 and 4, it is recommended to discontinue therapy immediately and permanently [21].

#### 7.3.3.8 Drug Interactions

Cetuximab in combination with platinum-based chemotherapy can lead to an increase in the frequency of severe leukopenia or neutropenia, which can lead to an increased rate of infectious complications, such as febrile neutropenia, pneumonia, and even sepsis, when compared to platinum-based chemotherapy alone. The association of cetuximab with fluoropyrimidines demonstrated that the frequency of cardiac ischemia and the frequency of hand-foot syndrome (palmar–plantar erythrodysesthesia) can be high when compared to the use of fluoropyrimidines alone. Cetuximab associated with capecitabine and oxaliplatin can lead to an increased frequency of severe diarrhea [16, 23].

#### 7.3.3.9 Dilution, Infusion Time, and Stability

Cetuximab must be diluted in a 0.9% sodium chloride solution; it is necessary to use a 0.22-micron in-line filter. The infusion time for the initial dose is 120 minutes, followed by 60 minutes for subsequent doses on a weekly basis. After dilution in sodium chloride solution, bag stability is 8 hours at room temperature [16].

#### 7.3.3.10 Main Adverse Reactions

The main adverse reactions are skin reactions, hypomagnesemia, severe skin rash, decreased heart rate, nausea, fever, chills, body aches, flu symptoms, bleeding, dizziness, dry mouth, diarrhea, headache, vomiting, pain stomach, loss of appetite, constipation, weight loss, and weakness, among others [22].

## 7.3.4 Durvalumab

### 7.3.4.1 Indication

It is indicated for the treatment of patients with locally advanced or metastatic urothelial carcinoma who had disease progression during or after the use of platinum-based chemotherapy and for those who had disease progression within 12 months with neoadjuvant or adjuvant treatment with chemotherapy of a platinum base. It is also indicated for the treatment of unresectable stage III non-small cell lung cancer, in addition to being indicated as the first line for the treatment of extensive stage small cell lung cancer [16, 24].

### 7.3.4.2 Pharmacokinetics

Steady state of durvalumab was reached in approximately 16 weeks. In addition, the geometric mean (% coefficient of variation [CV%]) of the stationary volume of distribution was 5.6 L. The main elimination pathways for durvalumab are protein catabolism through the reticuloendothelial system or therapeutic target-mediated arrangement [16]. The half-life elimination is about 18 days [26].

### 7.3.4.3 Dosage

The dosage of durvalumab is 10 mg/kg every 2 weeks applied intravenously, or 1500 mg every 4 weeks, until disease progression or in the maximum of 12 months [26].

### 7.3.4.4 Maximum Adult Dose

The maximum dose of durvalumab is 10 mg/kg every 2 weeks [16].

### 7.3.4.5 Pediatric Dose

In children and adolescents under the age of 18 years, safety and efficacy have not been established [26].

### 7.3.4.6 Maximum Dose in Geriatric Population

No dose adjustment is necessary for patients above the age of 65 years old [16, 24].

#### 7.3.4.7 Dose Adjustment

No dose adjustment is necessary in patients with renal and hepatic impairment. Therapy should be withheld for severe reactions (Grade 3) and permanently discontinued for life-threatening reactions (Grade 4) [26].

#### 7.3.4.8 Drug Interactions

Due to the potential of interaction with the pharmacodynamic activity and efficacy of durvalumab with systemic corticosteroids or immunosuppressants, their use is not indicated before starting durvalumab, except for physiological doses of systemic corticosteroids (≤10 mg/day). However, these medications can be used after starting durvalumab in order to treat adverse reactions [16, 24].

#### 7.3.4.9 Dilution, Infusion Time, and Stability

Durvalumab can be diluted in 0.9% sodium chloride solution or 5% glucose solution; it is necessary to use a 0.22-micron in-line filter. The infusion must be carried out within 60 minutes. The final concentration must be kept between 1 mg/ml and 15 mg/ml. The stability of durvalumab after dilution is 24 hours under refrigeration or 4 hours at room temperature [16].

#### 7.3.4.10 Main Adverse Reactions

The main adverse reactions are oral candidiasis, flu, cough, hypothyroidism, pneumonia, diarrhea, abdominal pain, pruritus, fever, dermatitis, skin rash, myalgia, myositis, nephritis, dysuria, peripheral edema, hyperglycemia, hyperkalemia, and fatigue, among others [25].

### 7.3.5 Panitumumab

#### 7.3.5.1 Indication

It is indicated for the first-line treatment of wild-type RAS metastatic colorectal cancer in adult patients, associated with oxaliplatin or irinotecan with 5-fluorouracil and leucovorin, and at the second-line, associated with irinotecan, 5-fluorouracil, and leucovorin in patients who had previously used first-line treatment excluding irinotecan. As monotherapy, it is indicated after failure with chemotherapy regimens that have fluoropyrimidine, oxaliplatin, and irinotecan in their treatment regimen [29].

#### 7.3.5.2 Pharmacokinetics

Regarding the pharmacokinetic properties of panitumumab, it is known that, when administered as a single agent or in combination with chemotherapy, it has nonlinear pharmacokinetics [29]. It has a half-life elimination of about 7.5 days (range 3.6–10.9 days) [27].

#### 7.3.5.3 Dosage

The recommended dose is 6 mg/kg intravenously over 1 hour on the first application (within 30 minutes in subsequent infusions if the first infusion is well tolerated) [27] given every 14 days [16].

#### 7.3.5.4 Maximum Adult Dose

The maximum dose is 6 mg/kg every 14 days [16].

#### 7.3.5.5 Pediatric Dose

Safety and efficacy for use in pediatric patients are not established [27].

#### 7.3.5.6 Maximum Dose in Geriatric Population

No dose adjustment is necessary in geriatric patients [16].

#### 7.3.5.7 Dose Adjustment

There are no reports of the need for dose adjustment in patients with renal and liver failure. However, for patients who have experienced a grade 1 or 2 infusion reaction without symptoms of anaphylaxis, the drug should be temporarily discontinued until the problems are resolved. If you experience a grade 3 or 4 reaction, panitumumab should be permanently discontinued [27, 28].

#### 7.3.5.8 Drug Interactions

Panitumumab has a drug interaction with aminolevulinic acid; this is because photosensitizing agents can potentiate the photosensitizing effects of aminolevulinic acid. Thus, it is necessary to avoid the combination. The same can happen when associated with methoxsalen and porfimer; the therapy must be monitored in this case [28].

#### 7.3.5.9 Dilution, Infusion Time, and Stability

It must be diluted in a 0.9% sodium chloride solution, not exceeding the maximum final concentration of 10 mg/mL. An in-line filter of 0.2 or 0.22 micrometers must be used. The recommended infusion time is 60 minutes for the first infusion; if well-tolerated, subsequent infusions can take 30–60 minutes. However, for doses above 1000 mg, it is recommended to infuse within 90 minutes [29]. Stability after dilution in 10 mg/mL concentration is 6 hours at room temperature or 24 hours refrigerated. If diluted at a concentration of 2.5 mg/mL, the stability is 14 days refrigerated [16].

#### 7.3.5.10 Main Adverse Reactions

The main adverse reactions are fatigue, skin toxicity, acneiform erythema, paronychia, rash, skin fissure, hypomagnesemia, nausea, diarrhea, vomiting, dyspnea, cough, and fever, among others [28].

### 7.3.6 Pertuzumab

#### 7.3.6.1 Indication

It is indicated for the treatment of HER2-positive, metastatic, or locally resectable breast cancer, in combination with trastuzumab and docetaxel, in patients who have previously received chemotherapy with anti-HER2 or also indicated for early breast cancer associated with trastuzumab [32].

#### 7.3.6.2 Pharmacokinetics

It is administered intravenously, and studies with other ways of administration have not been performed. The metabolism of pertuzumab has not been directly studied [32]. Pertuzumab has a total body clearance of 0.24 L/day, in addition to a half-life elimination of approximately 18 days [30, 31].

#### 7.3.6.3 Dosage

The initial dose of pertuzumab is 840 mg given over 60 minutes, followed by a maintenance dose of 420 mg, given over 30–60 minutes every 21 days until disease progression or acceptable toxicity [31].

#### 7.3.6.4 Maximum Adult Dose

The maximum dose of pertuzumab is 840 mg [16].

#### 7.3.6.5 Pediatric Dose

There are no studies that guarantee safety and efficacy in the use of pertuzumab in pediatric patients [30].

#### 7.3.6.6 Maximum Dose in Geriatric Population

No dose adjustment is necessary for elderly patients at the age of 65 years or older [31].

#### 7.3.6.7 Dose Adjustment

No dose adjustment is necessary for renal and hepatic impairment; no information was found from studies on the need for dose reduction [16, 31].

#### 7.3.6.8 Drug Interactions

Studies performed showed that there is no evidence of drug interactions between pertuzumab and trastruzumab or docetaxel. In addition, other studies were performed evaluating the effects of pertuzumab on the pharmacokinetics of some cytotoxic agents, such as paclitaxel, gemcitabine, erlotinib, capecitabine, and carboplatin, showing no interaction with these medications [32].

#### 7.3.6.9 Dilution, Infusion Time, and Stability

Pertuzumab should be diluted in 250 mL of 0.9% sodium chloride solution; it is not necessary to use a 0.2- or 0.22-micrometer in-line filter. The infusion time is 60 minutes for the initial dose, followed by 30 to 60 minutes for subsequent doses every 21 days [16]. After dilution in sodium chloride, it is stable for 24 hours at room temperature [33].

#### 7.3.6.10 Main Adverse Reactions

The most common adverse reactions are diarrhea, alopecia, neutropenia, nausea, fatigue, rash, and peripheral neuropathy [32]. In addition to laboratory changes, fever, shortness of breath, flu-like symptoms, and feeling of weakness, other reactions have also been reported [16].

### 7.3.7 Panitumumab

#### 7.3.7.1 Indications

Pembrolizumab is indicated as monotherapy for the treatment of advanced, metastatic, or unresectable melanoma. It is also indicated for adjuvant treatment in adults with melanoma with lymph node involvement, who have undergone surgical resection. It may also be indicated for non-small cell lung cancer in combination with platinum-based chemotherapy and pemetrexed and indicated for the treatment of locally advanced or metastatic urothelial carcinoma that has had disease progression during or after platinum-containing chemotherapy, as well as for a high-risk non-muscle-invasive bladder cancer [16].

In addition, it is indicated for recurrent, locally advanced, or metastatic gastric or gastroesophageal junction cancer, classic refractory or relapsed Hodgkin's lymphoma, renal cell carcinoma (in combination with axitinib), and unresectable or recurrent metastatic squamous cell head and neck cancer (as monotherapy). It is also indicated for local advanced cancer and recurrent or metastatic esophageal cancer, and finally, for metastatic colorectal cancer with high microsatellite instability or repair enzyme deficiency [34].

#### 7.3.7.2 Pharmacokinetics

It has complete and immediate absorption by the intravenous route and has a distribution volume of 6 L, with a half-life elimination of 22 days [35, 36]. As it is a monoclonal antibody, pembrolizumab does not bind to plasma proteins [16].

#### 7.3.7.3 Dosage

The recommended dose of pembrolizumab is 200 mg every 3 weeks or 400 mg every 6 weeks, until a disease progression or an acceptable toxicity [34, 36]. For non-small cell lung carcinoma previously treated with chemotherapy or for melanoma, it is indicated a dose of 2 mg/kg [16].

#### 7.3.7.4 Maximum Adult Dose

The maximum dose in adult patients is 200 mg intravenously every 3 weeks, or 400 mg every 6 weeks [16].

#### 7.3.7.5 Dose in Pediatrics

The recommended dose for the pediatric population, in children ≥2 years and adolescents, is 2 mg/kg/dose (maximum dose: 200 mg/dose) once every 3 weeks, until a disease progression, unacceptable toxicity, or for up to 24 months [35].

#### 7.3.7.6 Maximum Dose in Geriatric Population

No dose adjustment is required, and no overall differences in safety and efficacy have been reported between elderly and young patients [34, 35].

#### 7.3.7.7 Dose Adjustment

No dose adjustment is necessary in patients with renal and hepatic impairment [34]. However, for renal toxicity during treatment such as immune-mediated nephritis, it should be evaluated whether discontinuation of treatment or interruption is necessary. Therefore, it is recommended to administer systemic corticosteroids. In cases of grade 2 or 3 serum creatinine elevation, pembrolizumab should be discontinued and only resumed after complete or partial resolution within 12 weeks of starting corticosteroids. Grade 4 increase in serum creatinine implies permanent discontinuation of pembrolizumab [35].

#### 7.3.7.8 Drug Interactions

Axitinib: the use of axitinib can lead to potentiation of the hepatotoxic effect of pembrolizumab. The therapy must be monitored. Thalidomide analogs: pembrolizumab can lead to an increase in the toxic effect of thalidomide analogs. Mortality may increase when this combination is used for the treatment of refractory multiple myeloma. The combination must be avoided [35].

The use of systemic corticosteroids or immunosuppressants before starting treatment with pembrolizumab should be avoided as they have potential interferences with the pharmacodynamic activity and efficacy of pembrolizumab. However, they can be used after starting treatment with pembrolizumab to treat immune-mediated adverse reactions [34].

#### 7.3.7.9 Dilution, Infusion Time, and Stability

Pembrolizumab can be diluted in 0.9% sodium chloride solution or 5% glucose solution. The use of a 0.2- or 0.22-micrometer in-line filter is required. Administration should be carried out intravenously over 30 minutes. Once diluted, stability is 6 hours at room temperature or 24 hours under refrigeration [16].

#### 7.3.7.10 Main Adverse Reactions

The most common adverse reactions are hypertension, alopecia, pruritus, rash, hypercholesterolemia, hyperglycemia, hypertriglyceridemia, hyponatremia, constipation, decreased appetite, diarrhea, nausea, high alkaline phosphatase, musculoskeletal pain, neuropathy, cough, dyspnea, and fatigue [34, 36].

### 7.3.8 Ramucirumab

#### 7.3.8.1 Indications

It is indicated for gastric or gastroesophageal junction cancer in combination with paclitaxel, with advanced classification, or with disease progression after chemotherapy with platinum or fluoropyrimidine. For metastatic or locally advanced non-small cell lung cancer, it is used in combination with docetaxel for patients who have experienced disease progression or failure with prior platinum-based chemotherapy. It is also indicated for metastatic colorectal cancer in patients who have had disease progression after prior chemotherapy with chemotherapy, as well as for hepatocellular carcinoma as an isolated agent after previous chemotherapy with sorafenib [37].

#### 7.3.8.2 Pharmacokinetics

Ramucirumab is administered only intravenously and has a volume of distribution of 5.4 L. Elimination: the mean clearance of ramucirumab is 0.015 L/hour, and it has a mean half-life of 14 days [37–39].

#### 7.3.8.3 Dosage

Metastatic colorectal cancer: 8 mg/kg every 2 weeks in combination with irinotecan, leucovorin, and fluorouracil until a disease progression or an unacceptable toxicity. Gastric cancer, advanced or metastatic: 8 mg/kg every 2 weeks as a single agent or in combination with weekly paclitaxel until disease progression or an unacceptable toxicity. Hepatocellular carcinoma, advanced, relapsed, or refractory: 8 mg/kg every 2 weeks until a disease progression or an unacceptable toxicity. Metastatic, non-small cell lung carcinoma: 10 mg/kg every 2 weeks in combination with erlotinib or docetaxel until a disease progression or an unacceptable toxicity [38].

#### 7.3.8.4 Maximum Adult Dose

The maximum recommended dose is 10 mg/kg every 2 weeks [37].

#### 7.3.8.5 Dose in Pediatrics

The safety and efficacy of ramucirumab in pediatric patients are not established [39].

#### 7.3.8.6 Maximum Dose in Geriatric Population

No dose adjustment is necessary for elderly patients above 65 years old [38].

#### 7.3.8.7 Dose Adjustment

There are no reports of the need for dose adjustment in patients with renal and liver failure [38].

#### 7.3.8.8 Drug Interactions

Bisphosphonate derivatives: angiogenesis inhibitors may potentiate the toxic effects of bisphosphonate derivatives. The risk of osteonecrosis of the jaw may be increased. Monitor this therapy [38]. No drug interactions were observed between ramucirumab and paclitaxel, docetaxel, irinotecan, and erlotinib. The pharmacokinetics of these were not affected when administered together [37].

#### 7.3.8.9 Dilution, Infusion Time, and Stability

Ramucirumab should be diluted in 0.9% sodium chloride solution, and the final volume of the solution should be 250 mL; it should also be administered within 60 minutes [37]. After dilution, it is stable for 4 hours at room temperature or 24 hours under refrigeration [40].

#### 7.3.8.10 Main Adverse Reactions

The most common adverse reactions are hypertension, peripheral edema, hypoalbuminemia, hypocalcemia, hyponatremia, abdominal pain, decreased appetite, diarrhea, nausea, proteinuria, neutropenia, fatigue, headache, and insomnia [38].

### 7.3.9 Trastuzumab

#### 7.3.9.1 Indications

It is indicated for early, locally advanced, and metastatic breast cancer and inoperable, advanced, recurrent, or metastatic gastric cancer associated with capecitabine or 5-fluorouracil and a platinum agent [41].

#### 7.3.9.2 Pharmacokinetics

In most patients, trastuzumab has a concentration decrease of approximately 3% (approximately 97% clearance) within

7 months of discontinuation [42]. It has a volume of distribution of 44 mL/kg and a half-life elimination of 5.8 days (between 1 and 32 days) [43].

#### 7.3.9.3 Dosage

The indicated loading dose of trastuzumab is 8 mg/kg intravenously given over 90 minutes, followed by 6 mg/kg intravenously given between 30 and 90 minutes every 3 weeks for a total of 52 weeks [43].

#### 7.3.9.4 Maximum Adult Dose

The maximum indicated dose is 8 mg/kg every 21 days [16].

#### 7.3.9.5 Dose in Pediatrics

The safety and efficacy of using trastuzumab in pediatric patients are not established [43].

#### 7.3.9.6 Maximum Dose in Geriatric Population

No dose adjustment is necessary for elderly patients 65 years of age or older [42].

#### 7.3.9.7 Dose Adjustment

No dose adjustment is necessary in patients with impaired renal and hepatic function [42].

#### 7.3.9.8 Drug Interactions

Transtuzumab may increase the cardiotoxic effect of anthracyclines. Because of this, their use should be avoided for up to 7 months after stopping trastuzumab. If it is necessary to use them at the same time, cardiac dysfunction must be closely monitored [42].

#### 7.3.9.9 Dilution, Infusion Time, and Stability

Trastuzumab should be diluted in 250 mL of 0.9% sodium chloride solution and administered within 90 minutes in the first application. In the absence of reactions, it is administered between 30 and 60 minutes. After dilution, it is stable for 24 hours at room temperature [16].

#### 7.3.9.10 Main Adverse Reactions

The main adverse reactions are rash, abdominal pain, diarrhea, nausea, vomiting, infection, chills, dizziness, headache, insomnia, neuromuscular pain, cough, dyspnea, rhinitis, fever, reduced weight, and fatigue, among others [42, 43].

#### 7.3.9.11 Immune-Related Adverse Events (IRAEs)

The focus of immune coreceptor blockers is the immune system unfit and adaptive in the continuous process of surveillance of the organism, different from conventional cytotoxic chemotherapy, that is, the tumor cell.

Mechanisms of immunotherapy suppressors, CTLA 4 or PD-1/PDL-1, under physiological conditions are limited to immune response as a mechanism of tolerance and prevention of an exacerbated response. T lymphocytes are involved in the biological action of immunotherapeutics that have cytotoxic capacity. Cytotoxic responses occur more in the skin, gastrointestinal tract, liver, lung, and endocrine glands, but any organ may be the target of an immune-mediated response to more varied clinical presentations.

The incidence of immune-related events is most varied, both in frequency and manifestations, may occur in monotherapy and is associated with other immunoderivatives, and varies according to the neoplasm under treatment. It is important to note that IRAEs can occur after discontinuation of treatment, so prolonged surveillance is important [44].

The recommendation for patients receiving immunotherapy drugs is to be clinically evaluated with anamnesis, hematological, hepatic, renal, and thyroid function assessment, at each application, and in the segment every 6 to12 weeks in the first six months. For patients with preexisting autoimmune conditions such as vitiligo, hypothyroidism, systemic lupus erythematosus, rheumatoid arthritis, multiple sclerosis, HIV, and hepatitis B and C, who are candidates for immunotherapy, more attention is required from the health team regarding adverse events. Inclusion for treatment benefit should be greater than the risk to toxicity.

In an overview, the early diagnosis of potential AIS and differential not related to treatment-induced immune activation is

**Table 7.2** CTCAE v4

| S.No. | Immunotherapy | Directed treatment | Follow-up |
|---|---|---|---|
| 1 | Continue treatment | Symptoms; topical steroids | Stepping up surveillance |
| 2 | Consider temporary suspension | Symptoms; topical steroids; consider prednisone VO 0.5–1.0 mg/kg/day if persistent | Step up surveillance; in cases of suspension/ delay, reintroduce immunotherapy if grade 1 toxicity or resolved |
| 3 | Suspend; consider reintroduction only in selected situations | Prednisone VO 1-2 mg/kg/day or methylprednisone EV 1–2 mg/Kg/day | Reevaluations every 3–5 days; consider immunosuppressants if there is no improvement with steroids |
| 4 | Suspend permanently | Methylprednisone EV 1–2 mg/Kg/day; consider immunosuppressants | Reevaluations every 24–48 hours; consider the possibility of late recurrences |

indispensable for appropriate therapeutic guidance. Clinical manifestation should ideally be graded by the Common Terminology Criteria for Adverse Events (CTCAE) (Table 7.2), but adequacy and classification in degrees do not replace clinical judgment.

Discontinuation of treatment is recommended when grade 4 or 3 toxicities persist and are recurrent, without improvement after the indicated therapy. If another important immunotherapy is indicated, discuss with the patient the risks of AKI, and start treatment within 4 weeks

I would remind you that at discharge the patient should be followed up for 3 months in the first year, and every 6 months in the following years, due to the risk of late AKI [44]

### 7.3.10 Gastrointestinal Adverse Event and Its Management

The most common gastrointestinal adverse events are colitis, diarrhea, and pancreatitis. In clinical trials, it is believed that diarrhea is a result of colonic inflammation, so treatment of colitis and diarrhea are similar. For patients treated with ipilimumab for melanoma, the incidence of diarrhea (in any degree) is 30%, and 10% for grade 3 and 4. For colitis in grades 3 and 4, the incidence is 5%.

In patients treated with PD-1/PD-L1 inhibitors, the incidence of diarrhea is lower, any degree corresponds to 15%, and grade 3 and 4, about 2%. The frequency is higher in the combination of ipilimumab with nivolumab. However, the occurrence of intestinal perforation is a rare (<1%) event.

This toxicity starts from the sixth week after the beginning of immunotherapy. Early recognition is essential to minimize complications. There is no preventive treatment for diarrhea induced by these agents; the management of adverse events is based on the severity of symptoms and involves corticosteroids and/or immunosuppressants. In severe cases, treatment is discontinued.

Pancreatitis is diagnosed with high levels of lipase and amylase; in these cases, abdominal imaging is recommended to exclude actual pancreatitis.

### 7.3.11 Hepatic Adverse Event and Its Management

Liver AIS are usually asymptomatic, with laboratory alterations of AST, ALT, and GGT or bilirubins. The frequency is low from 2% to 7% in monotherapy and 15% to 30% in the double immune block. Main symptoms present asthenia and hyporexia. Symptoms may occur from 8 to 12 weeks of treatment.

The management of hepatoxicity involves systemic corticosteroids and mycophenolate of mofetil in the most severe cases [44].

### 7.3.12 Pulmonary Adverse Event and Its Management

Pulmonary toxicity is uncommon; it is more frequent in patients treated for non-small cell lung cancer. In monotherapy, the risk is 2.7%. Initial symptoms are cough, fever, or dyspnea to varying degrees and can occur in an unpredictable period during treatment from 9 days to 19 months. That is why systematic clinical evaluation is important. In the case of suspicion, computed tomography of the chest is indicated, the pneumonitis may appear in a radiological pattern of dull glass or infiltrated nodular, and there is no typical radiological pattern.

The management of pneumonitis is adequate according to the severity of the condition; immunosuppressives, infliximab, cyclophosphamide, and mycophenolate of mofetil are the recommendations for moderate to severe symptoms.

### 7.3.13 Cutaneous Adverse Event and Its Management

Cutaneous adverse events are more prevalent in combined immunotherapy treatments, anti-CTLA-4 agents, and in patients treated for melanoma. The main symptoms are itching, rash, maculopapular, and vitiligo. Other clinical manifestations with lower incidence are dry mouth, alopecia, stomatitis, and photosensitivity. Occurs in the first 3–4 weeks of treatment.

The management for this toxicity is hydration, photoprotection, topical steroids, and anti-histamines, and usually there is no need to discontinue treatment.

### 7.3.14 Endocrine Adverse Event and Its Management

Endocrine IRAEs can occur in 10% of cases. But keep constant surveillance. The occurrence of the event occurs in the 4–18 weeks of treatment and late. The endocrine event in any degree has been observed in all treated patients, affecting the thyroid gland and pituitary gland; manifestations such as type I diabetes mellitus and adrenalite may also occur. Symptoms include headache, fatigue, weight variations, hairloss, and constipation.

Management of endocrine IRAEs usually involves hormone replacement, anti-rheoid drugs, endocrine monitoring, and symptom control. Discontinuation of immunotherapy treatment is not recommended.

The least present AIS are myocarditis and myocardial dysfunction, described in patients using ipilimumab and anti-PD-1 agents; hematological dysfunction associated with ipilimunab with rapid response to improvement with venous immunoglobulin therapy; and neurological events such as Guillain–Barré syndrome and myasthenia gravis, which has been described more frequently. The use of corticosteroid therapy, immunosuppressants, and immunoglobulin are considered exceptional in the control of such events. Finally, ophthalmological IRAEs such as uveitis, conjunctivitis, and episclerites are associated with CTLA-4 inhibitors.

## 7.4 Conclusion

The use of immunotherapies, anti-CTLA-4, PD-1, and PDL-1, resulted in an advanced treatment of solid neoplasms. For a successful management of toxicities, an early diagnosis, a high degree of suspicion in the face of symptoms, efficient patient medical communication, and a rapid targeted treatment are necessary. In this context, the multidisciplinary team should be well informed of immune-related adverse events, the relationship with the patient's clinic, and the medication used. The earlier the diagnosis of IRAEs, the less damage to the patient.

## References

1. Dobosz P, Dzieciątkowski T. The intriguing history of cancer immunotherapy. Frontiers in Immunology I www.frontiersin.org. 2019;10:Article 2965.
2. Pennock GK, Chow LQ. The evolving role of immune checkpoint inhibitors in cancer treatment. Oncologist. 2015;20(7):812–22. https://doi.org/10.1634/theoncologist.2014-0422.
3. Kelly J. Brassil, PhD, RN, AOCNS®, ACNS-BC Pamela K. Ginex, EdD, RN, OCN. Guide to cancer immunotherapy. Chapter one: History of immunotherapy. Oncology Nursing Society; 2018.

4. Oiseth S, et al. Cancer immunotherapy: a brief review of the history, possibilities, and challenges ahead. J Cancer Metastasis Treat. 2017;3:250–61. https://doi.org/10.20517/2394-4722.2017.41. www.jcmtjournal.com.
5. Jorge JJ. Imunoterapia no tratamento do cancer Immunotherapy in cancer treatment. Arq Asma AlergImunol. 2019;3(2). https://doi.org/10.5935/2526-5393.20190023
6. Montfort A, Colacios C, Levade T, Andrieu-Abadie N, Meyer N, Ségui B. The TNF paradox in cancer progression and immunotherapy. Front Immunol. 2019;10:1818. https://doi.org/10.3389/fimmu.2019.01818.
7. Mellman I. The immunotherapy of cancer: past, present & the next frontier. Genentech, South San Francisco, California. Cancer Immunology.
8. Safety and tumor responses with lambrolizumab (Anti–PD-1) in melanoma. N Engl J Med. 2013;369:134–44. https://doi.org/10.1056/NEJMoa1305133.
9. Abril-Rodriguez G, Ribas A, Shot S. Immune checkpoint inhibitors. Cancer Cell. 2017;31(6):848–848.e1. ISSN 1535-6108. https://doi.org/10.1016/j.ccell.2017.05.010.
10. Brunet J-F, Denizot F, Luciani M-F, et al. A new member of the immunoglobulin superfamily—CTLA-4. Nature. 1987;328:267–70.
11. Keir ME, Butte MJ, Freeman GJ, et al. PD-1 and its ligands in tolerance and immunity. Annu Rev. Immunol. 2008;26:677–704.
12. Kulangara K, Zhang N, Corigliano E, et al. Clinical utility of the combined positive score for programmed death ligand-1 expression and the approval of pembrolizumab for treatment of gastric cancer. Arch Pathol Lab Med. 2019;143:330–7.
13. Tecentriq [Drug description leaflet]. Rio de Janeiro: ROCHE. Available in: https://consultas.anvisa.gov.br/#/bulario/q/?nomeProduto=tecentriq. Accessed in: 15 Sept 2021.
14. Atezolizumab. Micromedex solutions. Available in: https://www.micromedexsolutions.com/micromedex2/librarian/PFDefaultActionId/evidencexpert.DoIntegratedSearch?navitem=topHome&isToolPage=true#. Accessed in: 15 Sept 2021.
15. Atezolizumab. Up To Date. Available in: https://www.uptodate.com/contents/atezolizumab-drug-information?search=atezolizumabe&source=panel_search_result&selectedTitle=1~86&usage_type=panel&kp_tab=drug_general&display_rank=1. Accessed in: 15 Sept 2021.
16. Souza GB. Medicamentos Oncológicos na Prática Clínica. 2nd ed. São Paulo: Editora Farmacêutica; 2019.
17. Bevacizumab. Micromedex solutions. Available in: https://www. micromedexsolutions.com/micromedex2/librarian/CS/20CFB6/ND_PR/evidencexpert/ND_P/evidencexpert/DUPLICATIONSHIELDSYNC/C66F71/ND_PG/evidencexpert/ND_B/evidencexpert/ND_AppProduct/evidencexpert/ND_T/evidencexpert/PFActionId/evidencexpert.DoIntegratedSearch?SearchTerm=Bevacizumab&fromInterSaltBase=true&User

MdxSearchTerm=%24userMdxSearchTerm&false=null&=null#. Accessed in: 16 Sept 2021.
18. Bevacizumab. Up To Date. Available in: https://www.uptodate. com/contents/bevacizumab-including-biosimilars-of-bevacizumab-drug-information?search=BEVACIZUMABE&source= panel_search_ result&selectedTitle=1~148&usage_type=panel&kp_tab=drug_general&display_rank=1. Accessed in: 16 Sept 2021.
19. Bevacizumab. [Drug description leaflet]. Rio de Janeiro: ROCHE. Available in: https://consultas.anvisa.gov.br/#/bulario/q/?nomeProduto=Avastin. Accessed in: 16 Sept 2021.
20. Bevacizumab. Stabilis. Available in: https://www.stabilis.org/Monographie.php?IdMolecule=538. Accessed in: 17 Sept 2021.
21. Cetuximab. Micromedex solutions. Available in: https://www. micromedexsolutions.com/micromedex2/librarian/CS/C9B859/ND_PR/evidencexpert/ND_P/evidencexpert/DUPLICATIONSHIELDSYNC/1045FA/ND_PG/evidencexpert/ND_B/evidencexpert/ND_AppProduct/evidencexpert/ND_T/evidencexpert/PFActionId/evidencexpert.DoIntegratedSearch?SearchTerm=cetuximab#. Accessed in: 18 Sept 2021.
22. Cetuximab. Up To Date. Available in: https://www.uptodate.com/contents/cetuximab-drug-information?search=CETUXIMAB&source=panel_search_result&selectedTitle=1~107&usage_type=panel&kp_tab=drug_general&display_rank=1. Accessed in: 18 Sept 2021.
23. Erbitux. [Drug description leaflet]. Rio de Janeiro: MERK. Available in: https://consultas.anvisa.gov.br/#/bulario/q/?nomeProduto=ERBITUX. Accessed in: 18 Sept 2021.
24. IMFINZI. [Drug description leaflet]. São Paulo: AstraZeneca do Brasil Ltda. Available in: https://consultas.anvisa.gov.br/#/bulario/q/?nomeProduto=IMFINZI. Accessed in: 20 Sept 2021.
25. Durvalumab. Up To Date. Available in: https://www.uptodate.com/ contents/durvalumab-drug-information?search=DURVALUMAB&source=panel_search_result&selectedTitle=1~35&usage_type=panel&kp_tab=drug_general&display_rank=1. Accessed in: 20 Sept 2021.
26. Durvalumab. Micromedex solutions. Available in: https://www.uptodate.com/contents/durvalumab-drug-information?search=DURVALUMAB&source=panel_search_result&selectedTitle=1~35&usage_type=panel&kp_tab=drug_general&display_rank=1. Accessed in: 20 Sept 2021.
27. Panitumumab. Micromedex solutions. Available in: https://www.micromedexsolutions.com/micromedex2/librarian/CS/849129/ND_PR/evidencexpert/ND_P/evidencexpert/DUPLICATIONSHIELDSYNC/E11A38/ND_PG/evidencexpert/ND_B/evidencexpert/ND_AppProduct/evidencexpert/ND_T/evidencexpert/PFActionId/evidencexpert.DoIntegratedSearch?SearchTerm=PANITUMUMAB&UserSearchTerm=PANITUMUMAB&SearchFilter=filterNone&navitem=searchALL#. Accessed in: 21 Sept 2021.

28. Panitumumab. Up To Date. Available in: https://www.uptodate.com/contents/panitumumab-drug-information?search=panitumumab&source=panel_search_result&selectedTitle=1~38&usage_type=panel&kp_tab=drug_general&display_rank=1. Accessed in: 21 Sept 2021.
29. Vectibix. [Drug description leaflet]. São Paulo: AMGEM. Available in: https://consultas.anvisa.gov.br/#/bulario/q/?nomeProduto=vectibix. Accessed in: 21 Sept 2021.
30. Pertuzumab. Micromedex solutions. Available in: https://www.micromedexsolutions.com/micromedex2/librarian/CS/849129/ND_PR/evidencexpert/ND_P/evidencexpert/DUPLICATIONSHIELDSYNC/E11A38/ND_PG/evidencexpert/ND_B/evidencexpert/ND_AppProduct/evidencexpert/ND_T/evidencexpert/PFActionId/evidencexpert.DoIntegratedSearch?SearchTerm=PERTUZUMAB&UserSearchTerm=PERTUZUMAB&SearchFilter=filterNone&navitem=searchALL#. Accessed in: 22 Sept 2021.
31. Pertuzumab. Up To Date. Available in: https://www.uptodate.com/contents/pertuzumab-drug-information?search=PERTUZUMAB&source=panel_search_result&selectedTitle=1~49&usage_type=panel&kp_tab=drug_general&display_rank=1. Accessed in: 22 Sept 2021.
32. Perjeta. [Drug description leaflet]. Rio de Janeiro: ROCHE. Available in: https://consultas.anvisa.gov.br/#/bulario/q/?nomeProduto=perjeta. Accessed in: 22 Sept 2021.
33. Pertuzumab. Stabilis. Available in: https://www.stabilis.org/Monographie.php?IdMolecule=909. Accessed in: 24 Sept 2021.
34. Keytruda. [Drug description leaflet]. São Paulo: MERK. Available in: https://consultas.anvisa.gov.br/#/bulario/q/?nomeProduto=keytruda. Accessed in: 23 Sept 2021.
35. Pembrolizumab. Up To Date. Available in: https://www.uptodate.com/contents/pembrolizumab-drug-information?search=PEMBROLIZUMAB&source=panel_search_result&selectedTitle=1~148&usage_type=panel&kp_tab=drug_general&display_rank=1. Accessed in: 23 Sept 2021.
36. Pembrolizumab. Micromedex solutions. Available in: https://www.micromedexsolutions.com/micromedex2/librarian/PFDefaultActionId/evidencexpert.DoIntegratedSearch?navitem=topHome&isToolPage=true#. Accessed in: 23 Sept 2021.
37. Cyramza. [Drug description leaflet]. São Paulo: Eli Lilly. Available in: https://consultas.anvisa.gov.br/#/bulario/q/?nomeProduto=CYRAMZA. Accessed in: 25 Sept 2021.
38. Ramucirumab. Up To Date. Available in: https://www.uptodate.com/contents/ramucirumab-drug-information?search=RAMUCIRUMAB&source=panel_search_result&selectedTitle=1~30&usage_type=panel&kp_tab=drug_general&display_rank=1. Accessed in: 28 Sept 2021.

39. Ramucirumab. Micromedex solutions. Available. in: https://www.micromedexsolutions.com/micromedex2/librarian/PFDefaultActionId/evidencexpert.DoIntegratedSearch?navitem=topHome&isToolPage=true#. Accessed in: 28 Sept 2021.
40. Ramucirumab. Stabilis. Available in: https://www.stabilis.org/Monographie.php?IdMolecule=975. Accessed in: 04 Oct 2021.
41. Herceptin. [Drug description leaflet]. Rio de Janeiro: Roche. https://consultas.anvisa.gov.br/#/bulario/q/?nomeProduto=HERCEPTIN. Available in: https://consultas.anvisa.gov.br/#/bulario/q/?nomeProduto=HERCEPTIN. Accessed in: 28 Sept 2021.
42. Trastuzumab. Up To Date. Available in: https://www.uptodate.com/contents/trastuzumab-intravenous-including-biosimilars-of-trastuzumab-drug-information?search=trastuzumab&selectedTitle=1~128&usage_type=panel&display_rank=1&kp_tab=drug_general&source=panel_search_result. Accessed in: 30 Sept 2021.
43. Trastuzumab. Micromedex solutions. Available in: https://www.micromedexsolutions.com/micromedex2/librarian/CS/4E6188/ND_PR/evidencexpert/ND_P/evidencexpert/DUPLICATIONSHIELDSYNC/99C06B/ND_PG/evidencexpert/ND_B/evidencexpert/ND_AppProduct/evidencexpert/ND_T/evidencexpert/PFActionId/evidencexpert.DoIntegratedSearch?SearchTerm=Trastuzumab&fromInterSaltBase=true&UserMdxSearchTerm=%24userMdxSearchTerm&false=null&=null#. Accessed in: 30 Sept 2021.
44. Franco AO, Christmas SL. Immunorelated adverse events and their management in immunotherapy in cancer patients. Oswaldo Cruz Magazine. Issue 19.
45. Lewis AL, Chaft J, Girotra M, Fischer GW. Immune checkpoint inhibitors: a narrative review of considerations for the anaesthesiologist. Br J Anaesth. 2020;124(3):251e260.

**Cristiane Souza de Agostinho** Graduated in Nursing (Jorge Amado University, Brazil). Specialist in Oncology by the Brazilian Society of Oncology Nursing. MBA in Health Services Management. Postgraduate Professor of the Multidisciplinary Course in Oncology at Universidade Salvador and Courses in the areas of Health. Member of the Nursing Research Group at the Federal University of Bahia.

**Flávia Mendes Leite** Graduated in Pharmacy (Federal University of Bahia, Brazil). MBA in Quality Management (Unifacs, Bahia, Brazil). Specialist in Clinical and Hospital Oncology. Professional

Pharmacist in Oncology, Oncohematology, Bone Marrow Transplantation, and CAR-T Cell Therapy at a particular hospital in Brazil. Reference Professor in Oncology Studies at Sanar Saúde. Professor in Multidisciplinary Postgraduate Program in Oncology at Unifacs. Author and Reviewer of books about pharmaceutical issues at Sanar Saúde. Member of Educational Committee at Brazilian Society of Oncology Pharmacy. Chairman of the Oncology Commission at Pharmacy Regional Conseil, Bahia State Office.

**Marlize Brandão Ribeiro Cardoso** Master in Human Development and Social Responsibility. Specialist in Oncology and Bone Marrow Transplantation. MBA in Health Management. Coordinator of Oncology Nursing. Postgraduate Teacher. Organizer of the book Nursing Treaty in oncology.

**Priscila Pinto Costa** Graduated in Pharmacy (State University of Feira de Santana, Bahia, Brazil). Specialist in Clinical Pharmacy in Oncology (Estacio de Sá University, Bahia, Brazil). Professional Pharmacist in Oncology, at a particular hospital in Brazil.

# CAR-T Cells and Other Related Technologies

# 8

Marcus Rafael Lobo Bezerra, Larissa Queiroz Pontes, Igor Cabral Studart, Bruna de Sousa Lima, and Gilvan Pessoa Furtado

## 8.1 Conventional CAR Structure and Its Variations

Immunotherapy using chimeric antigen receptors (CARs) is based on the transfer of autologous T cells, genetically modified to express CAR, receptors developed based on TCRs (T cell receptors). A conventional TCR allows detection and destruction of cells by T cells after the presentation of tumor-associated antigens

M. R. L. Bezerra (✉) · L. Q. Pontes · I. C. Studart
Postgraduate Program in Biotechnology and Natural Resources, Federal University of Ceará, Fortaleza, Brazil

Fiocruz Ceará, Precabura, Eusébio, Brazil
e-mail: marcus.lobo@fiocruz.br

B. de Sousa Lima
Fiocruz Ceará, Precabura, Eusébio, Brazil

Undergraduate Program in Pharmacy, Federal University of Ceará, Fortaleza, Brazil

G. P. Furtado
Fiocruz Ceará, Precabura, Eusébio, Brazil
e-mail: gilvan.furtado@fiocruz.br



C. W. P. Schmidt, K. M. Otoni (eds.), *The Golden Guide to Oncologic Pharmacy*, https://doi.org/10.1007/978-3-030-98596-7_8

(TAAs) or tumor-specific antigens (TSAs) by the major histocompatibility complex class I (MHC I).

Alternative strategies addressing the use of modified TCRs have been studied previously. However, one of the main limitations of this therapy was the dependence of the TCR on MHC. This is relevant, primarily because one of the mechanisms of tumor evasion is a reduction of MHC expression in the cancer cell.

The classical CAR design has in its structure an extracellular domain, composed of a specific binding moiety and a hinge region (flexible moiety), a transmembrane domain, and an intracellular signaling and activation domain [32].

The specific binding moiety is usually formed by a single-chain variable fragment (scFv) of an antibody specific for tumor antigen recognition. The use of an scFv as a recognition region for TAAs allows a wide variety of CAR applications. Unlike TCR, CAR does not require the MHC I to present the antigen to recognize it. For this reason, it also enables the identification of antigens of another nature since the MHC only processes and presents protein-derived peptides. Thus, carbohydrate and glycolipid structures can also be used as potential targets. Another advantage is the possibility of carrying out mutations in the scFv moiety to modify its affinity for the target antigen, one of the factors that affect CAR-T cell activity (CAR-T). The magnitude of the cellular response of CAR-T cells against tumor cells depends, in addition to the binding affinity of scFv for its target, on the efficacy of CAR expression on the surface of the effector cell, the density of antigen on the tumor cell, and the accessibility of the epitope in the target cell [32].

One of the difficulties of CAR development is selecting a target since most of the antigens used are also expressed in healthy tissues and organs, which increases the risk of complications. Based on the binding affinity between antibody and antigen, it is possible to facilitate the differentiation between normal and tumor tissue when there is a difference in antigen density. Studies indicate that an scFv with low affinity for a target can destroy cells where the antigen is abundantly expressed but cannot cause the death of healthy cells where the target is expressed at low or normal levels [35, 40]. A CAR with low-affinity scFv against

EGFR (epidermal growth factor receptor) demonstrated an effect on cells overexpressing the target and no response to cells with lower EGFR levels [33]. Studies have also been done with trastuzumab-based CAR-T cells, where scFv with reduced affinity showed reactivity only to HER2 (human epidermal growth factor receptor-type 2) of breast cancer cells, with no effect against normal cells expressing the antigen [47]. These results illustrate the versatility of scFv usage, which can be designed and manipulated to influence specificity and differentiate tissues.

The spacer region, also called the hinge, is placed in most CARs between the binding domain and the transmembrane domain. Its function is to improve the flexibility and access of the binding moiety to the target antigen, so it should be planned in accordance with the epitope. Concerning its length, the longer the spacer, the easier it is to access epitopes proximal to the membrane or antigens surrounded by the glycocalyx. In contrast, CARs with shorter hinges are more efficient for binding epitopes distal to the membrane [32]. In addition to spacer length, its sequence also needs to be optimized to enhance the CAR. The hinges of most CARs are based on immunoglobulins or are derived from membrane receptor ligands such as CD8α and CD28. Human IgG-derived spacers (IgG1, IgG2, or IgG4) may have two domains, CH2 and CH3, similar to IgG. However, several studies have indicated that the CH2 domain preserves its ability to bind to Fc gamma receptors (FcγR), even when inserted into CAR [51]. This triggers the activation of other immune cells, reducing the persistence of CAR-T cells in the body. An alternative to circumvent this situation is modifying or deleting the CH2 domain, thus avoiding FcγR binding activity. These longer spacers are ideal for reaching epitopes proximal to the membrane. In contrast, hinges such as CD8α and CD28 have been widely employed since they do not interact with FcγR, especially for epitopes distal to the membrane, as these are shorter spacers. IgG-derived hinges without the CH2 and CH3 domains are also very useful in these cases.

The transmembrane domain has the function of anchoring the CAR to the cell membrane and is usually composed of a derivative of a membrane protein, such as CD4, CD8, CD28, CD3ζ, or

FcεRIγ [32]. CD8 and CD28 are used in most CARs. This domain is one of the least characterized. Still, some studies suggest that it may be relevant for CAR-T cell activity, influencing the activation signal transmitted from the extracellular domain to the intracellular domain [28]. CARs with ICOS (inducible T cell costimulator) as co-stimulatory in the intracellular domain showed better results when incorporated into ICOS as transmembrane domain, instead of CD8α [43]. These results suggest that the transmembrane domain of some co-stimulatory molecules may be involved in CAR-T cell signaling. The generations of CAR are distinguished by alterations in this signaling moiety, progressively intensifying the activity of these cells. Immunotherapy with CARs is widely studied and has shown several positive results in clinical trials. Some of these therapies have already been approved by the Food and Drug Administration (FDA), such as tisagenlecleucel (Kymriah®), axicabtagene ciloleucel (Yescarta®), and brexucabtagene autoleucel (Tecartus®) [44].

### 8.1.1 Source of Co-stimulatory Domains

Co-stimulatory domains are generally derived from the B7-CD28 family, composed of CD28 and ICOS, in addition to suppressor molecules, such as CTLA-4 and PD-1, or from the tumor necrosis factor receptor (TNFR) gene family, consisting of 4-1BB (CD137), OX40 (CD134), and CD27 [40].

The B7-CD28 family molecules perform their signals through the phosphatidylinositol 3-kinase (PI3K)-Akt pathway, with ICOS being able to induce a more intense activation than CD28 [38, 43]. In contrast, CD28 can recruit Grb2 and Lck in its intracellular domain, leading to the recruitment of Itk, increasing IL-2 levels and cell proliferation [29]. The TNFR family molecules, on the other hand, activate TRAF (TNF receptor-associated factor) proteins, being related to the modulation of T cell proliferation, differentiation, and survival [52]. Most CARs use CD28 and 4-1BB as co-stimulatory molecules in the three FDA-approved second-generation CAR-T models [44]. Third-generation CARs usually combine one co-stimulatory domain from the B7-CD28 family and another from the TNFR family to activate two different signaling pathways.

Clinical trials performed with CARs containing CD28 or 4-1BB domains have shown that both present a similar antitumor response. However, the cellular persistence between the two is quite different. Studies using these CARs in B-cell malignancies indicate that CAR-Ts with CD28 are eliminated from the body in about three months, while CAR-Ts with 4-1BB remain for years [31, 48]. Studies suggest that this is because activation through CD28 leads to a high initial effector function, triggered by IL-2 secretion, which accelerates the proliferation process but reduces the persistence of these cells due to exhaustion [42]. On the other hand, 4-1BB induces a slower effector response that sustains T-cell persistence for a longer time [43]. Combining the CD28 and 4-1BB domains into a single third-generation CAR demonstrated enhanced functionality and persistence [55]. In comparison, the incorporation of ICOS as a co-stimulatory domain showed greater cell persistence than CD28 or 4-1BB, as well as enabling polarization of Th17 effector T cells, which potentiates T helper functions [41, 43].

Researchers found that the motif responsible for interacting with the SH2 fraction of PI3-K of CD28 and ICOS is different by only one amino acid. For ICOS, the motif is YMFM composed of phenylalanine (F). In CD28, it corresponds to YMNM with an asparagine (N) [42]. The asparagine present in YMNM interacts with Grb2 causing NFAT (nuclear factor of activated T cells) activation and stimulating IL-2 production. An asparagine switch to phenylalanine at this CD28 motif blocks this binding to Grb2, reducing NFAT activation and increasing Akt activation. In vivo tests [42] compared the activity of native CAR-T CD28 cells and CAR-T CD28-YMFM cells and observed an improved tumor response and increased persistence of the mutated cells. An assay was also performed with native CAR-T ICOS cells and CAR-T ICOS-YMNM cells, where mutated cells had reduced cell persistence and antitumor activity compared to native cells. Other important motifs for CD28 signaling can also be explored as possible targets for mutations, such as PYAPP, which has also been studied [30].

In addition to studies using point mutations, the employment of other co-stimulatory domains, such as OX40 in association with CD28 demonstrated an increase in T cell survival compared to second-generation CAR-T CD28 [45]. The CD27 domain also showed better cell survival than CD28 [49].

New advances have addressed the use of other molecules as CD3ζ substitutes, such as DAP12 (DNAX-activating protein of 12 kDa) for application in ACT with NK cells, or DAP12 together with KIR2DS2 (killer immunoglobulin-like receptor) as a transmembrane domain, both showing positive results of antitumor activity and good expression [50].

### 8.1.2 Generations of CAR

The first proposals of CAR cells were composed of a single-chain fragment variable (scFv), a spacer, a transmembrane region, and an intracellular domain, based on the zeta chain of CD3 complex (CD3ζ). This structure was initially called first-generation CAR, which uses only CD3ζ as a co-stimulatory molecule of activation signal (Fig. 8.1).

CD3ζ chain has three domains called immunoreceptor tyrosine-based activation motifs (ITAMs), composed of an amino

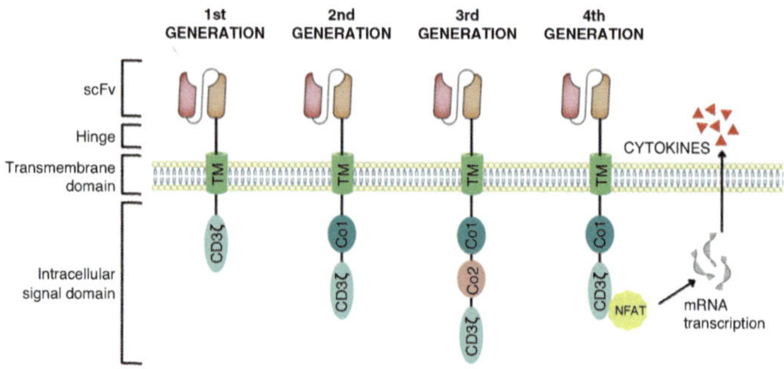


**Fig. 8.1** Four generations of chimeric antigen receptors (CARs)

acid sequence. When anscFv recognizes an epitope, a signaling cascade is triggered, phosphorylating ITAMs and causing an effector cell activation and tumor cell death [27]. Despite the proven antitumoral activity, first-generation CARs have shown some downsides regarding therapeutic efficacy and persistence in clinical trials [32, 37].

In addition, T cells need two-activation signaling, one MHC-dependent and the other via co-stimulatory molecules. Throughout time, CAR structure has been improved to add activation routes, which is possible by increasing co-stimulatory signals on the intracellular domain. Second-generation CAR presents the addition of CD28 as a co-stimulatory molecule (Fig. 8.1). Other molecules have also been tested, such as CD27, CD134 (OX-40), CD137 (4-1BB), and ICOS [43].

The addition of other co-stimulatory signals brought a better signaling cascade, improving cytokine production and proliferation in vivo on CAR-T cells [43]. After promising results from second-generation CAR co-stimulatory signals, a third-generation CAR is the one that presents a further signaling molecule on its intracellular structure (Fig. 8.1). In many studies, third-generation CARs have shown improvement regarding persistence, proliferation, and antitumor activities compared to second-generation CARs [43]. However, it is crucial to investigate superactivation signaling phenomena, which can exacerbate collateral damages and tonic signaling, an uncontrolled and sustained activation that causes CAR-T cell burnout.

Fourth-generation CARs, also known as T-cell redirected for antigen-unrestricted cytokine-initiated killing (TRUCKs), combine second-generation receptors with an efficacy boost through cytokine release (Fig. 8.1). Thus, this generation of CARs pursues CD3ζ as an intracellular signaling domain, a co-stimulatory molecule, and a pro-inflammatory factor, such as IL-7, IL-12, and IL-15 for CAR-T activity improvement and immunosuppressive tumor activity reduction. Thereby, the transgenic cytokine is released after CAR activation and will be placed on the target tissue, decreasing its systemic side effects [34, 75].

The first generation of CARs consisted of an scFV as a binding domain, a hinge, a transmembrane region, and a single intracellular signaling domain (CD3ζ). The second generation included a new co-stimulatory molecule (CD28, 4-1BB, ICOS, OX40, or CD27). The third generation has two co-stimulatory molecules, in addition to CD3ζ, usually CD28 or ICOS as Co1 and 4-1BB, OX40 or CD27 as Co2. The fourth generation, also called TRUCK, combines second-generation CARs with a molecule that induces the expression of transgenic cytokines (NFAT).

Recently, new CAR configurations have been developed to reduce tumor evasion and toxicity and increase its versatility, such as recognizing a broad antigen spectrum. Those new receptors may be considered the next generation of CARs [37, 40]. One of the main evasion mechanisms is CAR-T cell loss, mutation, or down expression of target antigens, bringing about a discussion of CARs that recognize more than one epitope. Thus, tandem CARs (TanCAR) are engineered to present a sequence of two scFv binding to two different epitopes [39]. TanCAR development is complex and needs a few more receptor optimizations, aided by computational modeling and other bioinformatics tools.

Another approach is double CARs, where two different CARs are expressed in the same cell. Preferentially, both CARs should be cloned using the same vector to guarantee the simultaneous expression of both molecules. Tandem CARs and double CARs are also known as CAR OR-gate because any scFv interaction to its epitope triggers CAR-T cell activation, which might be even more intense when both antigens are recognized [37, 40].

A conventional CAR-T cell limitation targets antigens expressed both in healthy and tumor cells, leading to "off-tumor" effect. New strategies have been developed to reduce toxicity, such as CAR-T cells activated only when both epitopes are recognized (AND-gate) [46]. An alternative is CAR combination, where the first CAR uses a CD3ζ domain while the second one uses another co-stimulatory domain. Thus, CAR-T cell activation is effectively triggered only when both epitope recognitions lead to reactivity reduction when there is interaction with only one epitope.

The CARs ON-switch have an extracellular domain dissociated from the extracellular signaling domain. In this case, even if there is one domain recognition, the receptor does not trigger a signaling cascade [53]. The activation happens through a small heterodimer molecule administered to the patient, allowing in situ dose control.

A more recent approach combines the AND-gate system with the synthetic Notch receptors (synNotch). Its activation leads to the expression of another CAR, responsible for CAR-T cell activation by binding to the target antigen [81]. The combination of activation CARs to inhibitory CARs (iCARs) has also been investigated, and it is commonly constructed using CTLA-4 or PD-1 receptors [82]. As a result, T cells are activated only in the presence of the corresponding antigen of conventional CAR and the absence of iCAR antigen.

Universal CARs have been studied to reduce tumor evasion and toxicity. In one of the possible conformations, CARs expressing cells have no specificity and bind to antibody-based conjugated to biotin or fluorescein isothiocyanate (FITC) [27, 54]. This approach allows different antibody binding and CAR substitution, allowing diverse antigen recognition into the same CAR.

Another conformation that has been studied is SUPRA CAR (split universal, programmable chimeric antigen receptor) through a zipCAR receptor (leucine-zipper conjugated to an intracellular signaling domain) and a zipFv domain (leucine-zipper bound to an scFv complementary to zipCAR) [36]. Therefore, different zipFv might be used with different targets. If "off-tumor" reactivity is observed, one might use competitive zipFv with a high affinity to zipCAR to compete with the target cell and block CAR activity.

Besides structural modifications, gene editing could be used to optimize CAR-T cells concerning efficacy and safety. There are works with suicidal genes, gene-insertion with endonucleases, and CRISPR/Cas9 system, among others [37, 40].

## 8.2 Lymphocyte Activation and Cell Death Signals Promoted by CAR Cells

When T lymphocytes interact with antigen/MHC receptors on antigen-presenting cells, many signal pathways are activated, such as Ras-extracellular signal-related kinase (EKR)-activator protein (AP)-1 pathway, inositol triphosphate (IP3)-$Ca^{2+}$-nuclear factor of activated T cell (NFAT) pathway, protein kinase C (PKC) θ-IκB kinase (IKK)-nuclear factor (NF)-κB pathway, the tuberous sclerosis complex (TSC)1/2-mammalian target of rapamycin (mTOR) pathway, and others, culminating in T cell activation to exert its cytotoxic effects. The TCR complex plays an essential role in T cell activation and thus cytotoxic effects. It is comprised of TCRα/β chains and CD3γ/δ/ε/ζ subunits. CD3 transmits the TCR activation signal to the cell cytoplasm, phosphorylating ITAM (immunoreceptor tyrosine-based activation motif) residues, thus activating protein tyrosine kinases, leading to cell death induction. This mechanism is dependent on TCR activation, and CAR-T cells overcome the use of TCR with the combination of the target-specific extracellular domain (i.e., scFv) and the intracellular domains of the TCR, which are the TCR's domains involved in cell signaling. Therefore, chimeric antigen receptors dismiss the necessity of antigen presentation by MHC I. Both strength and length of stimulation affect the intensity by which the cell will be activated and its differentiation patterns, such as the generation or enhancement of memory CD8+ T cells, proliferation, and survival [23]. Therefore, the extracellular domain's affinity is an essential factor when designing new CAR cells and the type of intracellular co-stimulatory domains. These features affect clinical outcome and toxicity by influencing the cell death capacity and release of cytokines, respectively.

CAR-T cell activation results in their proliferation, as demonstrated by Chen et al. [24], where CAR-T cells make 1–5% of total T cells within the tumor microenvironment (TME) after one week of infusion of axicabtagene ciloleucel. Their presence induces the production of IL-6 by non-CAR cells within the TME. Therefore, antitumor activity promoted by CAR seems to be performed by complementary mechanisms of cell death induction and local immune response. Their work also shows a continuous increase of CAR-T cells after the first two weeks of infusion, reaching 50–100 cells/μL by day 14 (2–60% of all peripheral T cells). The work performed by Blache et al. [25] shows an increased expression of CD-45 (exhaustion of T cells), inhibitory checkpoint molecules (LAG3, PD-1, and TIM3, suggesting T cell post-activation/exhaustion), granzyme B/perforin, and IFN-y and a decrease in the CD4/CD8 ratio, indicating that the cell will be active, and under intense proliferation, at the rate they express exhaustion-related molecules that will result in their decrease in cytotoxic effects.

## 8.3 Immunological Synapse Quality

### 8.3.1 Molecular Mechanisms of Cell Death Induction

When CAR cells find their target, they activate a set of signals that induce the target cell to death. These signals are intrinsically dependent on immunological synapse formation. As previously discussed, many signals are activated, promoting a set of morphological and physiological changes in the CAR-T cell. This activation's strength depends on both scFv affinity (extracellular) and co-stimulatory domains (intracellular), which will affect the degree to which death signals are released. Liu et al. [26] reviewed parameters and assays used to evaluate what might be considered a "good" or "bad" CAR cell, such as the expression rate of CD8 receptor in the batch to be infused (suggesting that the transformed cell has cytotoxic potential), the release of interleukins linked to cytotoxic effects (IL-1, IL-6, IFN-γ, IL-10), $^{51}$Cr release assay, and evidence of synapse formation, indicated by the polarization of granzymes/perforin granules (apoptosis inductors), accumulation and reorganization of F-actin (involved in cytoskeleton stabilization), and clusterization of CAR and other death receptors (such as Fas), among others. Such parameters may be examined by standard techniques such as flow cytometry [25], where up to 15 parameters (13 colors) were analyzed in a single flow cytometry experiment to follow CAR-T treated patients for both surface and intracellular markers. As the first sign of CAR-T cell activation, the number of CD8+ cells in treated patients increases at day-9 post-infusion, followed by several activations of molecular mechanisms at synapse formation.

When CAR cells approximate, besides the release of granzymes A and B, trimerization of FasL/TRAIL receptors induces apoptosis through different pathways. The trimerization of these receptors are necessary to recruit FADD, leading to procaspase-8 activation into caspase-8, followed by activation of two distinct pathways: (1) activation of Bid (BH3-interaction domain death agonist), leading to the mitochondrial release of cytochrome c and Smac/Diablo, culminating in the activation of the apoptosome and (2) activation of pro-caspases 3/6/7, all two paths leading to apoptosis, as described in Fig. 8.2.

Molecular mechanisms induced by CAR-T cell. Several caspases are activated, culminating in apoptosis induction from perforin/granzymes release and trimerization of cell death receptors, such as Fas. All those mechanisms are activated when the immunological synapse is formed.

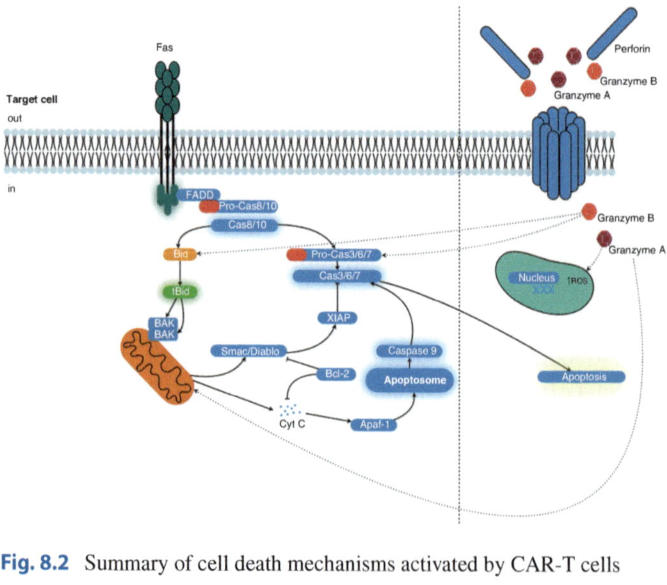


**Fig. 8.2** Summary of cell death mechanisms activated by CAR-T cells

### 8.3.2 Morphological Changes

A good CAR-T cell and target cell approximation will induce morphological changes that might determine a quality CAR [26]. The favorable formation of immunological synapses will cause the induction of signals previously mentioned. Therefore, synapse formation might be a predictor that can correlate to efficient clinical outcome with cytotoxic effect against a cancer cell. Engineering of the extracellular portion of the receptor aiming to obtain high-affinity binders might favor stronger interactions between cells, inducing a more protracted and closer communication channel. Even though this interface between cells is essential to set up the CAR's mechanisms, it is also known that overactivation of this cell might lead to critical cytotoxic events, suggesting that an optimal range of affinity would give a proper balance of T cell activation and controlled adverse events.

A CAR cell, such as CAR-T or CAR-NK, will form an immunological synapse when interacting with its target cell. That interaction is induced by approximation between the extracellular domain of the CAR (scFv) and its surface target. When this synapse is formed, accumulation of both CAR and cell death receptors (such as Fas) and cytoskeleton reorganization will occur, leading to lytic granule polarization (Fig. 8.3).

Cytoskeleton reorganization, the polarization of receptors (CAR and death induction), and perforin/granzymes are hallmarks of the immunological synapse.

## 8.4 Overview of CAR Cell Clinical Targets

Target selection is the most fundamental factor determining the potential of CAR-T therapy, and its selection criteria are not ordinary [18]. One of the major hurdles in cell-based therapy is the identification of appropriate targets that result in disease regression, sparing healthy tissues unharmed [1]. The majority of tumor antigens are proteins, but other biomolecules, such as carbohydrates and lipids, could be potential targets [18].

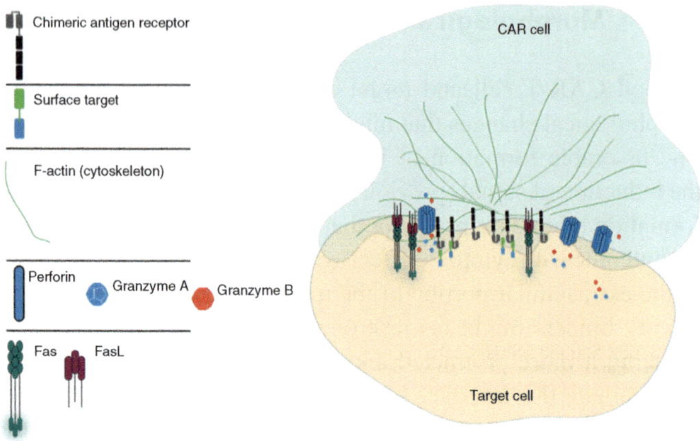


**Fig. 8.3** Morphological changes on CAR-mediated immune synapse

Some features might be considered when choosing a target, such as coverage and specificity. They refer to antigen distribution throughout the cell surface, besides the specific interaction between the CAR cell and its target. Both of these features guarantee the effectiveness and safety of the CAR-T cell. Another characteristic that should be evaluated is stability, which is related to target expression recurrence. In CAR-T cell treatment, losing targets is a common mechanism for treatment failure [18].

Tumor antigens have been largely restricted to cell surface proteins. There are three main types of cancer antigen:

- Tumor-specific antigens (TSAs): expressed only on malignant cells, which reduces the possibility of on-target/off-tumor effect. However, tumor heterogeneity among patients could make identification difficult.
- Tumor-associated antigens (TAAs): expressed at different levels on healthy and tumor tissues. Its increment might be a target identification, even though there is a high possibility of an on-target/off-tumor effect.

- ·Cancer germline antigens (CGAs): minimally expressed on healthy cells but frequently expressed on malignant cells and embryonic tissues. The major downside of this approach is that CARs could destroy healthy reproductive tissue.

Identifying antigens expressed in heterogeneous solid cancers that are not expressed in critical healthy tissues is one of the biggest challenges for the field of CAR-T cell therapy [1]. Despite these hurdles, some studies have had success in vitro in solid tumor treatments with CAR-T cells.

There are few targets in promising studies for solid tumors, such as gp100, an intracellular tumor-associated glycoprotein involved in melanin synthesis, which is 60% expressed in melanoma cells [17]. In vitro, gp100-specific TCR and chondroitin sulfate proteoglycan 4 (CSPG4)-specific CAR showed potent antitumor cytotoxicity against melanoma cells. Another target is GD2 ganglioside, a glycosphingolipid involved in signal transduction, cell–cell recognition, and tumor cell metastasis and is known to be overexpressed in solid tumors. GD2-specific CAR-T lymphocytes exhibit potent anti-melanoma activity in vitro and in vivo. Moreover, CAR-T cells directed to the GD2 antigen in neuroblastoma induced tumor responses and low-level persistence in patients, which was associated with more prolonged survival [17].

There are a plethora of cell-based immunotherapy approaches for multiple myeloma in preclinical and clinical trials. B-cell maturation antigen (BCMA) is a membrane bound of the tumor necrosis factor receptor superfamily expressed primarily by plasma cells [3]. Some of its ligands are B-cell activating factor (BAFF) and a proliferation-inducing ligand (APRIL) [16]. BCMA expression in multiple myeloma patients is almost universal, but the density of antigen expression in the cell surface is highly variable and affects CAR's overall success.

CD19 is the most well-established target for B-cell treatment using CAR-T cell technology. It is expressed only on B cells and B lymphoid progenitors but not on progenitor stem cells [13].

Clinical trials of CAR-T cell-targeting CD19 have shown significant responses in acute lymphoblastic leukemia (ALL), chronic lymphocytic leukemia (CLL), diffuse large B-cell lymphoma (DLBCL), and follicular lymphoma (FL). The US FDA approves two CD19 CAR-T cell products, and they have different CAR backbones, different gene transduction, and different culture conditions. Kymriah, which Novartis manufactures, uses 4-1BB as the co-stimulatory domain, whereas, Yescarta (Kite's product) uses a CAR construct with CD28 as the co-stimulatory domain [11]. The design of CAR has been constantly reviewed to achieve a better effect. A set of new scFv fragments has been constantly screened to get better clinical outcomes for the affinity and specificity of CAR-T cell therapy [9]. A new human scFv anti-CD19 was obtained by Gu et al. by using bioinformatics tools, such as structural modeling and docking [5]. Another study developed new CD19-CAR-T cells, which produced lower levels of cytokines, expressed higher levels of antiapoptotic molecules, and proliferated more slowly than the other CAR-T in comparison [22].

As with CD19, CD20 and CD22 are B-lineage markers and should be considered candidates for CAR cell therapy, even though targeting these molecules will probably result in an "on-target/off-tumor" effect on nonmalignant cells, leading to B-cell aplasia [10]. Those two markers are expressed in most mature B-cells but not on B-cell progenitors and plasma cells. CD20 is expressed in 50% and CD22 80–90% of B-acute lymphoblastic leukemia (B-ALL) cases [2].

CD47 is a cell surface glycoprotein of the immunoglobulin superfamily that is often overexpressed in both hematological and solid cancers such as ovarian, small cell lung cancer, pancreatic, glioma, glioblastoma, pediatric brain tumors, and other types of cancers. Its signaling plays a crucial role in maintaining tumor initiation or cancer stem cells [4]. Recently, Golubovskaya et al. have developed a humanized CD47-CAR-T cell, which effectively and specifically killed cancer cell lines and produced cytokines in a CD47-dependent manner. In addition, they demonstrated in the ovarian SKOV-3 cancer cell line that CD47-CAR-T cells could be used to target cancer stem cells, paving new roads to solid tumor therapies [4].

Recent studies have developed, using CD38, a glycoprotein detectable in B-ALL, as a target to CAR-T cell therapy. However, further experiments, including experiments optimizing the affinity of CD38-CAR-T cells to reduce target-mediated toxicity and knocking out the CD38 gene in CAR-T-38 cells by using gene-editing technology, such as CRISPR/Cas9, to avoid the "self-lysis" of CAR-T-38 cells, are required to improve the safety and persistence of these cells in future clinical studies, even though the potent and specific antitumor activity of CAR-T-38 cells is established in a relapsed B-ALL patient [6].

Some other targets, such as CD138 (a member of the syndecan family involved in cell–cell and cell–matrix interactions), CD229 (strongly expressed in multiple myeloma cells and their precursors), CD44v6 (expressed on keratinocytes, monocytes, epithelial, and hematologic tumors), and SLAMF7 (signaling lymphocytic activation molecule F7) have been investigated to elucidate their efficacy and safety in CAR-T cell therapy against multiple myeloma in vitro and in vivo [12].

## 8.5 Toxicological and Adverse Events Related to CAR-T Cell Therapies

Despite the extraordinary advances that adoptive genetically engineered immune cell therapy already represents for fighting, above all, hematological malignancies, challenges regarding safety and predictability of therapeutic outcome still impose limitations both on expanding the eligibility of patients who could benefit from therapy with CAR-T cells and their variants and on establishing their applicability to solid tumor cancers and autoimmune, metabolic, and infectious diseases.

Given that the basic principle of the method, in the oncological context, is deliberately applying cells with high destructive power (cytotoxicity) and promoting a robust immune response in an inexorably debilitated patient, the risks of occurrence of adverse events due to its level of toxicity are among the main concerns associated with CAR cell therapy. Although the idea is to restrict, when possible, the action of adoptive cells only to target tissues, the expression of the CAR-specific antigen in nontarget tissues or healthy cells, even in low amounts, as well as the excessive release of immune mediators, can lead to severe toxicity.

### 8.5.1 "On-Target Off-Tumor" Toxicity

It is not by chance that the FDA-approved CAR-T products so far are directed to hematological cancers of B cells [56], being restricted to patients that either have not responded or have relapsed after multiple standard treatments. In this context, as already mentioned, the antigen that is best characterized and used in the majority of cell therapies already available is the CD19 protein, expressed on B cells, in different development stages, but not in stem cells, which are critical for hematopoiesis. Patients can tolerate the complete depletion of B cells (B cell aplasia) through the temporary administration of immunoglobulins [58]. Still, humoral immunosuppression resulting from B cell depletion contributes to the risk condition of the patient that has just undergone anti-CD19 CAR cell therapy. Most patients stay in the hospital for weeks following treatment, allowing for close monitoring and care of the possible adverse effects [57].

Besides the search for new hematological targets, finding safe antigens expressed only and homogeneously on solid tumor cells or their microenvironment is one of the biggest obstacles to developing and approving CAR cells against this type of malignancy. The occurrence of cognate targets on cells of crucial healthy tissues is a source of so-called "on-target off-tumor" toxicity, which, ideally, must be detected early in the preclinical stages of the therapy development.

Most of the antigens targeted by the current CAR-T cells are not exclusively expressed on cancer cells. Although their off-tumor toxicity can be acceptable in some situations, they can be clinically manageable as in the cases of anti-CD19 and anti-BCMA—other examples have shown severe acute toxicity. An example of a disastrous outcome related to CAR-T cell-mediated "on-target off-tumor" toxicity happened in the clinical trial of an ErBB2-directed CAR-T cell administered to a patient with ErBB2 overexpressing metastatic colon cancer. Even though low, the level of target-antigen on healthy lung epithelial cells was probably enough to activate CAR-T cells, leading to tissue damage that resulted in the patient's death soon after infusion [59]. In another study with CAR-T cells in patients with metastatic renal cell carcinoma, the expression of targeted antigen, carboxy-anhydrase-IX (CAIX), on healthy bile-duct cells demonstrated unacceptable toxicity, rendering this CAR-T not feasible for further exploration [60].

Curiously, engaging antigen on healthy tissues can be a way of stimulating CAR-T cells repeatedly and, thereby, providing long-term on-tumor responses by more persistent CAR-T cells [75]. This, combined with other engineering strategies, has been explored in new CAR designing ideas to overcome toxicity issues and efficiency constraints. For example, short-term low-proliferative CAR cells could benefit from this fact and be safer at the same time through the targeting of multiple antigens. By recognizing more than one antigen, activation of CAR cell can be modulated by the signaling combinations of the different parts in a logic-gated manner. The function and outcome of these combinations can vary immensely and depend on each construction goal [76]. Other approaches involve targeting tumor-restricted post-translational modifications [61, 62] and improving selectivity for the tumor by decreasing CAR's affinity for antigens that are expressed at low levels on healthy tissues but densely expressed on the tumor [47].

### 8.5.2 Overactivation of Immune Effector Cells and Cytokine Release Syndrome

The exacerbation of a systemic pro-inflammatory environment due to the activation and proliferation of CAR-T cells can lead to a scenario in which native immune effector cells, such as macrophages, T-lymphocytes, and NK-cells, are overactivated. This, associated with a massive release of immunological mediators, ends up causing life-threatening damage. This common side-effect, known as cytokine release syndrome (CRS) or cytokine storm, is the main toxicity event following CAR-T cell treatment. CRS has been the most frequent cause of death related to anti-CD19 CAR-T cell therapy [63]; thus, several molecular engineering strategies for the generation of improved CAR cells are oriented to face this issue. Some clinical manifestations are flu-like symptoms, high fever, encephalopathy, rashes, arthralgia, myalgia, hypotension, cardiac complications, multiorgan system failure, and neurological disorders [65]. CRS's monitoring and mitigation strategies are essential parts of the mandatory risk management plan of any CAR-T cell therapy [57].

Although many other factors are also involved, cytokine IL-6 plays a central role in mediating CRS. IL-6 has both anti-inflammatory and pro-inflammatory activity. Its pro-inflammatory response is associated with high cytokine levels and, likely, as a result of a trans-signaling route mediated by a soluble IL-6 receptor, which reaches a wider range of cells than the classical anti-inflammatory IL-6 signaling route. On the other hand, the anti-inflammatory route is mediated by membrane IL-6 receptor (CD126), which is expressed on macrophages, neutrophils, hepatocytes, and some T cells, being associated with low levels of IL-6 [66]. Emerging evidence implicates non-CAR cells of the tumor microenvironment (TME) as the primary source of IL-6 following local CAR-T cell activation [24]. Many details on the pathophysiology of CRS remain yet to be better characterized. The blockade of IL-6 receptor with an anti-IL-6 mAb tocilizumab, which is approved by the FDA for severe cases, is not always effective for CRS [64]. TME profile and predisposition factors may also play crucial roles in the occurrence of CRS and other CAR-mediated toxicities.

Next-generation CAR cells have been engineered to improve their antitumor activity without increasing associated toxicity. Along with modulating activation and cytokine secretion profile by modifying the parts of the CAR (hinge, transmembrane region, and co-stimulatory domains) in a tailored way [22, 68], another promising strategy is focused on modulating the trafficking and regulatory functions not only of CAR-T cells but also of non-CAR-T cells in TME. The so-called "armored CAR-T cells" are modified to co-express interleukins, trafficking molecules (chemokines, chemokine receptors), and other effectors that might improve the CAR-T cell performance [67]. Expression of a defective IL-6 receptor capable of sequestering local IL-6 without promoting massive cytokine liberation is an example of an approach to mitigate CAR-T cell-mediated CRS [24].

CRS does not always necessarily accompany CAR cell-mediated neurotoxicity as well as macrophage massive activation. Both immune effector cell-associated syndrome (ICANS) and macrophage activation syndrome (MAS) are associated with a massive expansion of T cells and supraphysiologic cytokine production. ICANS and MAS overlap with many CRS symptoms and consequences; however, neurotoxicity following CAR-T cell therapy might occur even in the absence of CRS [69]. A different mechanism for CAR-mediated neurotoxicity might explain why anti-IL-6 therapy is usually not effective for neurotoxicity and, thus, it is often managed with corticosteroids [70].

### 8.5.3 Graft-Versus-Host Disease

Graft-versus-host disease (GVHD) is a life-threatening condition characterized by the cytotoxic activity of the transferred cells against the host healthy tissues. GVHD is commonly related to the context of allogeneic hematopoietic stem cell transplant (HSCT) [69] and, similarly, is one of the most significant issues of allogeneic T cells. The endogenous TCR on allogeneic T cells may recognize the alloantigens of the recipient, promoting GVHD. Allogeneic T cells are a promising alternative to circumvent some of the drawbacks of autologous T cells, thus having the potential to generate the so-called "off-the-shelf-CAR-T cells" [72].

A modality of adoptive genetically engineered immune cells is the TCR-T cells (TCR-engineered T cells). The idea was initially based on using natural T cells that were specific to intracellular tumor antigens. However, this kind of T cell tends to be naturally rare and small in activity since tumor-associated antigens are often similar to nonmutated versions of self-antigens. Furthermore, there is a natural TCR affinity limit related to avoiding severe cellular autoimmunity. In other words, natural T cells with potential high cytotoxic activity for tumor cells are negatively selected in the thymus. Thus, the TCR-T cells are like CAR cells. Still, instead of having antigen-binding regions from an antibody (VH-VL), TCR-T is genetically modified to express TCR (α and β chains) specific to a defined intracellular tumor target with high affinity [71]. While conventional CARs are restricted to cell-surface proteins in their native conformation, TCR-T cells can recognize intracellular antigens through its peptides presented on MHC molecules.

Despite several examples of efficient application of TCR-T cells [73], the concern is a possibility that the assembly of TCR engineered and endogenous TCR chains would generate self-reactive T cells with mixed TCR dimer, having the potential to lead to GVHD. In addition, it has been demonstrated that high-affinity engineered TCR may also lead to GVHD by cross recognition of self peptide-MHC [74], which corroborates the importance of that thymus' natural function of eliminating high-affinity TCRs.

The most efficient solution to avoid this problem is deleting endogenous TCR chain genes of the adoptive cells with CRISPR-Cas9 gene-editing system. Other genes, either related to further toxicity events or to activity, may also be precisely engineered in a multiplex gene editing approach [72]. Moreover, donor T cells expressing herpes simplex virus thymidine kinase (HSV-tk) suicide gene have long been used to control already established GVHD in the set of HSCT. The nucleoside analog prodrug ganciclovir is phosphorylated by the HSV-tk, forming a compound that inhibits DNA synthesis and, in turn, leads to cell death [77].

## 8.6 Design of New CAR Cells—scFv, VHH, and Other Specificity Domains

CAR configuration consists of an extracellular molecule (responsible for target specificity) coupled to the transmembrane and intracellular regions, responsible for propagating signaling in tumor cells, creating a modular molecular system. Each evolution regarding the intracellular domains rendered a new generation of CAR-T cells.

The display of antibody libraries on phage is a powerful technique to isolate human antibodies for cancer antigens [86]. Ochi et al. constructed an scFv library to produce new anti-CD19 fragments used in CAR-T cell therapy. Their T-cell-based scFv generation system may be of value for optimal tuning of an immunological synapse formed between CAR-T cell and tumoral antigen [15].

Another approach to improve specificity, avidity, and coverage is to construct a CAR with a bispecific, instead of only one scFv, once called TanCAR. A bispecific or biepitopic antibody binds to two different antigens in the same molecule. A proof-of-concept molecule of TanCAR simultaneously binds to CD19 and HER2/neu. It induced distinct T cell reactivity against two target molecules and produced synergistic enhancement of effector functions when both antigens were simultaneously encountered. Unfortunately, bispecifics face obstacles with manufacturing feasibility and some limitations regarding pharmacokinetics and stability [39].

A study aiming at two different BCMA epitope CAR-T cells obtained an overall response rate (ORR) of 82% compared to the BCMA-CAR-T cell in multiple myeloma patients [21]. A second-generation bispecific CAR-T cell containing a fully human anti-BCMA and a humanized anti-CD38 was developed and passed through a phase I clinical trial achieving an ORR of 73%. However, this synergistic binding had shown enhanced cytotoxicity [14].

There are preclinical models of TanCAR targeting HER2 and IL13Rα2 against glioblastoma. These CAR-T cells could be relevant for small-cell and non-small cell lung cancer, colon cancer, and breast cancer. Cotargeting both HER2 and IL13Rα2 results in better tumor control, evidenced by smaller tumor volumes, increased time to tumor progression, and a better ability to eliminate established tumors [8].

Single domain antibodies (nanobodies) are camelid-derived fragments presenting only variable regions of the heavy chain, pursuing the antigen recognition portions. They are suitable in CAR-T cells and have been used in preclinical trials. Xie et al. [20] generated CAR-T cells using a VHH that recognizes EIIIB, a splice variant of fibronectin strongly expressed in both the tumor extracellular matrix and the neovasculature in the tumor microenvironment. Targeting the tumor neovasculature and stroma with EIIIB-targeted CAR-T cells may not only compromise the tumor's blood supply, but it might also be a means for improving tumor accessibility for small-molecule drugs and other therapies that can be used in combination with the CAR-T cells, even if only transiently. A study with VHH-directed-BCMA CAR-T demonstrated safety and efficacy in multiple myeloma patients with no toxicity response presented [7]. An anti-CD47-CAR-T cell showed engagement of the innate immune system, which improved the antitumor effect.Treatment with an anti-CD47 VHH-secreting CAR-T cell enhanced survival over treatment with systemically delivered anti-CD47 VHH along with a CAR-T cell. Localized secretion of VHHs and VHH-Fc fusions by CAR-T cells results in an improved safety profile compared with systemic administration of these antibody derivatives and can contribute to enhanced persistence of CAR-T cells [19].

## 8.7 Future Perspectives

Despite the remaining hurdles, especially related to safety issues, several creative and exciting strategies have been proposed to overcome toxicity adverse events and provide CAR cells with improved therapeutic efficacy and enhanced applicability. CAR-based cell therapy is one of the most cutting-edge achievements in cancer therapy, having great potential to contribute on many other fronts. Virtually all molecular engineering approaches that emerged throughout the still brief and recent history of the different generations of CAR cells illustrate the level of technological inventiveness linked to the field and what is to come.

### 8.7.1 Switchable CAR Cells

Several approaches address either activity or toxicity challenges by precisely controlling CAR cell activation, inhibition, and self-destruction ideally at any time, location, and in a reversible manner. This rather diverse modality of constructions takes advantage of sequential and specific molecular interactions that occur depending either on the administration of an exogenous inducing agent or upon an endogenous molecule, which might be restricted to some tissue or expressed only after a prior signaling event.

Examples of these strategies are the inducible suicide genes, such as HSV-tk [78] and modified caspase 9 (iCasp9), which are used as safety switches to stop unacceptable toxicity by eliminating CAR-T cells [79], and the on-switch CARs, which have receptors that fully assemble or activate only in the presence of a small priming molecule that must be administered to the patient [80].

Combining different signaling events by engineering the adoptive cell with multiple receptors has also modulated CAR cell activity. Inspired by Boolean logic gates, the result of the signaling interaction transduced by both receptors will depend on their design. For example, dual antigen AND-gate CAR-T cells are logic-gated CAR-T cells to overcome the common lack of an antigen exclusively expressed on tumor cells, thereby attenuating "on-target off-tumor" toxicity. Dual AND-gate CAR-T cells are so called because they recognize two different antigens. Their activation depends on the synergy of the two signals transduced by both receptors, preserving healthy cells that express only one of the two antigens [83]. In the case of NOT-gate CAR-T cells, one of the co-expressed CARs recognizes an antigen expressed exclusively in normal cells. It has an inhibitory signaling domain derived from immune-checkpoint proteins [82]. These logic circuits are also explored with the so-called synthetic Notch (synNotch) receptors, which, after recognizing a first antigen, releases a transcriptional regulator that may be involved in the expression of either a CAR that targets a second antigen in an AND-gate manner, for example, or another effector molecule such as a cytokine [81].

### 8.7.2 CAR Cells in Solid Tumors

In addition to the difficulty of finding exclusive tumor antigens, the heterogeneity of solid tumor cell subpopulations and antigen escape tends to lead to refractory and relapsing neoplastic cells that do not express the target and, therefore, are prone to restart the tumor. Furthermore, limited penetrability and immunosuppressive microenvironment are also crucial challenges yet to be overcome so that CAR-T cell therapy becomes safe and efficient for treating solid tumors.

Many of the mentioned switchable, combinatorial multi-antigen and logic-gated signaling strategies have been explored to improve CAR-T cell performance in the context of solid malignancies. A CAR-T cell that is fully activated only after the engagement of a SynNotch receptor specific to a local TME (tumor microenvironment) antigen is one among several examples. Another interesting approach is focused on converting inhibitory signaling mediated by immunosuppressive checkpoint proteins present on TME into co-stimulatory signals. A fusion receptor made of the extracellular PD-1 domain and CD28-transmembrane and intracellular domains demonstrated enhanced activity in the presence of PDL1 in the xenograft model [84].

### 8.7.3 CAR-NK Cells

To overcome some of the intrinsic limitations of CAR-T cells, another promising strategy developed is based on NK cells that express CARs. As well as not inducing CRS, due to a less pro-inflammatory cytokine production profile, NK cells have a much restricted circulating life-span, which is also related to less off-tumor toxicity than CAR-T cells. Furthermore, NK cells can recognize a variety of ligands to naturally chase malignant and infected cells, being rather heterogeneous in the TME of solid malignancies, which can further enhance CAR cells' performance [85].

Since non-MHC-specific receptors mediate NK cell activation, HLA serotype matching is not a requirement, thus allowing allogeneic NK cell application [85]. This opens the door to the development of off-the-shelf products, which could make cell therapy much more accessible, less expensive, and readily available to debilitated patients in need of urgent care.

**Acknowledgments** The authors thank Connie McManus for the English review of the manuscript.

## References

1. Abbott RC, Cross RS, Jenkins MR. Finding the keys to the CAR: identifying novel target antigens for T cell redirection immunotherapies. Int J Mol Sci. 2020;21:515. MDPI AG.
2. Fousek K, Watanabe J, Joseph SK, et al. CAR T-cells that target acute B-lineage leukemia irrespective of CD19 expression. Leukemia. 2021;35(1):75–89. Springer Nature..
3. Gagelmann N, Ayuk F, Atanackovic D, Kröger N. B cell maturation antigen-specific chimeric antigen receptor T cells for relapsed or refractory multiple myeloma: a meta-analysis. Eur J Haematol. 2020;104(4):318–27. Blackwell Publishing Ltd.
4. Golubovskaya V, Berahovich R, Zhou H, et al. CD47-CAR-T cells effectively kill target cancer cells and block pancreatic tumor growth. Cancers. 2017;9:139. MDPI AG.
5. Gu R, Liu F, Zou D, et al. Efficacy and safety of CD19 CAR T constructed with a new anti-CD19 chimeric antigen receptor in relapsed or refractory acute lymphoblastic leukemia. J Hematol Oncol. 2020;13:122. BioMed Central Ltd.
6. Guo Y, Feng K, Tong C, et al. Efficiency and side effects of anti-CD38 CAR T cells in an adult patient with relapsed B-ALL after failure of bi-specific CD19/CD22 CAR T cell treatment. Cell Mol Immunol. 2020;17(4):430–2. Springer Nature.

7. Han L, Zhang JS, Zhou J, et al. Single VHH-directed BCMA CAR-T cells cause remission of relapsed/refractory multiple myeloma. Leukemia. 2021;35(10):3002–6. Springer Nature.
8. Hegde M, Mukherjee M, Grada Z, et al. Tandem CAR T cells targeting HER2 and IL13Rα2 mitigate tumor antigen escape. J Clin Investig. 2016;126(8):3036–52. American Society for Clinical Investigation.
9. Hyrenius-Wittsten A, Roybal KT. Paving new roads for CARs. Trends in Cancer:1–10. Elsevier Inc. 2019. Available from: https://doi.org/10.1016/j.trecan.2019.09.005.
10. Jackson HJ, Rafiq S, Brentjens RJ. Driving CAR T-cells forward. Nat Rev Clin Oncol. 2016;13(6):370–83. Nat Publ GroupNature Publishing Group.
11. Kang CH, Kim Y, Lee HK, et al. Identification of potent cd19 scFv for CAR T cells through scfv screening with NK/T-cell line. Int J Mol Sci. 2020;21(23):1–12. MDPI AG.
12. Kriegsmann K, Kriegsmann M, Cremer M, et al. Cell-based immunotherapy approaches for multiple myeloma. Br J Cancer. 2019;120(1):38–44. Nat Publ GroupNature Publishing Group.
13. Lorentzen CL, Straten PT. CD19-chimeric antigen receptor T cells for treatment of chronic lymphocytic leukaemia and acute lymphoblastic leukaemia. Scand J Immunol. 2015;82(4):307–19. Blackwell Publishing Ltd.
14. Mei H, Li C, Jiang H, et al. A bispecific CAR-T cell therapy targeting BCMA and CD38 in relapsed or refractory multiple myeloma. J Hematol Oncol. 2021;14(1):161. Available from: https://jhoonline.biomedcentral.com/articles/10.1186/s13045-021-01170-7.
15. Ochi T, Maruta M, Tanimoto K, et al. A single-chain antibody generation system yielding CAR-T cells with superior anti-tumor function. Commun Biol. 2021;4:273. Nature Research.
16. Rodríguez-Otero P, Prósper F, Alfonso A, Paiva B, San Miguel JF. Car T-cells in multiple myeloma are ready for prime time. J Clin Med. 2020;9(3577):1–16. MDPI.
17. Strobel SB, Machiraju D, Hülsmeyer I, et al. Expression of potential targets for cell-based therapies on melanoma cells. Life. 2021;11:269. MDPI AG.
18. Wei J, Han X, Bo J, Han W. Target selection for CAR-T therapy. J Hematol Oncol. 2019;12:62. BioMed Central Ltd.
19. Xie YJ, Dougan M, Ingram JR, et al. Improved anti-tumor efficacy of chimeric antigen receptor T cells that secrete single-domain antibody fragments. Cancer Immunol Res. 2020;8(4):518–29. American Association for Cancer Research Inc.
20. Xie YJ, Dougan M, Jailkhani N, et al. Nanobody-based CAR T cells that target the tumor microenvironment inhibit the growth of solid tumors in immunocompetent mice. Proc Natl Acad Sci U S A. 2019;116(16):7624–31. National Academy of Sciences.

21. Xu JIE, Chen LJ, Yang SS, et al. Exploratory trial of a biepitopic CAR T-targeting B cell maturation antigen in relapsed/refractory multiple myeloma. Proc Natl Acad Sci U S A. 2019;116(19):9543–51. National Academy of Sciences.
22. Ying Z, Huang XF, Xiang X, et al. A safe and potent anti-CD19 CAR T cell therapy. Nat Med. 2019;25(6):947–53. Nat Publ GroupNature Publishing Group.
23. Hwang J-R, Byeon Y, Kim D, Park S-G. Recent insights of T cell receptor-mediated signaling pathways for T cell activation and development. Exp Mol Med. 2020. Springer Science and Business Media LLC.;52(5):750–61. https://doi.org/10.1038/s12276-020-0435-8.
24. Chen P-H, Lipschitz M, Weirather JL, Jacobson C, Armand P, Wright K, Hodi FS, Roberts ZJ, Sievers SA, Rossi J. Activation of CAR and non-CAR T cells within the tumor microenvironment following CAR T cell therapy. JCI Insight. 2020. American Society for Clinical Investigation. PMID: 32484797; PMCID: PMC7406247.;5(12):1–12. https://doi.org/10.1172/jci.insight.134612.
25. Blache U, Weiss R, Boldt A, Kapinsky M, Blaudszun AR, Quaiser A, Pohl A, Miloud T, Burgaud M, Vucinic V, Platzbecker U, Sack U, Fricke S, Koehl U. Advanced flow cytometry assays for immune monitoring of CAR-T cell applications. Front Immunol. 2021;12:658314. https://doi.org/10.3389/fimmu.2021.658314.
26. Liu D, Badeti S, Dotti G, Jiang J-G, Wang H, Dermody J, Soteropoulos P, Streck D, Birge RB, Liu C. The role of immunological synapse in predicting the efficacy of chimeric antigen receptor (CAR) immunotherapy. Cell Commun Signal. 2020. 25 ago. Springer Science and Business Media LLC.;18(1):1–20. https://doi.org/10.1186/s12964-020-00617-7.
27. Abate-Daga D, Davila ML. CAR models: next-generation CAR modifications for enhanced T-cell function. Mol Ther Oncolytics. 2016;3:16014.
28. Alabanza L, Pegues M, Geldres C, Shi V, Wiltzius JJW, Sievers SA, et al. Function of novel anti-CD19 chimeric antigen receptors with human variable regions is affected by hinge and transmembrane domains. Mol Ther. 2017;25(11):2452–65.
29. Boomer JS, Green JM. An enigmatic tail of CD28 signaling. Cold Spring Harb Perspect Biol. 2010;2:8.
30. Boucher JC, Li G, Kotani H, et al. CD28 costimulatory domain–targeted mutations enhance chimeric antigen receptor T-cell function. Cancer Immunol Res. 2021;9:62–74.
31. Brentjens RJ, Rivière I, Park JH, Davila ML, Wang X, Stefanski J, Taylor C, Yeh R, Bartido S, Borquez-Ojeda O. Safety and persistence of adoptively transferred autologous CD19-targeted T cells in patients with relapsed or chemotherapy refractory B-cell leukemias. Blood. 2011;118:4817–28.
32. Cartellieri M, et al. Chimeric antigen receptor-engineered T cells for immunotherapy of cancer. J Biomed Biotechnol. 2010;2010:956304.

33. Caruso HG, Hurton LV, Najjar A, et al. Tuning sensitivity of CAR to EGFR density limits recognition of normal tissue while maintaining potent antitumour activity. Cancer Res. 2015;75(17):3505–18. American Association for Cancer Research Inc.
34. Chmielewski M, Abken H. TRUCKS, the fourth-generation CAR T cells: current developments and clinical translation. Adv Cell Gene Ther. 2020;3:e84.
35. Chmielewski M, Hombach A, Heuser C, Adams GP, Abken H. T cell activation by antibody-like immunoreceptors: increase in affinity of the single-chain fragment domain above threshold does not increase T cell activation against antigen-positive target cells but decreases selectivity. J Immunol. 2004;173:7647–53. American Association of Immunologists Inc.
36. Cho JH, Collins JJ, Wong WW. Universal chimeric antigen receptors for multiplexed and logical control of T cell responses. Cell. 2018;173(6):1426–38.
37. Chu F, Cao J, Neelalpu SS. Versatile CAR T-cells for cancer immunotherapy. Contemp Oncol (Pozn). 2018;22:73–80.
38. Fos C, Salles A, Lang V, Carrette F, Audebert S, Pastor S, Ghiotto M, Olive D, Bismuth G, Nunès JA. ICOS ligation recruits the p50alpha PI3K regulatory subunit to the immunological synapse. J Immunol. 2008;181(3):1969–77.
39. Grada Z, Hegde M, Byrd T, Shaffer DR, Ghazi A, Brawley VS, Corder A, Schönfeld K, Koch J, Dotti G. TanCAR: a novel bispecific chimeric antigen receptor for cancer immunotherapy. Mol Ther Nucleic Acids. 2013;2:7.
40. Guedan S, Calderon H, Posey AD Jr, Maus MV. Engineering and design of chimeric antigen receptors. Mol Ther Methods Clin Dev. 2018;12:145–56.
41. Guedan S, Chen X, Madar A, Carpenito C, Mcgettigan SE, Frigault MJ, Lee J, Posey AD Jr, Scholler J, Scholler N, Bonneau R, June CH. ICOS-based chimeric antigen receptors program bipolar TH17/TH1 cells. Blood. 2014;124(7):1070–80.
42. Guedan S, Madar A, Casado-Medrano V, Shaw C, Wing A, Liu F, Young RM, June CH, Posey AD Jr. Single residue in CD28-costimulated CAR-T cells limits long-term persistence and anti-tumor durability. J Clin Invest. 2020;130(6):3087–97.
43. Guedan S, Posey AD, Shaw C, Wing A, Da T, Patel PR, et al. Enhancing CAR T cell persistence through ICOS and 4-1BB costimulation. JCI Insight. 2018;3:1.
44. Han D, et al. Current progress in CAR-T cell therapy for hematological malignancies. J Cancer. 2021;12(2):326–34.
45. Hombach AA, Heiders J, Foppe M, Chmielewski M, Abken H. OX40 costimulation by a chimeric antigen receptor abrogates CD28 and IL-2

induced IL-10 secretion by redirected CD4(+) T cells. Oncoimmunology. 2012;1(4):458–66.
46. Kloss CC, Condomines M, Cartellieri M, Bachmann M, Sadelain M. Combinatorial antigen recognition with balanced signaling promotes selective tumor eradication by engineered T cells. Nat Biotechnol. 2013;31(1):71–5.
47. Liu X, Jiang S, Fang C, Yang S, Olalere D, Pequignot EC, Cogdill AP, Li N, Ramones M, Granda B. Affinity-tuned ErbB2 or EGFR chimeric antigen receptor T cells exhibit an increased therapeutic index against tumors in mice. Cancer Res. 2015;75:3596–607.
48. Milone MC, Fish JD, Carpenito C, Carroll RG, Binder GK, Teachey D, Samanta M, Lakhal M, Gloss B, Danet-Desnoyers G, Campana D, Riley JL, Grupp SA, June CH. Chimeric receptors containing CD137 signal transduction domains mediate enhanced survival of T cells and increased antileukemic efficacy in vivo. Mol Ther. 2009;17(8):1453–64.
49. Song DG, Ye Q, Poussin M, Harms GM, Figini M, Powell DJ Jr. CD27 costimulation augments the survival and anti-tumor activity of redirected human T cells in vivo. Blood. 2012;119(3):696–706.
50. Wang E, Wang LC, Tsai CY, Bhoj V, Gershenson Z, Moon E, Newick K, Sun J, Lo A, Baradet T, Feldman MD, Barrett D, Puré E, Albelda S, Milone MC. Generation of potent T-cell immunotherapy for cancer using DAP12-based, multichain, chimeric immunoreceptors. Cancer Immunol Res. 2015;3(7):815–26.
51. Watanabe N, Bajgain P, Sukumaran S, Ansari S, Heslop HE, Rooney CM, et al. Fine-tuning the CAR spacer improves T-cell potency. OncoImmunology. 2016;5:12.
52. Watts TH. TNF/TNFR family members in costimulation of T cell responses. Annu Rev Immunol. 2005;23:23–68.
53. Wu CY, Roybal KT, Puchner EM, Onuffer J, Lim WA. Remote control of therapeutic T cells through a small molecule-gated chimeric receptor. Science. 2015;350:6248.
54. Zhao J, Lin Q, Song Y, Liu D. Universal CARs, universal T cells, and universal CAR T cells. J Hematol Oncol. 2018;11:1–9.
55. Zhong XS, Matsushita M, Plotkin J, Riviere I, Sadelain M. Chimeric antigen receptors combining 4-1BB and CD28 signaling domains augment PI3kinase/AKT/Bcl-XL activation and CD8+ T cell-mediated tumor eradication. Mol Ther. 2010;18:413–20.
56. OSHU Knight Cancer Institute: CAR T-cell therapy for cancer 2021. Accesses 22 Oct 2021. https://www.ohsu.edu/knight-cancer-institute/car-t-cell-therapy-cancer.
57. Immunotherapy side effects: CAR T-cell therapy. National Comprehensive Cancer Center. 2020. Accessed 22 Oct 2021. https://www.nccn.org/patients/guidelines/content/PDF/immunotherapy-se-car-tcell-patient.pdf.
58. Maude SL, Frey N, Shaw PA, Aplenc R, Barrett DM, Bunin NJ, Chew A, Gonzalez VE, Zheng Z, Lacey SF, Mahnke YD, Melenhorst JJ, Rheingold

SR, Shen A, Teachey DT, Levine BL, June CH, Porter DL, Grupp SA. Chimeric antigen receptor T cells for sustained remissions in leukemia. N Engl J Med. 2014;371(16):1507–17.
59. Morgan RA, Yang JC, Kitano M, et al. Case report of a serious adverse event following the administration of T cells transduced with a chimeric antigen receptor recognizing ERBB2. Mol Ther. 2010;18:843–51.
60. Lamers CHJ, Sleijfer S, Van Steenbergen S, Van Elzakker P, Van Krimpen B, Groot C, Vulto A, Den Bakker M, Oosterwijk E, Debets R, Gratama JW. Treatment of metastatic renal cell carcinoma with CAIX CAR-engineered T cells: clinical evaluation and management of on-target toxicity. Mol Ther. 2013;21(4):904–13.
61. Steentoft C, et al. Glycan-directed CAR-T cells. Glycobiology. 2018;28:656–69.
62. Murad JP, et al. Effective targeting of TAG72+ peritoneal ovarian tumors via regional delivery of CAR-engineered T cells. Front Immunol. 2018;9:2268.
63. Cai C, Tang D, Han Y, Shen E, Ahmed OA, Guo C, Shen H, Zeng S. A comprehensive analysis of the fatal toxic effects associated with CD19 CAR-T cell therapy. Aging (Albany NY). 2020;12(18):18741–53. https://doi.org/10.18632/aging.104058. Epub ahead of print. PMID: 32973124; PMCID: PMC7585129.
64. Sterner RC, Sterner RM. CAR-T cell therapy: current limitations and potential strategies. Blood Cancer J. 2021;11:69. https://doi.org/10.1038/s41408-021-00459-7.
65. Santomasso BD, et al. Clinical and biological correlates of neurotoxicity associated with CAR T-cell therapy in patients with B-cell acute lymphoblastic leukemia. Cancer Discov. 2018;8:958–71.
66. Lee DW, et al. Current concepts in the diagnosis and management of cytokine release syndrome. Blood. 2014;124:188–95.
67. Park JH, Palomba ML, Batlevi CL, Riviere I, Wang X, Senechal B, Furman RR, Bernal Y, Hall M, Pineda J, Diamonte C, Halton E, Brentjens RJ, Sadelain M. A phase I first-in-human clinical trial of CD19-targeted 19-28z/4-1BBL "armored" CAR T cells in patients with relapsed or refractory NHL and CLL including Richter's transformation. Blood. 2018;132(1 Suppl):224.
68. Salter AI, et al. Phosphoproteomic analysis of chimeric antigen receptor signaling reveals kinetic and quantitative differences that affect cell function. Sci Signal. 2018;11:544.
69. Brudno JN, Kochenderfer JN. Toxicities of chimeric antigen receptor T cells: recognition and management. Blood. 2016;127(26):3321–30. https://doi.org/10.1182/blood-2016-04-703751. Epub 2016 May 20. PMID: 27207799; PMCID: PMC4929924.
70. Davila ML, et al. Efficacy and toxicity management of 19-28z CAR T cell therapy in B cell acute lymphoblastic leukemia. Sci Transl Med. 2014;6:224ra25.

71. Bendle GM, Linnemann C, Hooijkaas AI, Bies L, De Witte MA, Jorritsma A, Kaiser ADM, Pouw N, Debets R, Kieback E, Uckert W, Song JY, Haanen JBAG, Schumacher TNM. Lethal graft-versus-host disease in mouse models of T cell receptor gene therapy. Nat Med. 2010;16(5):565–70.
72. Ren J, Liu X, Fang C, Jiang S, June CH, Zhao Y. Multiplex genome editing to generate universal CAR T cells resistant to PD1 inhibition. Clin Cancer Res. 2017;23(9):2255–66.
73. Zhang J, Wang L. The emerging world of TCR-T cell trials against cancer: a systematic review. Technol Cancer Res Treat. 2019;18:1–13.
74. Holler PD, Chlewicki LK, Kranz DM. TCRs with high affinity for foreign pMHC show self-reactivity. Nat Immunol. 2003;4(1):55–62.
75. Chmielewski M, Abken H. TRUCKs: the fourth generation of CARs. Expert Opin Biol Ther. 2015;15(8):1145–54. https://doi.org/10.1517/14712598.2015.1046430.
76. Lima SCG, Fantacini DMC, Batista LC, Silveira RM, Furtado IP, Rossetti R, Brand H, Covas DT, de Souza LEB. Strategies to enhance the therapeutic efficacy, applicability, and safety of genetically engineered immune cells. Crit Rev Immunol. 2021;41(1):41–67. https://doi.org/10.1615/CritRevImmunol.2021037437.
77. Ciceri F, Bonini C, Marktel S, Zappone E, Servida P, Bernardi M, et al. Anti-tumor effects of HSV-TK-engineered donor lymphocytes after allogeneic stem-cell transplantation. Blood. 2007;109(11):4698–707.
78. Casucci M, Falcone L, Camisa B, Norelli M, Porcellini S, Stornaiuolo A, et al. Extracellular NGFR spacers allow efficient tracking and enrichment of fully functional CAR-T cells co-expressing a suicide gene. Front Immunol. 2018;9:507.
79. Gargett T, Brown MP. The inducible caspase-9 suicide gene system as a "safety switch" to limit on-target, off-tumor toxicities of chimeric antigen receptor T cells. Front Pharmacol. 2014;5:235.
80. Juillerat A, Marechal A, Filhol JM, Valton J, Duclert A, Poirot L, et al. Design of chimeric antigen receptors with integrated controllable transient functions. Sci Rep. 2016;6:18950.
81. Roybal KT, Williams JZ, Morsut L, Rupp LJ, Kolinko I, Choe JH, et al. Engineering T cells with customized therapeutic response programs using synthetic notch receptors. Cell. 2016;167(2):419–432.e416.
82. Fedorov VD, Themeli M, Sadelain M. PD-1- and CTLA-4-based inhibitory chimeric antigen receptors (iCARs) divert off-target immunotherapy responses. Sci Transl Med. 2013;5(215):215ra172.
83. Wilkie S, Van Schalkwyk MCI, Hobbs S, Davies DM, Van der Stegen SJC, Pereira ACP, Burbridge SE, Box C, Eccles SA, Maher J. Dual targeting of ErbB2 and MUC1 in breast cancer using chimeric antigen receptors engineered to provide complementary signaling. J Clin Immunol. 2012;32(5):1059–70.

84. Kobold S, Grassmann S, Chaloupka M, Lampert C, Wenk S, Kraus F, Rapp M, Düwell P, Zeng Y, Schmollinger JC, Schnurr M, Endres S, Rothenfußer S. Impact of a new fusion receptor on PD-1-mediated immunosuppression in adoptive T cell therapy. J Natl Cancer Inst. 2015;107(8):djv146.
85. Marofi F, Al-Awad AS, Sulaiman Rahman H, Markov A, Abdelbasset WK, Ivanovna Enina Y, Mahmoodi M, et al. CAR-NK cell: a new paradigm in tumor immunotherapy. Front Oncol. 2021;11:art. no. 673276.
86. Leyton-Castro NF, Brígido MM, Maranhão AQ. Selection of Antibody Fragments for CAR-T Cell Therapy from Phage Display Libraries. In: Swiech K, Malmegrim KCR, Picanço-Castro V, organizators. Chimeric Antigen Receptor T Cells - Development and Production. São Paulo: Springer; 2020. p. 13–26.

# Intrathecal Chemotherapy 9

Breno Magalhães Gomes

## 9.1 Introduction

Improvements in the treatment of leukemia and solid malignant tumors had a positive impact on overall disease-free survival with the results of new studies. However, there is currently an increase in the incidence of diseases with recurrence in the leptomeninges. This condition was first reported in childhood with acute lymphoblastic leukemia [1] and consequently has been observed in a variety of nonhematological malignancies, most common in solid tumors with lung cancer, breast cancer, ovarian cancer, melanoma, and gastrointestinal cancer [2]. The understanding of the central nervous system (CNS) as a unique site, where blood tissue is extremely filtered, protected from the effects of systemic administration of chemotherapy has resulted in the development of therapeutic strategies specifically directed to leptomeninges, including cranial or craniospinal irradiation, high-dose systemic chemotherapy, and intrathecal chemotherapy [3].

These therapeutic protocols, alone or in combination, have been reflected in successful outcomes in the prevention and treatment of CNS leukemia [4]. However, effective treatment options for patients with neoplastic spread of solid tumors or for patients

B. M. Gomes (✉)
Fortaleza, Ceara, Brazil



C. W. P. Schmidt, K. M. Otoni (eds.), *The Golden Guide to Oncologic Pharmacy*, https://doi.org/10.1007/978-3-030-98596-7_9

with recurrent CNS leukemia are very limited or nonexistent in part due to the small number of chemotherapeutic agents available for safe intrathecal administration. It is evident that new intrathecal drugs and intrathecal drug combinations must be developed for patients in these poor prognostic groups [5].

Intrathecal chemotherapy is a form of cancer treatment in which a healthcare professional injects chemotherapy drugs into the cerebrospinal fluid. This colorless fluid surrounds the brain and spinal cord, which form the central nervous system (CNS), to protect them from injuries. A doctor might recommend intrathecal chemotherapy if cancer affects the CNS [6].

During intrathecal chemotherapy, a healthcare professional will administer the chemotherapy drugs into the fluid around the spinal cord during a lumbar puncture or spinal tap. The person will usually receive a local anesthetic before the healthcare professional inserts a needle into the spinal area [3, 7].

In the intrathecal route, the drug is administered in the fluid around the spinal cord, and in the epidural route, the drug is administered in the space around the spinal cord; therefore, because they are different routes, each item is displaced at a different point [3].

One measure of CNS exposure to administered chemotherapy would be the ratio of steady-state concentration or the area under the concentration–time curve in cerebrospinal fluid (CSF) compared to plasma. The CSF exposure of most commonly used anticancer agents is less than 10% of the plasma exposure [8].

The reason for using this therapeutic strategy is that a protective layer called the blood–brain barrier surrounds the CNS. This barrier allows nutrients and oxygen to enter the brain, preventing the entry of toxins and harmful substances. The blood–brain barrier also blocks the passage of oral or intravenous cancer drugs, making them much less effective [9].

So the goal of intrathecal chemotherapy is to maximize CNS drug exposure in the CSF while reducing or eliminating systemic drug toxicity. Intrathecal administration of anticancer agents via the intralumbar route or the intraventricular route is successful with the fact that the CSF volume of distribution is much smaller than that of plasma (140 vs. 3500 ml); however, a drug with a high concentration can be reached in the CSF using a lower dose [10,

11]. In fact, the terminal half-life of most drugs is longer in CSF than in plasma. This prolonged exposure to the drug in the CSF is quite important for specific cell cycle agents, such as some cytostatic agents including methotrexate and cytarabine [12]. Even with the pharmacological advantages of using intrathecal chemotherapy, there are some disadvantages; for example, intralumbar drug administration can be associated with inconvenience and pain, radioisotope studies have shown that in up to 10% of lumbar punctures, drug use can be inadvertently administered in the epidural or subdural space, rather than the intended subarachnoid space, and drug distribution within the neuraxis after intralumbar infusion may not be homogeneous as it varies with CSF bulk flow and patient position and following intrathecal drug administration, penetration into tissue is minimal, thereby limiting potential efficacy in patients who have bulky leptomeningeal or parenchymal tumors [13, 14].

The manifestations of neoplastic meningitis vary according to each individual, which prevents recommendations for a single treatment approach; that is, there is no way to standardize this type of treatment. Essential factors to consider when taking a specific treatment recommended for an individual patient include the histology of the underlying primary malignancy, the patient's age, previous history of targeted CNS therapy, the extent of the leptomeningeal, and the underlying systemic disease and the dynamics of the LCR flow [15].

The American Cancer Society notes that healthcare professionals may also administer the chemotherapy drugs through a long-term catheter and port that sits under the skin on the head. The port is called an Ommaya reservoir [16].

The Ommaya reservoir has a small tube attached that enters the CSF through a cavity in the brain. A healthcare professional will remove the port once the person has completed their treatment [17].

## 9.2 Procedures

The preparation of the patient for the intrathecal chemotherapy procedure must be planned in advance, and the patient needs to be informed about all the risks. After the doubts are clarified, the patient will need to give informed consent for the treatment to proceed. The keywords for this consultation would be lumbar puncture, chemotherapy treatment, what the treatment involves, the risks, and side effects of intrathecal chemotherapy [6, 18].

Intrathecal chemotherapy can be administered in three different ways.

### 9.2.1 Lumbar Puncture

This procedure involves a doctor inserting a needle into the spinal canal and injecting the drug into the CSF between two vertebrae at the bottom of the spine.

Before a person has a lumbar puncture, they will have laboratory tests to make sure they have enough platelets for their blood to clot effectively afterward.

If platelet levels are sufficient, the person will either lie on their side (fetal position) or sit with their head and chest resting on a surface to expose their spine. A doctor or nurse will administer a local anesthetic to numb the area. The individual may feel some pressure, but the procedure is usually not painful [18–20].

The treatment takes about 20 minutes. The person will need to remain immobile for 1 hour or more to allow the drug to move through the CSF [7].

### 9.2.2 Ommaya Reservoir

A healthcare provider may recommend the placement of an Ommaya reservoir if a person needs multiple intrathecal chemotherapy treatments. This door will provide the healthcare team with safe, repeatable access to the LCR.

An Ommaya reservoir is a small plastic device that the surgeon places under the scalp. It connects to a catheter tube that allows the drug to reach an open area in the brain where there is CSF.

When a doctor injects a chemotherapy drug into the reservoir, it moves into the CSF without the doctor having to administer a lumbar puncture each time. It also allows the doctor to take CSF samples from the person to monitor how well the treatment is going. Furthermore, since CSF flow proceeds in a ventricular-lumbar direction, distribution throughout the neuraxis may be more uniform than after intralumbar administration. The disadvantage of an intraventricular device is that placement requires a neurosurgical procedure. With catheter placement, there is also the potential risk of infection or obstruction of the catheter. Thus, the use of intraventricular catheters is generally reserved for patients with recurrent CNS leukemia or for the treatment of neoplastic meningitis due to solid tumors [17].

### 9.2.3 Intralumbar Catheter

Another method of intrathecal drug administration involves the use of an intralumbar catheter connected to a reservoir with implanted access to a subcutaneous device. The prosaic advantage of subcutaneously implanted lumbar catheters is that, like Ommaya reservoirs, drug delivery to the CSF is guaranteed, but it also shares the same disadvantages as the risk of infections. But there is still not enough experience in cancer patients, either with regard to the feasibility of maintaining long-term catheter patency or in relation to the potential long-term complications of these devices. Thus, the use of such devices is generally limited to patients with overt neoplastic meningitis who, for a variety of reasons, may refuse the placement of an Ommaya reservoir or an intralumbar catheter, even though the patient prefers additional therapy without the associated pain and the inconvenience of repeated sessions with lumbar perforations [21].

## 9.3 Dosage

According to Bleyer's studies that were instrumental in demonstrating the dose for intrathecal administration, medications should be based on the patient's age and not on body size or surface area. In pediatrics, children and adolescents grow, increasing much faster in CSF volume than in body surface area (BSA) [14].

An interesting result would be that at age three the adult and child CSF volumes are equivalent. Because there is no correlation between CSF volume and BSA, there is no consistent relationship between drug dose and CSF concentration if the dose is based on BSA. In contrast, age-based dosing provides more uniform CSF drug concentrations. After implementing age-based intrathecal methotrexate dosing for methotrexate, neurotoxicity in adults and adolescents decreased, as did CNS relapse rates for younger children and infants with leukemia. Age-based dosing regimens for chemotherapeutic agents are often used [6, 14].

Patient position may affect drug exposure following intrathecal delivery. Pharmacokinetic studies in nonhuman primates kept in a flat or upright position for one hour following intralumbar methotrexate administration showed that the distribution of the drug was better in animals that were consistently maintained in the flat versus the upright position [22]. There was also less variability in the ventricular methotrexate concentrations in animals maintained in the prone position. In addition, peak ventricular methotrexate drug concentrations and drug exposure were consistently higher in animals that were kept prone. Therefore, it appears that uniformity of CSF drug distribution can be improved by maintaining patients in a prone position for at least 1 h after intralumbar drug administration [18].

A variety of circumstances can affect CSF drug release. As an example, delayed release of intrathecal methotrexate has been documented in conditions that interfere with CSF flow; another example is the presence of neoplastic meningitis, segregated from the CSF from CSF flow or communicating hydrocephalus [2]. When there is a delay in drug clearance, it can lead to increased neurotoxicity, so it is essential to recognize conditions that may impede drug elimination [22]. Studies have shown that CSF flow in patients with leptomeningeal spread of solid tumors may reflect marked changes in flow dynamics without evidence of obstruction or other flow abnormality on computed tomography or magnetic resonance imaging. Therefore, radionuclide flux in CSF studies (e.g., 111In-DTPA) should be strongly considered before starting intrathecal therapy in all patients with neoplastic meningitis due to a solid tumor picture, as well as when clinically indicated in patients with leukemia of the CNS [23]. If there is evidence of obstruction of the CSF flow, an attempt to alleviate the obstruction with local radiation recommended prior to initiating intrathecal drug therapy should be considered as an alternative [24].

The presence of a ventriculoperitoneal (VP) or ventriculoatrial (VA) shunt may also create difficulty in the use of intrathecal chemotherapy. In contrast to patients who are at increased risk of toxicity from delayed drug clearance, patients with functioning VP or VA shunts may be at risk of inadequate drug exposure if the drug is rapidly cleared from the CSF space by the shunt (in essence, defeating the attempt at regional therapy). The use of an on–off valve in the shunt may circumvent this problem. However, caution must be utilized in assessing a patient's tolerance to having the shunt closed for an extended period of time. In addition, the optimal duration for shunt closure after intrathecal dosing is not known [25].

## 9.4 Standard Cytostatic Agents for Intrathecal Administration

There are few effective chemotherapeutic agents that are currently available for intrathecal delivery. Methotrexate and cytarabine, administered either alone or in combination with hydrocortisone or dexamethasone, are extensively utilized for the treatment and prevention of leptomeningeal leukemia or lymphoma. However, the role of these agents in the treatment of solid tumors is limited because they have a restricted spectrum of antitumor activity [26–27].

The use of these glucocorticoids maintains the stability of the combined drugs, even if, according to stability studies, it is recommended for immediate use after preparation. The safe order of homogenization would be to intersperse the two cytostatics with the available glucocorticoid in order to avoid incompatibility. This concomitant use has two objectives: increasing the effectiveness of IT therapy and reducing the incidence of meningeal irritation. In some services, drugs are delivered separately and homogenized at the time of administration. Thus, there is a risk of exposure to cytostatic by professionals involved in the administration [28, 29].

## 9.5 Methotrexate

Intralumbar methotrexate, either as a single agent or in combination with cytarabine and hydrocortisone or dexamethasone, is the most commonly used drug for the prevention and treatment of CNS leukemia. As outlined above, improvements in both the efficacy and toxicity profiles of this agent are a direct result of age-based dosing. Elimination of methotrexate from the CSF is biphasic with terminal half-lives of 4.5 and 14 h. Clearance is primarily by bulk CSF resorption, although a nonspecific transport system has also been identified. Mean methotrexate levels in the lumbar CSF exceed 10 mM at 6 h and are approximately 0.1 mM at 48 h [14]. Ventricular CSF methotrexate concentrations after an intralumbar dose can be quite variable and are approximately only 10% of the simultaneous lumbar CSF levels. Administration of methotrexate via the intraventricular route, rather than the intralumbar route, should be considered for patients who have refractory or recurrent CNS leukemia. As previously discussed, direct intraventricular administration of methotrexate provides higher and more consistent ventricular CSF methotrexate concentrations than intralumbar dosing, although interpatient variability still occurs [30]. Ventricular access devices such as Ommaya reservoirs permit greater flexibility in dosing schedules. These devices facilitate drug administration using the "concentration times time" (C × T) approach, which involves the administration of frequent small doses of methotrexate and/or cytarabine. "C × T" therapy results in increased duration of CSF exposure to cytotoxic drug concentrations while avoiding excessively high peak concentrations and results in the delivery of a lower total cumulative methotrexate dose over time. Since methotrexate-associated neurotoxicity has been correlated with both high concentrations and total dose, the "C × T" approach provides a means of simultaneously increasing potential efficacy and decreasing toxicity [17]. Moser et al. recently reported that "C × T" methotrexate alternated with "C × T" cytarabine provided a sustained complete response (median duration 15 month) in 14 of 15 patients with recurrent CSF leukemia or lymphoma [31].

Systemic toxicity is usually minimal after intralumbar methotrexate because plasma exposure is approximately 100-fold less than CSF exposure. However, systemic exposure after intrathecal methotrexate is prolonged relative to an equivalent intravenous dose, with plasma levels of methotrexate above 0.01 mM for twice as long after the intrathecal dose compared with the intravenous dose. Potential neurotoxicities after intrathecal methotrexate are generally categorized as acute, subacute, or late. Acute toxicity, i.e., toxicity that occurs within days of drug administration, is the most commonly observed toxicity after intrathecal methotrexate. Acute toxicity presents as a chemical arachnoiditis, with symptoms of headache, nuchal rigidity, back pain, vomiting, fever, and CSF pleocytosis. Subacute toxicities may occur within days to weeks of intrathecal methotrexate administration. Rarely, patients develop reversible or irreversible paraplegia, myelopathy, or encephalopathy characterized by limb weakness, ataxia, cranial nerve palsies, visual impairment, seizures, or coma. Late (chronic) neurotoxicity, or leukoencephalopathy, may occur months to years after treatment and is most common after combined modality therapy with craniospinal irradiation and intrathecal methotrexate [30, 32]. The pathophysiology of methotrexate-induced neurotoxicity is an ongoing focus of clinical and laboratory research. Predominant theories, based on methotrexate-induced alterations in folate metabolic pathways, include adenosine accumulation in the CNS; perturbations of biopterin recycling with resultant impairment in dopamine and serotonin synthesis; and CNS homocysteine accumulation with the production of sulfur-containing excitatory amino acids. Elucidation of the etiology of the specific mechanism(s) of methotrexate-induced neurotoxicity will facilitate the development of preventative measures or antidotes. Preliminary studies of aminophylline as an antidote for adenosine-mediated toxicity have met with encouraging results [33].

Acute life-threatening neurotoxicity may occur after an inadvertent methotrexate overdose. Treatment for such a catastrophic event may include immediate CSF drainage, ventriculolumbar perfusion, systemic leucovorin administration, and systemic administration of steroids, although these measures are often ineffective. A more specific antidote is carboxypeptidase-G2, an enzyme that hydrolyzes methotrexate to an inactive metabolite. In nonhuman primate studies, administration of carboxypeptidase-G2 resulted in a more than a 400-fold decrease in CSF methotrexate concentrations within 5 min of carboxypeptidase administration. Carboxypeptidase-G2 is available to all pediatric cooperative group institutions in the United States and should be used in the acute management of this medical emergency. The potential benefit of this agent is greatest if administered immediately after recognition of the overdose. Therefore, it is recommended that the institutional hospital or clinic pharmacy have carboxypeptidase-G2 available if needed for immediate use [31].

## 9.6 Cytarabine

The antimetabolite cytarabine (Ara-C, cytosine arabinoside) is the second most commonly used agent for intrathecal administration. Cytarabine is primarily utilized in the treatment of CNS leukemias and lymphomas. A prospective randomized study with intrathecal methotrexate versus intrathecal methotrexate plus cytarabine demonstrated that the addition of cytarabine did not appear to improve results [34]. As with methotrexate, optimal dosing is based on age rather than body surface area. Elimination of cytarabine from CSF is biphasic with half-lives of 1 and 3.4 h. Peak CSF concentrations exceed 2 mM following a 30-mg intraventricular dose and remain above 1 mM for greater than 24 h. Plasma concentrations of cytarabine after an intraventricular dose are not detectable, minimizing the potential for systemic toxicity [35]. Unlike systemically administered cytarabine, which is rapidly converted to the inactive metabolite, ara-U, by cytidine deaminase, there is negligible conversion to ara-U after intrathecal dosing because there are extremely low levels of cytidine deaminase in the brain and CSF. As a result, the half-life of cytarabine is prolonged in CSF versus plasma, and clearance is similar to bulk CSF flow at a rate of 0.42 ml/min. As with methotrexate, an intraventricular access device facilitates cytarabine administration using the "C × T" approach. In a pharmacokinetic simulation of intrathecal cytarabine (30 mg) given daily for three days, cytotoxic concentrations are maintained for 72 h, compared to approximately 24 h after a single intraventricular 70-mg dose [31].

The most common toxicity associated with intrathecal cytarabine, like methotrexate, is a chemical arachnoiditis. Other observed, but less common, toxicities include seizures, transient paraplegia, peripheral neuropathy, myelopathy, and encephalopathy [35].

## 9.7 DepoCyt® (DTC101)

A liposomal formulation DTC101 is a sustained release formulation of cytarabine for intrathecal administration that has received US Food and Drug Administration approval for the treatment of lymphomatous meningitis in adult patients [36]. Because cytarabine is a cell-cycle specific agent, prolonged exposure to cytotoxic concentrations provides a pharmacokinetic advantage. After a single intrathecal DTC101 dose, the terminal half-life of free cytarabine was increased more than 40-fold versus conventional cytarabine, from 3.4 to 141 h. Drug distribution throughout the neuraxis is also improved with DTC101. Following a single intraventricular injection, lumbar drug concentrations were equal to those in the ventricle within 6 h of injection. Furthermore, cytotoxic concentrations in the lumbar CSF were maintained for an average of nine days. Randomized multicenter trials of intrathecal DepoCyt versus methotrexate have been reported for adults with lymphomatous meningitis and neoplastic meningitis due to an underlying solid tumor. In patients with lymphomatous meningitis, 7/17 (41%) patients treated with intrathecal DTC101 had a complete response (negative CSF cytology and no symptomatic worsening) compared with 1/16 (6%) patients treated with intrathecal cytarabine ($P = 0.04$). There was also a trend to improvement in time to neurologic progression (median 78.5 vs. 42 days) and median survival (99.5 vs. 63 days) for patients treated with DTC101. In adults with neoplastic meningitis due to solid tumors, the response rates in both arms were similar (26 vs. 20%). However, there appeared to be a trend toward increased time to neurologic progression in the DepoCyt treated group. Thus, the less demanding dose schedule of intrathecal DepoCyt, coupled with its similar toxicity profile and comparable or improved response rates, suggests that further studies should be performed to delineate the role of DTC101 in the treatment and prevention of neoplastic meningitis [13].

The toxicity profile of DTC101, when given with concomitant oral dexamethasone, is similar to that of unencapsulated cytarabine. Acute toxicities include fever, headache, back pain, nausea, and encephalopathy. It is too early to determine whether there is any delayed or chronic neurotoxicity associated with intrathecal DTC101 [37].

## 9.8 Thiotepa

Thiotepa, a lipid-soluble alkylating agent, is occasionally administered by the intrathecal route. Unlike methotrexate and cytarabine, there is not a significant pharmacological advantage for intrathecal versus systemic thiotepa. After systemic administration, both thiotepa and its active metabolite, TEPA, readily cross the blood–brain barrier, and CSF and plasma drug exposures are nearly identical. Since the CSF elimination of TEPA is slower than that of thiotepa, there is greater total exposure to TEPA. However, following intrathecal administration, thiotepa CSF clearance is nine times the rate of CSF bulk flow. The rapid diffusion of thiotepa out of the CSF limits drug distribution throughout the neuraxis. In addition, TEPA is not detectable in the CSF after intrathecal drug administration. Thus, overall CSF exposure to active species may be lower after intrathecal versus intravenous administration. A randomized prospective comparison of intraventricular methotrexate and thiotepa revealed that the efficacy and overall toxicity of these agents in the treatment of neoplastic meningitis were similar. The median survival for both treatment arms was short, 15.9 weeks for the methotrexate group and 14.1 weeks for thiotepa. Thus, there is little compelling evidence for the use of intrathecal thiotepa [23].

## 9.9 Topotecan

Topotecan is a water-soluble semisynthetic camptothecin analog that exerts its cytotoxic effect via inhibition of the enzyme topoisomerase I. Preclinical studies demonstrated that this agent has antitumor activity against both leukemias and solid tumors. Clinical studies of intravenous topotecan in humans have demonstrated objective clinical antitumor activity leading to US Food and Drug Administration approval for the treatment of non-small cell lung cancer and ovarian carcinoma. This antitumor activity coupled with the drug's novel mechanism of action, lack of neurotoxicity after intravenous administration, and results of preclinical studies demonstrating that there was a high degree of penetration into the CSF led to preclinical studies to evaluate the safety and feasibility of intrathecal topotecan administration. Following administration of a 0.1-mg intraventricular dose in the nonhuman primate, the ventricular CSF drug exposure was 450-fold greater than that following intravenous administration of a 40-fold higher dose (10 mg/m$^2$). In addition, peak lumbar levels approached 1 mM. The marked pharmacokinetic advantage of intrathecal versus systemic drug administration and the lack of observed toxicity following chronic dosing studies in the nonhuman primate model led to the development of a phase I trial of intrathecal topotecan for patients with neoplastic meningitis. Results to date demonstrate that intrathecal topotecan is well-tolerated. A phase II study of intrathecal topotecan in children with CNS leukemia or neoplastic meningitis due to solid tumors was recently initiated by the Children's Oncology Group [38].

## 9.10 Mafosfamide

Mafosfamide and 4-hydroperoxycyclophosphamide are cyclophosphamide derivatives that do not require hepatic microsomal activation for antineoplastic activity. Preclinical pharmacokinetic studies in the nonhuman primate model demonstrated that following intrathecal administration, ventricular CSF concentrations in excess of in vitro cytotoxic targets could be attained at doses not associated with systemic or neurologic toxicity. Clinical trials of intrathecal mafosfamide are now underway. Following an intraventricular dose of 5 mg, CSF levels in excess of target cytocidal levels could be achieved, but the lumbar CSF levels did not consistently exceed the target level even at the 5.0-mg dose level. With higher doses, headache became dose limiting following bolus administration. Therefore, mafosfamide is currently being administered as a 20-min intrathecal infusion after premedication with dexamethasone and a narcotic analgesic. Using a similar approach, they routinely administer mafosfamide doses of 20 mg in children with disseminated brain tumors [39].

## 9.11 Busulfan

Busulfan is a cell-cycle nonspecific alkylating agent primarily utilized in the treatment of chronic leukemias and in preparative regimens for bone marrow transplantation. Despite the wide spectrum of preclinical antitumor activity, routine clinical use of busulfan is limited because it causes profound and cumulative myelosuppression and may also produce pulmonary fibrosis. In an attempt to circumvent the toxicities associated with systemic drug delivery, preclinical studies to evaluate the feasibility of intrathecal administration of a microcrystalline busulfan formulation to nude rats with neoplastic meningitis were performed. These studies by Friedman et al. demonstrated that there was antitumor activity following intrathecal busulfan administration; however, there was also a narrow therapeutic dose range for toxicity [40].

## 9.12 Vincristine

Vincristine belongs to a group of drugs known as the vinca alkaloids. These drugs block cell growth by stopping mitosis by interfering with microtubule polymerization. The FDA-approved indications of vincristine are acute lymphocytic leukemia, lymphoid blast crisis of chronic myeloid leukemia, and Hodgkin and non-Hodgkin lymphoma. Vincristine also has several off-label uses that include central nervous system (CNS) tumors, Ewing sarcoma, gestational trophoblastic tumors, multiple myeloma, ovarian cancer, primary CNS lymphoma, small cell lung cancer, and advanced thymoma in adult patients. But when intrathecal administration occurs, potential neurotoxicities may cause coma, motor dysfunction, paralysis, neuralgia, peripheral neuropathy, sensory disturbances, dizziness, muscle impairment, and decreased tendon reflex. Its use via intralumbar is not recommended [22, 41, 42].

## 9.13 Monoclonal Antibodies: Rituximab and Trastuzumab

There has been recent research into the administration of two monoclonal antibodies; this represents an innovative targeted therapy for the treatment of leptomeningeal carcinomatosis: trastuzumab for HER2 positive breast cancer and rituximab for the treatment of B-cell lymphoma. Trastuzumab is highly effective in the treatment of breast cancer with HER2 overexpression; however, despite its efficacy, patients treated with trastuzumab and chemotherapy will experience an incidence of CNS metastasis ranging from 28% to 42%. The concentration of trastuzumab in the CSF after intravenous administration was 300 or 400 times lower than its concentration in plasma; therefore, in order to achieve therapeutic concentrations of trastuzumab in the CSF, it has been considered to use IT administration. This drug has been used in a series of cases, alone or in combination with intrathecal methotrexate or thiotepa, at doses between 12.5 and 25 mg administered with a frequency ranging from 3 days to 3 weeks. The most typical regimen used was 20–25 mg once a week, and all dosing regimens were well tolerated. With these regimens, there have been responses at the CSF level and even an increase in survival without toxic effects [43]. Rituximab is an anti-CD20 antibody; over 90% of B-cell non-Hodgkin lymphomas (NHLs) and primary CNS lymphomas express the CD20 marker, but healthy brain tissue does not express it. Like trastuzumab, rituximab has a low penetration in the CSF; its concentration in CSF after systemic administration represents 0.1% of concentrations in blood serum. The doses used for rituximab were 10 mg, 25 mg, and 50 mg, and toxic effects appeared with the 50-mg dosing (hypertension, nausea, vomiting, and double vision). The median survival was 21 weeks, six patients experienced meningeal response, and two of the three patients with intraocular disease experienced a local response. The combination of liposomal cytarabine with IT rituximab was tested by Chamberlain and colleagues in 14 patients with lymphoma and relapsing neoplastic meningitis. Each patient was administered an induction regimen including 25 mg of IT rituximab twice a week and liposomal cytarabine every 14 days, during 4 weeks. A maintenance stage was then conducted, including 50 mg of liposomal cytarabine and two doses of rituximab 25 mg administered in the same week, every 4 weeks, until disease progression. After the induction regimen, 10 patients experienced partial neurological response and received maintenance therapy. The probability of survival at 6 months was 29%, and toxic effects were moderate and expected, probably due to liposomal cytarabine. There is a lack of information about the way in which monoclonal antibodies should be prepared and administered for intrathecal administration; logically, the requirements for preparation for intrathecal use must be considered, always in a sterile and apyrogenic setting, and using dissolvents preservatives-free. In the case of trastuzumab, only one of the publications explained how it had been prepared: the usual reconstitution process (150 mg in 7.2 ml water for injection; pH 6), and administration of the adequate volume (20 mg in 0.95 mL), without additional dilution. For rituximab, one of the studies specified that it had been prepared by diluting rituximab with 0.9% sodium chloride solution on a 1:1 ratio for 10 and 25 mg doses, and without dilution for 50-mg doses, and administered over 1–5 minutes. It has not been established if intraventricular or intralumbar administration has any influence on the results [44].

## 9.14 Albumin-Bound Paclitaxel

Research has been conducted in the treatment of meningeal metastasis of lung cancer. But these studies are still very recent. The intrathecal injection chemotherapy can improve the clinical symptoms of patients, and the treatment is safe and effective. The patients with meningeal metastasis of lung cancer with combined EGFRTKI therapy, combined EGFR-TKI therapy, and a KPS score of ≥70 had a longer survival time. There are still no conclusive results [45].

## 9.15 Considerations

There is a wide variability in practice when using IT chemotherapy, despite being an effective therapy, accepted by all international groups, particularly for the treatment of acute leukemia and non-Hodgkin lymphomas. This variability and uncertainty are not limited to the drugs and doses administered, but it also includes the way of preparation and the administration technique. The treatment and prevention of neoplastic meningitis remain a significant challenge for clinical oncologists. We must continue our ongoing research efforts to identify new agents and treatment strategies to improve the quality of life and event-free survival of patients with this devastating disease. Even the use of good practices is still not enough to prevent failures or errors in the administration of chemotherapy from occurring. It is necessary to create a safety culture aimed at sharing responsibility and implementing institutional policies and standards in order to improve safety, created from a multidisciplinary team with interdisciplinary characteristics.

## References


1. Badell I, Munoz A, Estella J, Fernandez-Delgado R, Javier G, Verdeguer A, et al. Long-term results of two consecutive trials in childhood acute lymphoblastic leukaemia performed by the Spanish Cooperative Group for Childhood Acute Lymphoblastic Leukemia Group (SHOP) from 1989 to 1998. Clin Transl Oncol. 2008;10(2):117–24.
2. Treatment of leptomeningeal metastases. Uptodate 2014 (citado 13-06-2016). Available from: http://www.uptodate.com/contents/treatment-ofleptomeningeal-metastasescarcinomatousmeningitis?source=search_result&search=treatment+of+leptomeningeal+metastases&selectedTitle=1%7E54.
3. Pui CH, Thiel E. Central nervous system disease in hematologic malignancies: historical perspective and practical applications. Semin Oncol. 2009;36(4 Suppl 2):S2–S16.
4. Liu HC, Yeh TC, Hou JY, Chen KH, Huang TH, Chang CY, et al. Triple intrathecal therapy alone with omission of cranial radiation in children with acute lymphoblastic leukemia. J Clin Oncol. 2014;32(17):1825–9.
5. Matloub Y, Lindemulder S, Gaynon PS, Sather H, La M, Broxson E, et al. Intrathecal triple therapy decreases central nervous system relapse but fails to improve eventfree survival when compared with intrathecal methotrexate: results of the Children's Cancer Group (CCG) 1952 study for standard-risk acute lymphoblastic leukemia, reported by the Children's Oncology Group. Blood. 2006;108(4):1165–73.
6. Gil LG, Clemente BS, Oliveras AM, Cabanas Poy MJ, Hidalgo AE. Dosage of drugs for cerebrospinal administration. Farm Hosp. 2005;29(3):185–90.
7. Ellenby MS, Tegtmeyer K, Lai S, Braner DA. Videos in clinical medicine. Lumbar puncture. N Engl J Med. 2006;355(13):e12.
8. Vora A, Andreano A, Pui CH, Hunger SP, Schrappe M, Moericke A, et al. Influence of cranial radiotherapy on outcome in children with acute lymphoblastic leukemia treated with contemporary therapy. JCO. 2016;34(9):919–26.
9. Pascual JM, Gonzalez F, Prieto R, Celdran S, Roda JM. Blood brain barrier: development of a structure which supports the functional heterogeneity of the central nervous system. Rev Neurol. 2004;38(6):565–81.
10. Slevin ML, Piall EM, Aherne GW, Johnston A, Lister TA. The pharmacokinetics of cytosine arabinoside in the plasma and cerebrospinal fluid during conventional and high-dose therapy. Med Pediatr Oncol. 1982;10 Suppl 1:157–68.
11. Fleischhack G, Jaehde U, Bode U. Pharmacokinetics following intraventricular administration of chemotherapy in patients with neoplastic meningitis. Clin Pharmacokinet. 2005;44(1):1–31.
12. Jabbour E, O'Brien S, Kantarjian H, Garcia-Manero G, Ferrajoli A, Ravandi F, et al. Neurologic complications associated with intrathecal liposomal cytarabine given prophylactically in combination with high-dose

methotrexate and cytarabine to patients with acute lymphocytic leukemia. Blood. 2007;109(8):3214–8.
13. Phuphanich S, Maria B, Braeckman R, Chamberlain M. A pharmacokinetic study of intra-CSF administered encapsulated cytarabine (DepoCyt) for the treatment of neoplastic meningitis in patients with leukemia, lymphoma, or solid tumors as part of a phase III study. J Neurooncol. 2007;81(2):201–8.
14. Bleyer WA, Coccia PF, Sather HN, Level C, Lukens J, Niebrugge DJ, et al. Reduction in central nervous system leukemia with a pharmacokinetically derived intrathecal methotrexate dosage regimen. J Clin Oncol. 1983;1(5):317–25.
15. Hitchins RN, Bell DR, Woods RL, Levi JA. A prospective randomized trial of single agent versus combination chemotherapy in meningeal carcinomatosis. J Clin Oncol. 1987;5(10):1655–62.
16. American Society of Health-System Pharmacists. AHFS drug information. Bethesda, MD; 2008.
17. Sandberg DI, Bilsky MH, Souweidane MM, Bzdil J, Gutin PH. Ommaya reservoirs for the treatment of leptomeningeal metastases. Neurosurgery. 2000;47(1):49–54.
18. Pui CH. Central nervous system disease in acute lymphoblastic leukemia: prophylaxis and treatment. Hematology Am Soc Hematol Educ Program. 2006:142–146.
19. Administration of Chemotherapeutic Drugs. BC Cancer 2014 (citado 13-06-2016). Available from: http://www.bccancer.bc.ca/NR/rdonlyres/13EF6DF8-9F77-4B50-842A-0D3765B73103/73657/C252ChemotherapeuticAgentsAdministrationOf.pdf.
20. Lin WY, Liu HC, Yeh TC, Wang LY, Liang DC. Triple intrathecal therapy without cranial irradiation for central nervous system preventive therapy in childhood acute lymphoblastic leukemia. Pediatr Blood Cancer. 2008;50(3):523–7.
21. Blaney SM, Poplack DG, Godwin K, McCully CL, Murphy R, Balis FM. Effect of body position on ventricular CSF methotrexate concentration following intralumbar administration. J Clin Oncol. 1995;13(1):177–9.
22. Sempere AP, Berenguer-Ruiz L, Lezcano-Rodas M, Mira-Berenguer F, Waez M. Lumbar puncture: its indications, contraindications, complications and technique. Rev Neurol. 2007;45(7):433–6.
23. BCCA protocol summary for solid tumours using intrathecal methotrexate and/or thiotepa and/or cytarabine. BC Cancer 2015 (citado 11-06-2016). Available from: http://www.bccancer.bc.ca/NR/rdonlyres/42271735-B80E-435B-9F01-E11FB1320EF2/14239/MOIT_1Jul05.pdf.
24. Zimm S, Collins JM, Miser J, Chatterji D, Poplack DG. Cytosine arabinoside cerebrospinal fluid kinetics. Clin Pharmacol Ther. 1984;35(6):826–30.

25. Shapiro WR, Young DF, Mehta BM. Methotrexate: distribution in cerebrospinal fluid after intravenous, ventricular and lumbar injections. N Engl J Med. 1975;293(4):161–6.
26. Franklin JL, Finlay J. Leukemias and lymphomas: treatment and prophylaxis of the central nervous system. Curr Treat Options Neurol. 2006;8(4):335–45.
27. Shapiro WR, Johanson CE, Boogerd W. Treatment modalities for leptomeningeal metastases. Semin Oncol. 2009;36(4 Suppl 2):S46–54.
28. Zhang Y. Physical and chemical stability of methotrexate, cytarabine and hydrocortisone in Elliot's B solution. Hosp Pharm. 1996;31(8):965–970.
29. Trissel LA, King KM, Zhang Y, Wood AM. Physical and chemical stability of methotrexate, cytarabine and hydrocortisone in Elliot's B solution for intrathecal use. J Oncol Pharm Pract. 2002;8(1):27–32.
30. Mahoney DH, Shuster JJ, Nitschke R, Lauer SJ, Steuber CP, Winick N, et al. Acute neurotoxicity in children with B-precursor acute lymphoid leukemia: an association with intermediate-dose intravenous methotrexate and intrathecal triple therapy--a Pediatric Oncology Group study. J Clin Oncol. 1998;16(5):1712–22.
31. Moser A, Adamson P, Gillespie A, et al. Intraventricular concentration times time (C × T) methotrexate and cytarabine for recurrent meningeal leukemia and lymphoma. Cancer. 1999;85:511–6.
32. Cortes J, O'Brien SM, Pierce S, Keating MJ, Freireich EJ, Kantarjian HM. The value of high-dose systemic chemotherapy and intrathecal therapy for central nervous system prophylaxis in different risk groups of adult acute lymphoblastic leukemia. Blood. 1995;86(6):2091–7.
33. Rowe JM, Buck G, Burnett AK, Chopra R, Wiernik PH, Richards SM, et al. Induction therapy for adults with acute lymphoblastic leukemia: results of more than 1500 patients from the international ALL trial: MRC UKALL XII/ECOG E2993. Blood. 2005;106(12):3760.
34. Kim DY, Lee KW, Yun T, Park SR, Jung JY, Kim DW, et al. Comparison of intrathecal chemotherapy for leptomeningeal carcinomatosis of a solid tumor: methotrexate alone versus methotrexate in combination with cytosine arabinoside and hydrocortisone. Jpn J Clin Oncol. 2003;33(12):608–12.
35. Tomizawa D, Tabuchi K, Kinoshita A, Hanada R, Kigasawa H, Tsukimoto I, et al. Repetitive cycles of high-dose cytarabine are effective for childhood acute myeloid leukemia: long-term outcome of the children with AML treated on two consecutive trials of Tokyo Children's Cancer Study Group. Pediatr Blood Cancer. 2007;49(2):127–32.
36. Ficha tecnica Depocyte. Agencia Espanola de Medicamentos y Productos Sanitarios 2015 (citado 14-06-2016). Available from: http://www.ema.europa.eu/docs/es_ES/document_library/EPAR_-_Product_Information/human/000317/WC500035649.pdf.
37. Glantz MJ, Jaeckle KA, Chamberlain MC, Phuphanich S, Recht L, Swinnen LJ, et al. A randomized controlled trial comparing intrathecal sustained-release cytarabine (DepoCyt) to intrathecal methotrexate in

patients with neoplastic meningitis from solid tumors. Clin Cancer Res. 1999;5(11):3394–402.
38. Rowinsky E, Grochow L, Hendricks C, et al. Phase I and pharmacologic study of topotecan: a novel topoisomerase I inhibitor. J Clin Oncol. 1992;10:647–56.
39. Slavc I, Schuller E, Czech T, et al. Intrathecal mafosfamide therapy for pediatric brain tumors with meningeal dissemination. J Neurooncol. 1998;38:213–8.
40. Cokgor Ilkcan, Allan H. Friedman, and Henry S. Friedman. "Current options for the treatment of neoplastic meningitis." J neurooncology. 2002;79–88.
41. Golightly LK, Smolinske SS, Bennett ML, Sutherland EW III, Rumack BH. Pharmaceutical excipients. Adverse effects associated with inactive ingredients in drug products (Part I). Med Toxicol Adverse Drug Exp. 1988;3(2):128–65.
42. Hetherington NJ, Dooley MJ. Potential for patient harm from intrathecal administration of preserved solutions. Med J Aust. 2000;173(3): 141–3.
43. Stemmler HJ, Mengele K, Schmitt M, Harbeck N, Laessig D, Herrmann KA, et al. Intrathecal trastuzumab (Herceptin) and methotrexate for meningeal carcinomatosis in HER2-overexpressing metastatic breast cancer: a case report. Anticancer Drugs. 2008;19(8):832–6.
44. Stemmler HJ, Schmitt M, Willems A, Bernhard H, Harbeck N, Heinemann V. Ratio of trastuzumab levels in serum and cerebrospinal fluid is altered in HER2-positive breast cancer patients with brain metastases and impairment of blood-brain barrier. Anticancer Drugs. 2007;18(1):23–8.
45. Chamberlain MC, Johnston SK, Van HA, Glantz MJ. Recurrent lymphomatous meningitis treated with intra-CSF rituximab and liposomal ara-C. J Neurooncol. 2009;91(3):271–7.

## Suggested Reading

1. Giebel S, Krawczyk-Kulis M, Mczyk-Cioch M, Czyz A, Lech-Maranda E, Piatkowska-Jakubas B, et al. Prophylaxis and therapy of central nervous system involvement in adult acute lymphoblastic leukemia: recommendations of the Polish Adult Leukemia Group. Pol Arch Med Wewn. 2008;118(6):356–61.
2. Cradock JC, Kleinman LM, Rahman A. Evaluation of some pharmaceutical aspects of intrathecal methotrexate sodium, cytarabine and hydrocortisone sodium succinate. Am J Hosp Pharm. 1978;35(4):402–6.
3. Geiser CF, Bishop Y, Jaffe N, Furman L, Traggis D, Frei E. Adverse effects of intrathecal methotrexate in children with acute leukemia in remission. Blood. 1975;45(2):189–95.

4. Sullivan MP, Moon TE, Trueworthy R, Vietti TJ, Humphrey GB, Komp D. Combination intrathecal therapy for meningeal leukemia: two versus three drugs. Blood. 1977;50(3):471–9.
5. Beauchesne P. Intrathecal chemotherapy for treatment of leptomeningeal dissemination of metastatic tumours. Lancet Oncol. 2010;11(9): 871–9.
6. Kiewe P, Fischer L, Martus P, Thiel E, Korfel A. Meningeal dissemination in primary CNS lymphoma: diagnosis, treatment, and survival in a large monocenter cohort. Neuro Oncol. 2010;12(4):409–17.
7. Omura GA, Moffitt S, Vogler WR, Salter MM. Combination chemotherapy of adult acute lymphoblastic leukemia with randomized central nervous system prophylaxis. Blood. 1980;55(2):199–204.
8. Hill QA, Owen RG. CNS prophylaxis in lymphoma: who to target and what therapy to use. Blood Rev. 2006;20(6):319–32.
9. Camiener GW, Smith CG. Studies of the enzymatic deamination of cytosine arabinoside. I. Enzyme distribution and species specificity. Biochem Pharmacol. 1965;14(10):1405–16.
10. Saito T, Asai O, Dobashi N, Yano S, Osawa H, Takei Y, et al. Peripheral neuropathy caused by high-dose cytosine arabinoside treatment in a patient with acute myeloid leukemia. J Infect Chemother. 2006; 12(3):148.
11. Dunton SF, Nitschke R, Spruce WE, Bodensteiner J, Krous HF. Progressive ascending paralysis following administration of intrathecal and intravenous cytosine arabinoside. A Pediatric Oncology Group study. Cancer. 1986;57(6):1083–8.
12. Stary J, Zimmermann M, Campbell M, Castillo L, Dibar E, Donska S, et al. Intensive chemotherapy for childhood acute lymphoblastic leukemia: results of the randomized intercontinental trial ALL ICBFM 2002. J Clin Oncol. 2014;32(3):174–84.
13. Kamps WA, Bokkerink JP, Hakvoort-Cammel FG, Veerman AJ, Weening RS, van Wering ER, et al. BFM-oriented treatment for children with acute lymphoblastic leukemia without cranial irradiation and treatment reduction for standard risk patients: results of DCLSG protocol ALL-8 (1991–1996). Leukemia. 2002;16(6):1099–111.
14. Thomas X, Boiron JM, Huguet F, Dombret H, Bradstock K, Vey N, et al. Outcome of treatment in adults with acute lymphoblastic leukemia: analysis of the LALA-94 trial. J Clin Oncol. 2004;22(20):4075–86.
15. Huguet F, Leguay T, Raffoux E, Thomas X, Beldjord K, Delabesse E, et al. Pediatric-inspired therapy in adults with Philadelphia chromosome-negative acute lymphoblastic leukemia: the GRAALL-2003 study. J Clin Oncol. 2009;27(6):911–8.
16. Ortega JJ, Ribera JM, Oriol A, Bastida P, Gonzalez ME, Calvo C, et al. Early and delayed consolidation chemotherapy significantly improves the

outcome of children with intermediate risk acute lymphoblastic leukemia. Final results of the prospective randomized PETHEMA ALL-89 TRIAL. Haematologica. 2001;86(6):586–95.
17. Protocolo LAL SEHOP/PETHEMA 2013. Sociedad Espanola de Hematologia y Hemoterapia 2014 (citado 11-06-2016). Available from: http://www.sehh.es/images/stories/recursos/2014/noticias/LAL_SEHOP_PETHEMA_2013.pdf.
18. Sancho JM, Morgades M, Alonso N, Deben G, Fernandez de SA, Vazquez L, et al. Prospective study on the practice of central nervous system prophylaxis and treatment in non-Hodgkin's lymphoma in Spain. Med Clin (Barc). 2008;131(12):441–6.
19. Nagpal S, Recht L. Treatment and prophylaxis of hematologic malignancy in the central nervous system. Curr Treat Options Neurol. 2011;13(4):400–12.
20. Vagace JM, Caceres-Marzal C, Gonzalez de MS, Gervasini G. Central nervous system chemotoxicity during treatment of pediatric acute lymphoblastic leukemia/lymphoma. Crit Rev Oncol Hematol. 2012;84(2):274–86.
21. Ribera JM, Oriol A, Morgades M, Montesinos P, Sarra J, Gonzalez-Campos J, et al. Treatment of high-risk Philadelphia chromosome-negative acute lymphoblastic leukemia in adolescents and adults according to early cytologic response and minimal residual disease after consolidation assessed by flow cytometry: final results of the PETHEMA ALL-AR-03 trial. J Clin Oncol. 2014;32(15):1595–604.
22. Olmos-Jimenez R, Espuny-Miro A, Diaz-Carrasco MS, Fernandez-Varon E, Valderrey-Pulido M, Carceles-Rodriguez C. Stability of four standardized preparations of methotrexate, cytarabine, and hydrocortisone for intrathecal use. J Oncol Pharm Pract. 2015. pii: 1078155215600905.
23. Cheung YW, Vishnuvajjala BR, Flora KP. Stability of cytarabine, methotrexate sodium, and hydrocortisone sodium succinate admixtures. Am J Hosp Pharm. 1984;41(9):1802–6.
24. D'Hondt M, Vangheluwe E, Van DS, Boonen J, Bauters T, Pelfrene B, et al. Stability of extemporaneously prepared cytarabine, methotrexate sodium, and methylprednisolone sodium succinate. Am J Health Syst Pharm. 2012;69(3):232–40.
25. Guia de buenas practicas de preparacion de medicamentos en servicios de farmacia hospitalaria. Ministerio de Sanidad, Servicios Sociales e Igualdad (citado 12-11-2016). Available from: http://www.msssi.gob.es/profesionales/farmacia/pdf/GuiaBPP3.pdf.
26. Usarralde-Perez A, Toro-Chico P, Perez-Encinas M. Actualizacion de la estabilidad de los medicamentos citostaticos y otras mezclas intravenosas aplicando la metodologia de la matriz de riesgo para la elaboracion de medicamentos esteriles. Farm Hosp. 2016;40(4):260–71.

# Support Drugs

# 10

Gabriela Sandoval da Silva,
Lygia Leão Fernandes,
and Taynna Tatiane Pereira

## 10.1 Hypersensitivity Reaction

Hypersensitivity reactions can be induced by many drugs, including most chemotherapy drugs under clinical use. These reactions to chemotherapy drugs are generally characterized as being a type I hypersensitivity reaction; however, many appear not to be mediated by immunoglobulin E (IgE) [1].

Manifestations are generally associated with type I hypersensitivity reactions, such as urticaria, pruritus, abdominal cramps, dyspnea, and agitation; some cases may progress to laryngeal spasm, bronchospasm, and complete anaphylaxis [2]. The classic cancer drugs most likely to trigger hypersensitivity reactions are platinum derivatives (oxaliplatin and carboplatin) and taxanes (paclitaxel and docetaxel). The reported incidence of hypersensitivity of any degree of reactions to platinum derivatives is approximately 12–19%; for paclitaxel and docetaxel, the

G. S. da Silva (✉) · T. T. Pereira
Pharmacy, Hospital Israelita Albert Einstein, São Paulo, SP, Brazil

L. L. Fernandes
Pharmacy, Hospital Salvalus (Grupo NotreDame Intermédica), São Paulo, SP, Brazil



C. W. P. Schmidt, K. M. Otoni (eds.), *The Golden Guide to Oncologic Pharmacy*, https://doi.org/10.1007/978-3-030-98596-7_10

reported incidences are approximately 8–45% and 5–20%, respectively [3].

Immediate hypersensitivity reactions are common during monoclonal antibody (mAB) infusion and vary according to the infused agent, with occurrences reported for chimeric, humanized, and "totally human" mAbs [4]. Reactions include acute idiosyncratic infusion reactions, cutaneous, anaphylactic, and serum sickness type. Urticaria, for instance, has been reported in up to 15% of mAb infusions [5]. The rate of infusion reactions clinically consistent with immediate hypersensitivity is 5–10% for rituximab, 2– 3% for infliximab, and 0.6–5% for trastuzumab. Reactions of HSRws have also been reported for omalizumab, natalizumab, basiliximab, abciximab, and cetuximab [6].

### 10.1.1 Treatment and Monitoring of Hypersensitivity Reactions

Pharmacological prophylaxis with antihistamines, corticosteroids, or both is generally recommended to reduce the frequency and severity of hypersensitivity reactions [3]. Patients should be monitored frequently during and immediately after all infusions, particularly when the risk of hypersensitivity reactions is greater, such as the first infusion of taxanes and monoclonal antibodies, or after multiple cycles of platinum-derived therapy. Vital signs should be checked before, during, and after infusions [7].

Prompt medical care and recognition are essential to reduce the risk of severe symptoms, as described in Tables 10.1 and 10.2. When an infusion reaction occurs, it should be stopped and sup-

**Table 10.1** Main supportive drugs used as premedication for chemotherapy with potential for hypersensitivity reaction

| | | |
|---|---|---|
| Diphenhydramine | 25–50 mg intravenously | 30 minutes before infusion |
| Dexamethasone | 10–20 mg orally or intravenously | 30 minutes before infusion |
| H2-receptor antagonist (ranitidine) | 150–300 mg intravenously | 30 minutes before infusion |

**Table 10.2** Main drugs for managing hypersensitivity reactions

| | | |
|---|---|---|
| Epinephrine | 0.3–0.5 mg intramuscularly | Repeat it every 15 minutes if necessary |
| Oxygen | 8–10 L/minute | If necessary |
| Salbutamol | 2.5–5 mg in 3 mL of saline solution via nebulizer<br>or<br>2 or 3 puff | Cases of epinephrine-resistant bronchospasm |

portive care administered until symptoms go away [7]. In most cases, mild and moderate reactions will resolve after a brief interruption of the infusion and drug administration can be resumed at a slower infusion rate, but in cases of severe reactions, temporary interruption of the drug is recommended [3].

The need to develop institutional protocols for the management of hypersensitivity reactions in cancer patients is essential to ensure a quick and effective response [3].

## 10.2 Tumor Lysis Syndrome

Tumor lysis syndrome (TLS) is a metabolic oncological emergency and is characterized by acute cell destruction, leading to the release of its cellular content into the extracellular space, impairing homeostasis and causing a series of metabolic complications, such as hyperkalemia, hyperphosphatemia, hyperuricemia, hypocalcemia, and consequently, acute uric acid nephropathy, acute renal failure, and high mortality. Previous identification of patients at high risk for TLS can lead to prevention and prophylaxis strategies, reducing the risk of clinical complications [8].

The development of TLS is independent of the patient's gender and race. Related risk factors include tumor type and size, the type of chemotherapy used in the treatment and the stage of the chemotherapy cycle, and the patient's previous health condition. Dehydrated, hypotensive patients, with previous nephropathies, oliguria, acidic urine, and lactic dehydrogenase levels above 1500 IU are more likely to develop TLS [9]. Tumor lysis syndrome is more frequent in neoplasms with a high rate of cell proliferation and good response to treatment, occurring mainly in hematological patients, more frequently in acute lymphoblastic leukemia and in aggressive non-Hodgkin lymphomas [10]. It is also observed in solid tumors, especially those with high rates of proliferation and response to cytotoxic therapy [11].

Tumor lysis syndrome may occur spontaneously, but it usually occurs 42–78 hours after the start of cytotoxic chemotherapy treatment, as a consequence of accelerated cell lysis and release of intracellular components into the bloodstream, including anions, cations, and products resulting from the metabolism of proteins and nucleic acids [12].

The clinical manifestations of TLS are diverse and nonspecific, including nausea, vomiting, diarrhea, anorexia, and lethargy. Acute kidney injury can lead to fluid overload and pulmonary edema; calcium and phosphate abnormalities can lead to muscle cramps or seizures; hyperkalemia or hyperphosphatemia, intensified by renal failure, can induce cardiac arrhythmia and sudden death. Even though up to one-third of patients with TLS may have acute kidney injury, cardiac or neurological manifestations remain rare [13].

### 10.2.1 Treatment and Monitoring of Tumor Lysis

Recognition of the patient's risk factors, monitoring of high-risk patients, and prompt and appropriate intervention are essential factors to ensure prevention and adequate treatment of TLS [14]. Table 10.3 describes the supportive medications for the treatment of TLS and the respective indications. Three stages must be distinguished: prevention of TLS, prevention of clinical manifestations, and prevention of organ dysfunction, covering three main purposes: hydration, treatment of metabolic abnormalities, and renal replacement. The main purpose of preventive measures is to prevent the development of an acute kidney injury, which will increase the clinical manifestations of TLS [8].

Hydration allows increasing renal blood flow, glomerular filtration rate, and total urine volume, decreasing the probability of precipitation of uric acid and calcium phosphate. It should start 2 days before chemotherapy starts and continue for 2–3 days after

**Table 10.3** Drugs used in the treatment of tumor lysis syndrome

| | Drugs | Mechanism of action | Dosage |
|---|---|---|---|
| Hyperuricemia | Allopurinol | Xanthine oxidase inhibitor | Oral intake = 600–900 mg (maximum: 500 mg/m$^2$/dia) intravenous = 200–400/m$^2$/dia (maximum: 600 mg/day Dose adjustment for renal failure |
| | Rasburicase | Recombinant protein acting on the oxidation of enzymatic catalysis of uric acid to allantoin. Inactive and more soluble | Adult: 0.2 mg/kg/day for 5 days. Children: 0.15–0.2 mg/kg/dia intravenous Renal adjustment not required |
| Hypocalcaemia | Calcium | Calcium supplementation | Adult: 500–2000 mg orally or 3 g intravenously/day Children: 200–2000 mg orally or 100 mg/kg intravenously/day |
| Hypercalcemia | Calcium polystyrene sulfonate | Exchange of potassium for calcium | 30–60 g at intervals of 4–6 h |
| | Calcium gluconate 10% | Membrane stabilization | 1–2 |
| Hyperphosphatemia | Polarizing solution | Potassium cell translocation | Regular insulin 10 U + 50% intravenous glucose solution |
| Lactic acid | Sodium bicarbonate | Alkalization | 8.9%–1 mEq/kg |
| Kidney dysfunction | Furosemide | Increased renal tubular flow | 40 mg intravenously, as needed |

chemotherapy ends. In patients at high risk for TLS, it is recommended to administer high volumes, with the exception of those who are at risk of volume overload [15].

In addition to hydration, hypouric agents can reduce urate levels. The most used drug for patients with low and moderate risk of TLS is allopurinol, which prevents the formation of uric acid from xanthine and hypoxanthine. Rasburicase is a recombinant enzyme of the enzyme urate oxidase that converts uric acid to allantoin, a compound 5–10 times more soluble in urine, and is recommended as a first-line drug in patients at high risk of developing TLS [16].

The treatment of acute hyperkalemia consists of stabilizing the cardiac membrane, allowing potassium to enter the intracellular environment and reducing the total amount of potassium. The main treatments consist of hydration, administration of potassium exchange resins, and loop diuretics or thiazides [15].

Initial treatment for hyperphosphatemia consists of hydration and administration of phosphate binders, such as calcium carbonate and aluminum hydroxide. Asymptomatic hypocalcemia does not need treatment as it usually corrects with improvement in TLS. If there are symptoms, however, the recommended treatment is a single dose of 10% calcium gluconate [15].

The treatment of lactic acidosis is based on the correction of the condition responsible for the alteration of lactate metabolism. In patients with a pH of less than 7.15, that is, with severe acute acidosis, the recommended treatment is to supplement with sodium bicarbonate [16].

When standard electrolyte control therapies are not enough to prevent acute renal failure, it is necessary to perform renal replacement therapies with intermittent and continuous dialysis methods, such as hemodialysis, hemofiltration, and peritoneal dialysis [16].

## 10.3 Hematotoxicity

Most cytotoxic antineoplastic agents used in cancer treatment attack rapidly dividing cells in an undifferentiated way, resulting in cell death and toxic effects mainly on healthy cells in the membranes of the gastrointestinal tract, hair follicle, and bone marrow.

Myelosuppression associated with antineoplastic treatment can lead to neutropenia, anemia, thrombocytopenia, or both, increasing the risk of infection, fatigue, decreased quality of life, reductions and delays in treatment, and reduced survival [17].

Neutrophils are produced in the bone marrow, are the first line of defense against pathogens, and have a relatively short half-life of 7 or 8 hours in peripheral blood [18]. Neutropenic patients are particularly prone to serious and potentially fatal bacterial infections. Chemotherapy-induced severe neutropenia is defined by the National Comprehensive Cancer Network (NCCN) as less than 500 neutrophils/mcL or less than 1000 neutrophils/mcL with a progression of decline to 500 neutrophils/mcL over the next 48 hours. Infections in patients with neutropenia may be evident from fever alone. This febrile neutropenia is defined as an axillary temperature greater than 37.8 °C or a temperature persistence between 38 and 38.3 °C for more than 1 turn [18].

Risk assessments for neutropenia and infectious complications are important components of cancer patient care, considering the risk inherent in the chemotherapy regimen, the type of cancer, and the characteristics of the patient [18]. Another hematologic toxicity experienced by patients using cytotoxic chemotherapy is anemia. Defined by hemoglobin less than 12 g/dL, it is present in 20–60% of all patients at the time of diagnosis and treatment and is often undertreated, despite its prevalence [19]. The causes of anemia in cancer patients have been classified into three categories: anemia occurring as a result of the malignancy, anemia attributed to therapy for the malignancy, and anemia as a result of other contributing factors [20].

Fatigue is the clinical manifestation of anemia most commonly reported by patients, followed by tachycardia and headache. Hemoglobin levels have been shown to have a considerable impact on the incidence of fatigue and quality of life in multiple studies. Consistently, patients with a hemoglobin of 11–13 g/dL presented better quality of life [21].

Thrombocytopenia is defined as a decrease in the number of platelets, it is a myelotoxicity attributed to chemotherapy, but it can also be related to the disease itself. The main consequence of thrombocytopenia is bleeding, which can occur spontaneously when platelet counts are below 10,000/mcL. The incidence, severity, and duration of chemotherapy-related thrombocytopenia is quite variable and depends on the treatment that the patient is undergoing [22].

### 10.3.1 Treatment and Monitoring of Hematological Toxicities

In the period of neutropenia, the patient is at greater risk of developing infections; one option is to use prophylactic antimicrobials during periods of neutropenia. This option includes antibiotic coverage for gram-positive and gram-negative bacteria, antifungals, and/or antivirals, depending on the patient's history of infections, the type of malignancy, and the chemotherapy regimen [18].

It is recommended to use febrile neutropenia risk assessment models. The MASCC score index for risk assessment in patients with febrile neutropenia is the most used; risk stratification helps to establish the treatment of patients enabling the best choice of antimicrobial treatment (monotherapy or combinations), route of administration, and location treatment (home, outpatient, or inpatient) [23].

The current recommendation for prophylactic treatment for adults with an expectation of neutropenia greater than 7 days from the start of treatment until the recovery of granulocytes, or until the development of fever and initiation of empirical antimicrobial therapy, is described in Table 10.4.

If fever develops during neutropenia, the recommendation is to start empiric broad-spectrum antibiotics immediately. Therapeutic options include beta-lactams: cefepime, ceftazidime, piperacillin-tazobactam, and carbapenems in monotherapy [24].

Another option for the treatment of neutropenia due to antineoplastic agents is the use of granulocyte colony-stimulating factors (G-CSF) as an adjunct to chemotherapy to reduce the incidence, severity, and duration of neutropenia. The most used G-CSFs are filgrastim and pegylated filgrastim (pegfilgrastim) [18].

G-CSF can be administered as primary prophylaxis (with each chemotherapy cycle, starting from the first cycle) or secondary

**Table 10.4** Prophylaxis of main infections

| | Prophylaxis |
|---|---|
| Infection by pneumocystis Pneumocystis jirovecii | **First choice:**<br>Sulfamethoxazole + trimethoprim 400 + 80 mg orally 1×/day or 800 + 160 3×/week<br>**Alternatives:**<br>Dapsone 50 mg orally 2×/day or 100 mg 1×/day (first line in cases of confirmed allergy to sulfa drugs) or<br>Atovaquone 1500 mg orally 1×/day or<br>Pentamidine 300 mg inhaled for 21–28 days |
| Fungal infection | **First choice:**<br>Fluconazole 400 mg 1×/day orally or intravenously<br>**Alternatives:**<br>Micafungin 50 mg intravenously 1×/day or (first choice if *C. kruse*ior *C. glabrata* confirmed)<br>Posaconazole 200 mg orally 2×/day (first choice in the presence of severe graft versus host disease)<br>Voriconazole 200 mg orally 2×/day |
| Viral infection | **First choice:**<br>Acyclovir intravenously 250 mg/m$^2$ or 5 mg/kg 12/12 hours<br>Acyclovir orally 60 mg 8/8 hours or 400 mg 12/12 hours<br>**Alternative:**<br>Valaciclovir orally 500 mg 12/12 hours |
| Bacterial infection | **First choice:**<br>Ciprofloxacin 500 mg 12/12 hours orally<br>**Alternatives:**<br>Levofloxacin 500 mg 1×/day orally |
| Parasitic infection | **First choice:**<br>Ivermectin 200 µg/kg/day orally for 2 days; repeat it in 2 weeks |

Adjusted from NCCN Guidelines, 2016

prophylaxis (in all cycles remaining after a neutropenic event), the recommendations vary according to the chemotherapy protocol used [25].

The treatment of anemia in cancer patients will depend on the cause, severity, clinical status of the patient, and comorbidities. The therapeutic option is erythropoiesis-stimulating agents, responsible for cell proliferation, maturation, and differentiation, represented by erythropoietin alfa, erythropoietin beta, and darbepoetin. The main purpose of erythropoietin therapy is to prevent or eliminate the need for blood transfusion. There is no recommendation for prophylactic use to prevent anemia in patients undergoing chemotherapy or radiotherapy with normal hemoglobin values at the start of treatment [26].

Currently, there is no information enough in the literature to support the development of appropriate guidelines and approaches for the treatment of thrombocytopenia in cancer patients [22].

## 10.4 Nausea and Vomiting

Chemotherapy-induced nausea and vomiting (CINV) are very frequent adverse events, present in 70% of patients who do not receive prophylaxis and in 25–55% of patients even with adequate prophylaxis [27]. Tables 10.5 and 10.6 describe the grade of these adverse events.

It is one of the main factors leading to dose reduction or discontinuation of the treatment protocol, directly interfering with the patient's diet and quality of life, in addition to the high investment of time and savings for cancer treatment centers in its management and consequences [28, 29].

**Table 10.5** Grade of adverse events: Nausea

| Adverse event | Degree | | | |
|---|---|---|---|---|
| | 1 | 2 | 3 | 4 |
| Nausea | Loss of appetite without changing eating habits | Decrease in food intake without significant weight loss, dehydration, or malnutrition | Inadequate intake of fluids or caloric foods; tube feeding; hospitalization and parenteral nutrition indicated | – |

Adjusted from Grunberg et al. [35]; Guia para notificação de reaçõesadversasemoncologia / SociedadeBrasileira de FarmacêuticosemOncologia – SOBRAFO [36]

**Table 10.6** Grade of adverse events: Vomiting

| Adverse event | Degree | | | |
|---|---|---|---|---|
| | 1 | 2 | 3 | 4 |
| Vomiting | One to two episodes (separated by 5 minutes) in 24 hours | Three to five episodes (separated by 5 minutes) in 24 hours | Six or more episodes (separated by 5 minutes) in 24 hours; tube feeding; hospitalization and parenteral nutrition indicated | Risk of death; urgent medical intervention indicated |

Adjusted from Grunberg et al. [35]; Guia para notificação de reaçõesadversasemoncologia / SociedadeBrasileira de FarmacêuticosemOncologia – SOBRAFO [36]

For correct prophylactic treatment, not only the emetogenic potential of the protocol should be taken into account, which we will discuss in more depth shortly, but previous risk factors such as gender, age, alcohol consumption, experience of nausea and vomiting in previous chemotherapy protocols, anxiety, and fatigue [30].

### 10.4.1 Nausea

It is a stomach discomfort and a pre-vomiting sensation, a nonspecific symptom; that is, it can be caused by several reasons [31].

Nausea can occur at four different moments:

- Acute (it occurs within the first 24 hours after chemotherapy infusion)
- Late (24–120 hours after infusion, with the peak between 48 and 72 hours)
- Anticipatory (it occurs before and during chemotherapy infusion)
- Refractory (acute and late symptoms in all cycles, with increasing intensities, indicating a poor clinical prognosis) [31]

### 10.4.2 Emesis/Vomiting

Emesis is the result of multiple stimuli, summarized below:

- *Efferent*: The impulse is sent by the vomiting center of the brain to the center of saliva, abdominal muscles, and respiratory and cranial nerves; it prepares the body with physical stimuli so that the body expels the stomach contents toward the mouth [32–35].
- *Afferent:* The afferent impulse is coordinated by neurons spread throughout the spinal cord that indirectly stimulate the vomiting center (located in the medulla) or emotional factors directly stimulating it, so emesis can occur through some different routes [32–35].

Thus, after the confirmation of studies on the great influence of nausea and vomiting on the success of cancer treatment, a practice that is now standard began around the 1980s: using pre-chemotherapeutic drugs, such as antiemetics. The prescription follows the risk classification of emetogenic potential (Table 10.7) [34].

In order to standardize protocols and offer the best treatment to cancer patients, some international institutions provide guides with the best treatment practices, with one of them being the adequate prophylaxis of nausea and vomiting in chemotherapy, as is the case with the scheme described in Table 10.8, provided by the National Comprehensive Cancer Network (NCCN) [35].

**Table 10.7** Risk of chemotherapy-induced emetogenic potential

| Potential risk | Acute | Late |
|---|---|---|
| High (>90%) | ++ | ++ |
| Moderate (30–90%) | ++ | + |
| Low (10–30%) | + | – |
| Minimum (<10%) | – | – |

Adjusted from National Comprehensive Cancer Network (NCCN) Guidelines [34]

**Table 10.8** Protocols indicated for prophylaxis of nausea and vomiting

| High potential (select option A, B, or C) | Moderate potential (select option A, B, or C) | Low potential | Minimum potential |
|---|---|---|---|
| D1<br>Antagonist NK1 +<br>Antagonist 5HT3<br>OR<br>Olanzapine +<br>Palonosetron +<br>Dexamethasone<br>OR<br>Olanzapine +<br>Antagonist NK1 +<br>Antagonist 5HT3 +<br>Dexamethasone | D1<br>Dexamethasone +<br>Antagonist 5HT3<br>OR<br>Olanzapine +<br>Palonosetron +<br>Dexamethasone<br>OR<br>NK1 + Antagonist<br>5HT3 +<br>Dexamethasone | Dexamethasone<br>OR<br>Metoclopramide<br>OR<br>Prochlorperazine<br>OR<br>Antagonist<br>5HT3 | No prophylaxis |
| D2, 3, and 4<br>Aprepitant +<br>Dexamethasone<br>OR<br>Olanzapine<br>OR<br>Olanzapine +<br>Aprepitant +<br>Dexamethasone | D2 and 3<br>Dexamethasone<br>OR Antagonist<br>5HT3<br>OR<br>Olanzapine<br>OR<br>Aprepitant +<br>Dexamethasone | – | – |

Adjusted from National Comprehensive Cancer Network (NCCN) Guidelines [34]
*Abbreviations*: *D(1–4, or)* days of the chemotherapy protocol

## 10.5 Dermatological Adverse Events

The skin and its appendages, hair, and nails are components frequently affected by cancer therapies, as they are cells in constant activity and division [37]. Maintaining dermatological integrity is very important, as it is one of the main barriers against opportunistic infections and directly reflects on the quality of general health, in addition to its importance in the expression of personality and self-esteem [38]. Therefore, these changes must be observed, discussed with the patient, and managed early, avoiding complications that affect the quality of life.

To help us classify and handle it correctly, there is a "Guia para notificação de reaçõesadversasemoncologia" [Guide for the notification of adverse reactions in oncology], made available through a partnership between Anvisa and SOBRAFO [36]. Tables 10.9, 10.10, 10.11, 10.12, 10.13, and 10.14 describe the grade of each adverse event discussed in this topic.

Main involvements, management, and performance of the pharmacist are described below.

### 10.5.1 Exanthema

The rash (skin rash) presents as follicular papules and pustules and usually develops initially in areas with a high density of sebaceous glands, especially the face (forehead, nose, and cheeks), and can then progress to the chest and upper back [39].

The main associated symptoms are itching, burning, and pain. Although rash severity is generally classified according to the Common Terminology Criteria for Adverse Events (CTCAE) [40], the impact on patients is greater than suggested by the scores.

Infectious stimuli can then lead to skin inflammation, which requires additional treatment. One factor that can promote the development of rash is impaired skin barrier function mediated by epidermal ichthyosis (skin peeling) [41].

In short, papulopustular eruption/rash is an inflammatory process that can be secondarily infected. Controlling the inflammatory response is therefore the basis of therapy.

#### 5.1.1 Prevention

- Avoiding frequent washing with hot water (during hand washing, showers, and baths)
- Avoiding skin irritants such as anti-acne medications, cleansers, or over-the-counter disinfectants; OTC moisturizing lotions without alcohol or ointments, preferably with moisturizers containing urea (5–10%) for the body

**Table 10.9** Grading table of rash degrees in oncology

| | Degree | | | |
|---|---|---|---|---|
| Adverse event | 1 | 2 | 3 | 4 |
| Rash Acneiform | Papular eruption and/or pustules located in less than 10% of the body area, which may or may not be associated with itching or skin tenderness | Papular eruption and/or pustules located in 10% to 30% of the body area, which may or may not be associated with itching or skin tenderness; associated with psychosocial impact, limiting daily activities | Papular eruption and/or pustules located in more than 30% of the body area, which may or may not be associated with itching or skin sensitivity, limiting self-care; associated with local superinfection and with indication of oral antibiotics | Papular rash and/or pustules on any length of the body, which may or may not be associated with itching or skin tenderness; associated with extensive local superinfection, with an indication for intravenous antibiotics; risk of death |
| Maculopapular rash | Macules/papules located in less than 10% of the body area, which may or may not be associated with symptoms (e.g., itching, burning, or skin tenderness) | Macules/papules located in 10–30% of the body area, which may or may not be associated with symptoms (e.g., itching, burning or skin tenderness), limiting daily activities. | Macules/papules located in more than 30% of the body area, which may or may not be associated with symptoms, limiting self-care | – |

Adjusted from Guia para notificação de reaçõesadversasemoncologia / SociedadeBrasileira de FarmacêuticosemOncologia – SOBRAFO [36]

**Table 10.10** Grading table of hand-foot syndrome degrees in oncology

| Adverse event | Degree | | | |
|---|---|---|---|---|
| | 1 | 2 | 3 | 4 |
| Hand-foot syndrome | Minimal skin changes or dermatitis, unpainful (erythema, edema, or hyperkeratosis) | Skin changes with pain (blisters, peeling, wounds, edema, or hyperkeratosis), limiting daily activities | Skin changes, severe, with pain, limiting self-care | – |

Adjusted from Guia para notificação de reaçõesadversasemoncologia / SociedadeBrasileira de FarmacêuticosemOncologia – SOBRAFO [36]

**Table 10.11** Grading table of alopecia degrees in oncology

| Adverse event | Degree | | | |
|---|---|---|---|---|
| | 1 | 2 | 3 | 4 |
| Alopecia | Loss of up to 50% of the normal amount of hair | Loss of >50% of the normal amount of hair | – | – |

Adjusted from Guia para notificação de reaçõesadversasemoncologia / SociedadeBrasileira de FarmacêuticosemOncologia – SOBRAFO [36]

**Table 10.12** Grading table of degrees of pruritus in oncology

| Adverse event | Degree | | | |
|---|---|---|---|---|
| | 1 | 2 | 3 | 4 |
| Itching | Light or localized; indicated topical intervention | Intense or widespread; intermittent; skin changes due to exfoliation (edema, papulation, excoriations); limits daily activities; indicated oral interventions | Intense or widespread; constant, limiting self-care or sleep; indicated oral corticosteroids or immunosuppressants | – |

Adjusted from Guia para notificação de reaçõesadversasemoncologia / SociedadeBrasileira de FarmacêuticosemOncologia – SOBRAFO [36]

**Table 10.13** Grading table of paronychia degrees in oncology

| Adverse event | Degree | | | |
|---|---|---|---|---|
| | 1 | 2 | 3 | 4 |
| Paronychia | Edema or erythema of the nail fold; cuticle tear | Indicated local and oral intervention (antibiotic, antifungal, antiviral), nail fold edema or erythema with pain; associated with discharge or separation of the nail plate, limitation of daily activities | Indicated surgical intervention and use of IV antibiotics, limited self-care | – |

Adjusted from Guia para notificação de reaçõesadversasemoncologia / SociedadeBrasileira de FarmacêuticosemOncologia – SOBRAFO [36]

**Table 10.14** Grading table of diarrhea grade in oncology

| Adverse event | Degree | | | |
|---|---|---|---|---|
| | 1 | 2 | 3 | 4 |
| Diarrhea | Less than 4 bowel movements a day. | 4–6 bowel movements a day. | Greater than or equal to 7 bowel movements a day; incontinence; limitation for daily activities; indicated hospitalization | Risk of death: urgent intervention indicated |

Adjusted from Guia para notificação de reaçõesadversasemoncologia / SociedadeBrasileira de FarmacêuticosemOncologia – SOBRAFO [36]

- Avoiding excessive exposure to the sun; using sunscreen applied to exposed areas of the body and every 2 hours when outside
- Oral antibiotics for 6 weeks at the start of therapy with or without low/moderate strength topical steroid on face and chest [42]

### 5.1.2 Therapeutic Management

- For grade 1 and 2 rashes, initiation or increased potency of topical corticosteroids, and initiation of oral tetracycline antibiotics for at least 6 weeks [43].

- For the treatment of grade 3 rash, the use of systemic corticosteroids (e.g., prednisone 0.5–1 mg/kg body weight for 7 days with a weaning dose for 4–6 weeks) is suggested along with the interruption of EGFRis until the rash is grade 1. When infection is suspected (i.e., failure to respond to oral antibiotics covering gram-positive organs, presence of painful skin lesions, pustules on arms, legs, and trunk, yellow scabs, discharge), a bacterial culture should be obtained and antibiotics administered in at least 14 days based on sensitivities [43].
- Additional treatments include the use of oral retinoids (i.e., acitretin, isotretinoin) or dapsone [44].

### 10.5.2 Hand-Foot Syndrome

Described in 1974, hand-foot syndrome [45, 46] is defined as a disorder characterized by redness, severe discomfort, swelling, and tingling in the palms of the hands or the soles of the feet, which can worsen leading to severe pain, blisters, difficulty in performing daily activities and in more severe cases necrosis, strongly impacting the patient's quality of life, and even discontinuing treatment. Molecular and cellular mechanisms are still poorly understood [44].

Some examples of cytotoxic drugs that can influence the development of the syndrome are 5-fluorouracil (5-FU), capecitabine, sorafenib, sunitinib, doxorubicin [47], remurafenib, dabrafenib, or encorafenib, among others [48, 49].

The occurrence and severity of the syndrome were correlated with the response to therapy [50, 51], that is, the more severe the effects of the syndrome, the greater the therapeutic response, resulting in a paradox with the treatment, requiring a balance to ensure a minimum of quality of life. Diagnosis and pathology usually develop within days to weeks after initiation of therapy; however, depending on the pharmacokinetics of therapy, it can also take up to 6 months for the first symptoms to occur [38].

There is no treatment after symptoms start; the focus is to balance the treatment so that the dose of the cytotoxic drug has the expected effect causing the least discomfort. It is necessary to treat the predisposing factors before starting therapy, for example, dryness of the skin using cream with 10% urea three times a day, hyperkeratosis, for treatment with a taxane base, gloves and cooling socks can be used, and in this case of capecitabine, a personalized approach based on 200 mg celecoxib is recommended. In addition, it is recommended to avoid irritation and friction on hands and feet: long walks, unprotected weight carrying, chemical stress, irritants, solvents, or disinfectants [38].

### 10.5.3 Alopecia

Hair is an important element in image, self-esteem, and often synonymous with health. Chemotherapy-induced alopecia is defined as the spontaneous loss of hair and, less commonly, body hair [50] and is a common consequence during treatment, caused by several classes of drugs. It is usually reversible after the end of cytotoxic treatment; however, it can cause such a devastating psychological effect that it results in refusal and/or discontinuation of the treatment [38].

Alopecia can be caused by different mechanisms, depending on the drug used, but we can summarize the attack of the follicle in the anagen phase (phase of accelerated cell division, which results in hair growth); the process is called hair follicle dystrophy [52].

The fall usually starts between the second week to 4 weeks after the start of treatment, and the severity depends mainly on the type, dose, method of administration, and time interval between infusions. The hair will start to grow back 2–3 months after completion of the CT and often grows with characteristics different from the original, yet a small number of patients may develop scarring alopecia (when hair no longer grows) [38].

### 5.3.1 Therapeutic Management

- Scalp cooling is recommended for prevention, which usually starts 20–45 minutes before the infusion and continues during and for 20–150 minutes after the infusion.
- Biotin and orthosilicic can stimulate hair growth but are generally not recommended.
- Minoxidil may be considered to stimulate hair growth after cytotoxic treatment ends.
- Spironolactone is not recommended because the risk–benefit analysis does not justify its routine use.
- Bimatoprost ophthalmic solution may result in eyelash growth in some patients but is generally not recommended [38].

## 10.5.4 Itching

Drug-induced pruritus is an itch that usually becomes chronic, which, according to the International Forum on the Study of Itch, is defined as itching lasting 6 weeks [53].

The identification of the patient's history, which must include all current medications, transfusions, emotional components, correlation between the time of symptom onset and drug administration for cancer treatment, and clinical examination, is mandatory before starting any type of specific therapy, as it is the evaluation of pruritus including intensity, onset, evolution, quality, location, and triggering factors defining the treatment. Chronic pruritus, often associated with other types of skin manifestations (hence the importance related to the treatment of events such as rash), may be accompanied by behavioral disturbance and withdrawal from social life and work, so the psychosocial suffering involved [38].

There is still no standardized method to document and quantify pruritus, as it is a sensation subject to individual variations related to various factors such as tiredness, anxiety, and stress. Currently, the intensity of itching is assessed using a visual scale or a numerical rating scale [54]. There is a lack of studies that address effective strategies against pruritus, ensuring the quality of life and maintenance of treatment [38].

### 5.4.1 Therapeutic Management

- Dry skin can be a factor for pruritus [57], and in the case of mild to moderate pruritus, a topical antipruritic containing 0.5% menthol or a topical corticosteroid such as mometasone furoate 0.1% ointment, betamethasone valerate 0.1% ointment, and 2.5% hydrocortisone can be considered, in addition to lotions containing urea or polidocane [43].
- Antihistamines have been used to provide symptom relief in patients with mild to moderate pruritus of various etiologies, but evidence is weak in the treatment of targeted therapy-induced pruritus. Second-generation nonsedating antihistamines (loratadine, 10 mg daily) may be the first choice for daytime systemic therapy, as well as the use of first-generation antihistamines (such as diphenhydramine, 25–50 mg/day and hydroxyzine, 25–50 mg/day) can be considered based on its sedative properties in patients who suffer overnight [55, 56].
- The use of antiepileptic agents such as pregabalin (25–150 mg per day) and gabapentin (900–3600 mg per day) are considered second-line treatment in patients refractory to treatment with antihistamines and therapies against rash and/or xeroderma [58].
- The tricyclic antidepressant doxepin, which is also a potent histamine antagonist, has been used to relieve general itching in topical and oral preparations [59].
- Aprepitant, an NK-1 receptor antagonist, has been reported to reduce pruritus related to erlotinib, cetuximab, panitumumab, sunitinib, gefitinib, imatinib, and other EGF-Ris [59].
- Systemic corticosteroids (0.5–2 mg/kg daily) are considered for temporary relief of severe itching. [59]
- For severe or widespread pruritus, oral corticosteroids or immunosuppressive therapy are indicated [59].

## 10.5.5 Paronychia

Targeted therapy-induced paronychia develops gradually after several weeks of treatment. Lesions around the nails initially manifest acutely, corresponding to a painful erythematous inflammation with swelling and tenderness in the lateral folds of the nail, which may progress to the formation of granulation tissue, simulating ingrown nails. Usually, the thumbs and big toes are the most affected due to repeated trauma [38].

The pathogenesis of paronychia is believed to result from inhibition of EGFR and EGFR-dependent pathways in keratinocytes. This leads to altered differentiation and migration of epidermal cells associated with inhibition of keratinocyte proliferation and decreased cell survival through induction of apoptosis [43]. The periungual stratum corneum becomes thinner, which can lead to perionychium perforation by the nail plate (onychocryptosis) [38].

### 5.5.1 Prevention

- Gentle skin care instructions [38]
- Preventive correction of curvature of the nails with referral to the podiatrist (if necessary) [38]
- Avoiding repeated friction and trauma/excessive pressure
- Wearing gloves when cleaning [38]
- Avoiding biting or cutting nails too short [38]
- Using antimicrobial immersion and washing with soap and water [38]
- Regular cut of the nails ensuring they are straight and not too short [38]
- Daily application of topical emollients to cuticles and periungual tissues [38]
- Wearing comfortable, well-fitting shoes and cotton socks [38]

### 5.5.2 Therapeutic Management

- If self-limiting injuries, conservative management is chosen: high potency topical corticosteroids alone or combined with topical antibiotics, chemical cauterization with silver nitrate and elastic adhesive tape [56–58]

- For grade 1 and 2 paronychia, 2% topical povidone-iodine showed benefits in a controlled study [59, 60]
- Oral antibiotics [61].
- Recently, complete elimination of nail paronychia was reported with 0.5% topical timolol gel under occlusion for 1 month in eight patients treated with EGFRis [61].
- Cryotherapy may be considered in the treatment of pyogenic granuloma [62].
- Grade 2 or 3 intolerable pyogenic paronychia/granuloma is indicated surgical treatment with partial extraction of the nail plate (or removal of a longitudinal segment of the nail along with the matrix) with physical destruction of excessive granulation tissue [62].

### 10.5.6 Onycholysis

The impact of taxane-related onycholysis varies, but the lesions can be very painful and can affect patients both aesthetically and functionally, resulting in treatment interruption or discontinuation. In addition, chronic onycholysis can lead to keratinization of the nail bed and persistent subungual hyperkeratosis [53].

Onycholysis is defined as the separation of the nail plate from the underlying nail bed. It usually starts at the distal portion of the nail bed, progresses proximally, and may involve the entire nail with the formation of a new space [56]. Lesions are evident after several weeks of treatment [63] due to the slow growth rate of the nails, being more evident in the toenails due to friction. The signs for diagnosis are the following: the affected part of the nail becomes opaque, loses its transparency, and may take on a black, white, or reddish-brown color; the ventral part of the detached plaque can also accumulate debris and lead to a secondary bacterial or fungal infection [64] with the formation of painful abscesses, hemorrhages, and/or loss of the nail and consequently cause pain [53]. Lesions are evident after several weeks of treatment [63] due to the slow growth rate of the nail [47, 53].

Severe cases occur almost exclusively with taxanes and are one of the most common adverse events in the class [53, 65], while mild/moderate can also be seen with the use of other drugs (e.g., capecitabine, etoposide, cytarabine, cyclophosphamide, doxorubicin, or combination therapy) and, to a lesser extent, with some targeted therapies (mTOR, EGFRis, or MEKis inhibitors).

#### 5.6.1 Prevention

- Daily use of topical emollients, nail protection plates (to limit water loss from the nail plate), and cotton gloves [56, 66, 67].
- Avoid rubbing or irritating, including handling cuticles and biting nails, using nails as "tools," prolonged immersion in water, exposure to chemical solvents, and application of artificial nails [53, 56].
- The preventive use of frozen products such as gloves and/or socks allowed a significant reduction in nail changes from 51% to 11% in fingernails and from 21% to 0% in toenails [68, 69].

#### 5.6.2 Therapeutic Management

The management of nail onycholysis depends on clinical grade and impact on activities of daily living. The nail bed should be cleaned, and any infection should be promptly treated with appropriate topical/oral antibiotics and antiseptics. Nails should be trimmed regularly until the nail plate has grown and replaced [64].

### 10.5.7 Diarrhea

Diarrhea is commonly induced by oncologic treatment, mainly in pelvic region radiotherapy, fluoropyrimidines, and irinotecan. It is defined as three or more episodes of soft or liquid stools within 24 hours or a change in the patient's normal frequency of evacuation [70]. Table 10.15 describes the main causes of diarrhea in cancer patients.

This adverse event influences the adjustment of doses or interruption of the treatment protocol, as, depending on the severity, it has a great impact on quality of life, making it impossible to perform basic daily activities. Furthermore, it is directly associated with electrolyte disturbances and in the general state due to dehydration [70, 71].

### 10.5.8 Treatment

After initial assessment and classification of diarrhea severity [36], the conduct and treatment are defined. Treatment must be based on the cause and, when there is no response to specific therapy, treatment with a nonspecific antidiarrheal is started, as described in Table 10.16 [72].

**Table 10.15** Main causes of diarrhea in cancer patients

| Cause | Examples | Management |
|---|---|---|
| Drugs | Laxative, antibiotics, antidiabetics, antacids, iron, proton pump inhibitor, non-steroidal anti-inflammatory | Adjustment of medication |
| Local | Obstruction, constipation, late effect of radiotherapy, pancreatic insufficiency, reduction in the absorption area | Symptomatic therapy |
| Immunity | Late effect of graft-versus-host disease (GvHD) | Immunosuppression |

Adjusted from Bossi et al. [70]

**Table 10.16** Medicines used in the management of diarrhea

| Medicine | indication | Dose |
|---|---|---|
| Loperamide | First line of treatment | Initial dose of 4 mg followed by 2 mg every 2–4 h (higher frequency for persistent diarrhea) or after each soft stool (maximum 16 mg per day) |
| Codeine | Alternative to loperamide | 15–60 mg maximum four times a day |
| Ocreotide | High-risk grade 1–2 diarrhea or persistent diarrhea after loperamide/first-line treatment grade 3–4 | 100 μg three times a day; increase if there is no improvement after 24 h (maximum 500 μg per day) for intractable diarrhea; in critically ill patients, start with 500 μg three times a day |
| Budesonide | Second line of treatment for persistent grade 1–2 diarrhea, would refract to loperamide | 9 mg once a day for 3–5 days |

(continued)

**Table 10.16** (continued)

| Medicine | indication | Dose |
|---|---|---|
| Atropine | Acute diarrhea within 24 hours after irinotecan infusion caused by cholinesterase inhibition | 0.25 mg for prophylaxis or treatment of the cholinergic effects of irinotecan |
| Antibiotic | Grade 3–4 diarrhea associated with neutropenia | Prophylactic: oral ciprofloxacin 250–500 mg twice daily; Treatment: 400 mg norfloxacin twice daily, 600 mg rifaximin daily, 100–200 mg doxycycline daily or 400 mg metronidazole 3 times daily for 7–14 days |
| Bile acid sequestrant | Diarrhea or steatorrhea caused by malabsorption of bile acid | Cholestyramine initially 2–4 g daily with food (maximum dose 24 mg daily) or colesevelam up to 6 × 625 mg three times daily with food; follow up with a low-fat diet |
| Oral rehydration | Grade 1–2 diarrhea | Homemade serum |

Adjusted from Andreyev et al. [71]

## References

1. Weiss RB, Baker JR. Hypersensitivity reactions from antineoplastic agents. Cancer Metas Rev. 1987;6:413–32.
2. Weiss RB, Donehower RC, Wiernik PH, et al. Hypersensitivity reactions from taxol. J Clin Oncol. 1990;8(7):1263–1268 9782.
3. Lenz HJ. Management and preparedness for infusion and hypersensitivity reactions. Oncologist. 2007;12(5):601–9.
4. Calogiuri G, Ventura MT, Mason L, et al. Hypersensitivity reactions to last generation chimeric, humanized, and human recombinant monoclonal antibodies for therapeutic use. Curr Pharm Des. 2008;14:2883–91.
5. Dillman RO. Infusion reactions associated with the therapeutic use of monoclonal antibodies in the treatment of malignancy. Cancer Metastasis Rev. 1999;18:465–71.
6. Brennan PJ, Bouza TR, Hsu FI, Sloane DE, Castells MC. Hypersensitivity reactions to mABs: 105 desensitizations in 23 patients, from evaluation to treatment. J Allergy Clin Immunol. 2009;124(6):1259–66.

7. Ream MA, Tunison D. Hypersensitivity reactions. In: Yasko JM, editor. Nursing Management of Symptoms Associated with chemotherapy. Meniscus Health Care: Bala Cynwyd; 2001. p. 213–24.
8. Darmon M, Malak S, Guichard I, Schlemmer B. Acute tumor lysis syndrome: a comprehensive review. Rev Bras Ter Intensiva. 2008;20(3): 278–85.
9. Locatelli F, Rossi F. Incidence and pathogenesis of tumor lysis syndrome. Contrib Nephrol. 2005;147:61–8.
10. Montesinos P, Lorenzo I, Martín G, et al. Tumor lysis syndrome in patients with acute myeloid leukemia: identification of risk factors and development of a predictive model. Haematologica. 2008;93(1):67–74.
11. Hande KR, Garrow GC. Acute tumor lysis syndrome in patients with highgrade non-Hodgkin's lymphoma. Am J Med. 1993;94(2):133–9.
12. Howard SC, Jones DP, Pui CH. The tumor lysis syndrome. N Engl J Med. 2011;364(19):1844–54.
13. Tallo FS, Vendrame LS, Lopes RD, Lopes AC. Síndrome da lise tumoral: umarevisão para o clínico. Rev Bras Clin Med. São Paulo. 2013;11(2):150–4.
14. Solh M, Appel J. Tumor lysis syndrome. Hosp Physician. 2008;44: 25–9.
15. Tosi P, Barosi G, Lazzaro C, et al. Consensus conference on the management of tumor lysis syndrome. Hema. 2008;93(12):1877–85.
16. Coiffier BA, Altman A, Pui CH, Younes A, Cairo MS. Guidelines for the management of pediatric and adult tumor lysis syndrome: an evidence-based review. J Clin Oncol. 2008;26(16):2767–78.
17. Montoya L. Managing hematologic toxicities in the oncology patient. J Infus Nurs. 2007;30(3):168–72.
18. National Comprehensive Cancer Network. NCCN clinical practice guidelines in oncology: fever and neutropenia. Available at: http://www.nccn.org/professionals/physician_gls/PDF/fever.pdf. Accessed 13 June 2021.
19. Foubert J. Cancer-related anaemia and fatigue: assessment and treatment. Nurs Stand. 2013;20(36):50.
20. Miller CB, Jones RJ, Piantadosi S, Abeloff MD, Spivak JL. Decreased erythropoietin response in patients with the anemia of cancer. N Engl J Med. 1990;322(24):1689–92.
21. Cella D. The Functional Assessment of Cancer Therapy-Anemia (FACT-An) Scale: a new tool for the assessment of outcomes in cancer anemia and fatigue. Semin Hematol. 1997;34(3):13–9.
22. Kuter DJ. Managing thrombocytopenia associated with câncer chemotherapy. Oncology. 2015;29(4):282.
23. Klastersky J, Paesmans M, Rubenstein EB, et al. The multinational association for supportive care in cancer risk index: a multinational scoring system for identifying low-risk febrile neutropenic cancer patients. J Clin Oncol. 2000;18(16):3038–51.

24. Tomblyn M, Chiller T, Einsele H, et al. Guidelines for preventing infectious complications among hematopoietic cell transplant recipients: a global perspective. Bone Marrow Transplant. 2009;44(8):453–5.
25. Cooper KL, Madan J, Whyte S, Stevenson MD, Akehurst R. Granulocyte colony-stimulating factors for febrile neutropenia prophylaxis following chemotherapy: systematic review and meta-analysis. BMC Cancer. 2011;11(1):1–11.
26. Bokemeyer C, Aapro MS, Courdi A, et al. EORTC guidelines for the use of erythropoietic proteins in anaemic patients with cancer. Eur J Cancer. 2004;40(15):2201–16.
27. Organização Pan Americana de SaúdeBrasil. Folha informativa – Câncer. https://www.paho.org/bra/index.php?option=com_content&view=article&id=5588:folha-informativa-cancer&Itemid=1094. Acessoem 22 de julho.
28. O'Brien BJ, Rusthoven J, Rocchi A, Latreille J, Fine S, Vandenberg T, Laberge F. Impact of chemoterapy – associated nausea and vomiting on patients functional status and on costs: survey of five Canadian centers. Can Med Assocj. 1993;149(3):296–302.
29. Fresco DR, Suárez L. Recomendaciones para la prevención y eltratamento de náuseas y vómitosinducidos por quimioterapia. Revista Medica del Uruguay. 2004;20(2):120–9.
30. Hu Z, Liang W, Yang Y, et al. Personalized estimate of chemoterapy-induced nausea and vomiting: development and external validation of a nomogram in cancer patients receiving highly/moderately emetogenic chemoterapy. Medicine. 2016;95(2) https://journals.lww.com/md-journal/Fulltext/2016/01120/Personalized_Estimate_of_Chemotherapy_Induced.58.aspx Accessed July 22.
31. Becker J, Nardin JM. Use of antiemetics in the antineoplastic treatment of cancer patients. R Bras Farm Hosp Serv Saúde São Paulo. 2011;2(3):18–22.
32. Almeida RGL, Pontes ACAA, Cardoso DA, Carrera JS, Sousa MS, Maia SF. O Manejo da ÊmeseemumaUnidadeOncológica: a Necessidade da IntervençãoFarmacêuticaem Tempo Real. RevistaBrasileira de Cancerologia. 2015;61(2):115–21.
33. Aapro M, Jordan K, and Feyer P. 2013. Pathophysiology of chemotherapy-induced nausea and vomiting. https://link.springer.com/chapter/10.1007%2F978-1-907673-58-0_2.
34. National Comprehensive Cancer Network (NCCN) Guidelines. Antiemesis, version 1.2019, 2019.
35. Grunberg SM, Deuson RR, Mavros P, et al. Incidence of chemotherapy-induced nausea and emesis after modern antiemetics. Cancer. 2004;100(10):2261–8.
36. Guia para notificação de reaçõesadversasemoncologia/ SociedadeBrasileira de FarmacêuticosemOncologia – SOBRAFO, Agência Nacional de VigilânciaSanitária – ANVISA. 2. ed. São Paulo: ConectfarmaPublicaçõesCientíficas; 2011.

37. Barrios DM, Phillips GS, Freites-Martinez A, et al. Outpatient dermatology consultations for oncology patients with acute dermatologic adverse events impact anticancer therapy interruption: a retrospective study. J Eur Acad Dermatol Venereol. 2020;34(6):1340–7.
38. Lacouture ME, Sibaud V, Gerber PA, et al. ESMO Guidelines Committee. Electronic address: clinicalguidelines@esmo.org. Prevention and management of dermatological toxicities related to anticancer agents: ESMO Clinical Practice Guidelines☆. Ann Oncol. 2021;32(2):157–70.
39. Nardone B, Nicholson K, Newman M, et al. Histopathologic and immunohistochemical characterization of rash to human epidermal growth factor receptor 1 (HER1) and HER1/2 inhibitop.rs in cancer patients. Clin Cancer Res. 2010;16:4452–60.
40. Saad ED, Hoff PM, Carnelós RP, et al. Comun toxicity criteria of the National Cancer Institute. Revista Brasileira de Cancerologia. 2002;48(1):63–96.
41. Lichtenberger BM, Gerber PA, Holcmann M, et al. Epidermal EGFR controls cutaneous host defense and prevents inflammation. Sci Transl Med. 2013;5:111.
42. Roe E, Garcia Muret MP, Marcuello E, et al. Description and management of cutaneous side effects during cetuximab or erlotinib treatments: a prospective study of 30 patients. J Am Acad Dermatol. 2006;55: 429–37.
43. Lacouture ME, Anadkat MJ, Bensadoun RJ, et al. Clinical practice guidelines for the prevention and treatment of EGFR inhibitor-associated dermatologic toxicities. Support Care Cancer. 2011;19:1079–95.
44. Zhao CY, Liu RC, Consuegra G, et al. Epidermal growth factor receptor inhibitor-induced papulopustular eruption successfully treated with low-dose oral dapsone. Australas J Dermatol. 2018;59:219–20.
45. Jo SJ, Shin H, Jo S, et al. Prophylactic and therapeutic efficacy of pyridoxine supplements in the management of hand–foot syndrome during chemotherapy: a meta-analysis. Clin Exp Dermatol. 2015;40(3):260–70.
46. Zhang RX, Wu XJ, Wan DS, et al. Celecoxib can prevent capecitabine related hand-foot syndrome in stage II and III colorectal cancer patients: result of a single-center, prospective randomized phase III trial. Ann Oncol. 2012;23:1348–53.
47. Miller KK, Gorcey L, McLellan BN. Chemotherapy-induced hand-foot syndrome and nail changes: a review of clinical presentation, etiology, pathogenesis, and management. J Am Acad Dermatol. 2014;71:787–94.
48. Dummer R, Ascierto PA, Gogas HJ, et al. Overall survival in patients with BRAF-mutant melanoma receiving encorafenib plus binimetinib versus vemurafenib or encorafenib (COLUMBUS): a multicentre, openlabel, randomised, phase 3 trial. Lancet Oncol. 2018;19:1315–27.
49. Anforth R, Fernandez-Penas P, Long GV. Cutaneous toxicities of RAF inhibitors. Lancet Oncol. 2013;14:11–8.

50. Zielinski C, Lang I, Beslija S, et al. Predictive role of hand-foot syndrome in patients receiving first-line capecitabine plus bevacizumab for HER2-negative metastatic breast cancer. Br J Cancer. 2016;114:163–70.
51. Stintzing S, Fischer von Weikersthal L, Vehling-Kaiser U. et al., Correlation of capecitabine-induced skin toxicity with treatment efficacy in patients with metastatic colorectal cancer: results from the German AIO KRK-0104 trial. Br J Cancer. 2011;105(2):206–11.
52. Freites-Martinez A, Azael. The MASCC textbook of cancer supportive care and survivorship. New York: Springer International Publishing; 2018. p. 2018.
53. Sibaud V, Leboeuf NR, Roche H, et al. Dermatological adverse events with taxane chemotherapy. Eur J Dermatol. 2016;26:427–43.
54. Stander S, Weisshaar E, Mettang T, et al. Clinical classification of itch: a position paper of the international forum for the study of itch. Acta Derm Venereol. 2007;87:291–4.
55. Monroe EW. Relative efficacy and safety of loratadine, hydroxyzine,and placebo in chronic idiopathic urticaria and atopic dermatitis. ClinTher. 1992;14:17–21.
56. Robert C, Sibaud V, Mateus C, et al. Nail toxicities induced by systemic anticancer treatments. Lancet Oncol. 2015;16:181–9.
57. Kiyohara Y, Yamazaki N, Kishi A. Erlotinib-related skin toxicities: treatment strategies in patients with metastatic non-small cell lung cancer. J Am Acad Dermatol. 2013;69:463–72.
58. Piraccini BM, Bellavista S, Misciali C, et al. Periungual and subungual pyogenic granuloma. Br J Dermatol. 2010;163:941–53.
59. Capriotti K, Capriotti JA. Chemotherapy-associated paronychia treated with a dilute povidone-iodine/dimethylsulfoxide preparation. Clin CosmetInvestig Dermatol. 2015;8:489–91.
60. Capriotti K, Capriotti J, Pelletier J, et al. Chemotherapy-associated paronychia treated with 2% povidone-iodine: a series of cases. Cancer Manag Res. 2017;9:225–8.
61. Cubiro X, Planas-Ciudad S, Garcia-Muret MP, et al. Topical timolol for paronychia and pseudopyogenic granuloma in patients treated with epidermal growth factor receptor inhibitors and capecitabine. JAMA Dermatol. 2018;154:99–100.
62. Mirshams M, Daneshpazhooh M, Mirshekari A, et al. Cryotherapy in the treatment of pyogenic granuloma. J Eur Acad Dermatol Venereol. 2006;20:788–90.
63. Winther D, Saunte DM, Knap M, et al. Nail changes due to docetaxelda neglected side effect and nuisance for the patient. Support Care Cancer. 2007;15:1191–7.
64. Garden BC, Wu S, Lacouture ME. The risk of nail changes with epidermal growth factor receptor inhibitors: a systematic review of the literature and meta-analysis. J Am Acad Dermatol. 2012;67:400–8.
65. Minisini AM, Tosti A, Sobrero AF, et al. Taxane-induced nail changes: incidence, clinical presentation and outcome. Ann Oncol. 2003;14:333–7.

66. Thomas R, Williams M, Cauchi M, et al. A double-blind, randomised trial of a polyphenolic-rich nail bed balm for chemotherapy-induced onycholysis: the UK polybalm study. Breast Cancer Res Treat. 2018;171:103–10.
67. Kim JY, Ok ON, Seo JJ, et al. A prospective randomized controlled trial of hydrating nail solution for prevention or treatment of onycholysis in breast cancer patients who received neoadjuvant/adjuvant docetaxel chemotherapy. Breast Cancer Res Treat. 2017;164:617–25.
68. Scotte F, Tourani JM, Banu E, et al. Multicenter study of a frozen glove to prevent docetaxel-induced onycholysis and cutaneous toxicity of the hand. J Clin Oncol. 2005;23:4424–9.
69. Scotte F, Banu E, Medioni J, et al. Matched case-control phase 2 study to evaluate the use of a frozen sock to prevent docetaxel-induced onycholysis and cutaneous toxicity of the foot. Cancer. 2008;112:1625–31.
70. Bossi P, Antonuzzo A, Cherny NI, et al. ESMO guidelines committee. Electronic address: clinicalguidelines@esmo.org. Diarrhea in adult cancer patients: ESMO clinical practice guidelines. Ann Oncol. 2018;29(4):126–42.
71. Andreyev J, Ross P, Donnellan C, et al. Guidance on the management of diarrhoea during cancer chemotherapy. Lancet Oncol. 2014;15(10):447–60.
72. Benson AB III, Ajani JA, Catalano RB, et al. Recommended guidelines for the treatment of cancer treatment-induced diarrhea. J Clin Oncol. 2004;22(14):2918–26.

# 11 Managing Issues: Tumor Lysis, Extravasation, Adverse Effects, and Others

Lucio Frigo,
Guilherme Aparecido Monteiro Duque da Fonseca,
Giovani Marino Favero,
and Durvanei Augusto Maria

## 11.1 Adverse Effects

Modern medicine has contributed to enhance human longevity and quality of life. On the other hand, an elderly population inhabiting a continuously polluted environment certainly contributes to the raise of cancer development.

L. Frigo (✉)
Associação Paulista de Cirurgiões Dentistas School of Dentistry (FAOA), São Paulo, Brazil

G. A. M. D. da Fonseca
Periodontology Department, School of Dentistry, Universidade Guarulhos, São Paulo, Brazil

G. M. Favero
General Biology Department, Universidade Estadual de Ponta Grossa, Parana, Brazil

D. A. Maria
Molecular Biology Laboratory, Instituto Butantan, São Paulo, Brazil
e-mail: durvanei.maria@butantan.gov.br


C. W. P. Schmidt, K. M. Otoni (eds.), *The Golden Guide to Oncologic Pharmacy*, https://doi.org/10.1007/978-3-030-98596-7_11

In this context, anticancer drugs are in high demand in recent decades, and oncology pharmacology is one of the medical fields experiencing a remarkable research activity and development of new drugs [6, 8].

However, anticancer drugs are among the more toxic drugs legally available. The National Cancer Institute's Common Terminology Criteria for Adverse Events (NCICTCAE), which is responsible to classify the grade seriousness of adverse reactions, lists more than 750 different types of adverse reactions related to cancer treatments [8].

The balance of the expected benefits and the potential adverse drug reactions is the frequent challenge faced by clinicians [8, 11].

Adverse drug reactions (ADRs) are among the leading concerns when drug research and development are considered once they are potentially related to therapeutic failures, and consequently, drugs withdraw from the market.

ADRs have been estimated to contribute up to 60% of the total costs involved in chemotherapy [8].

The economic impact of cancer therapy is, generally, relegated to second plane due to population willingness to pay for to resolve this feared disease. However, the treatment costs are relevant information to decision makers in health-care system.

Literature approach used to take two routes are (1) cost-effectiveness analysis of the anticancer treatment and (2) cost-effectiveness analysis of the ADRs related to anticancer treatment [7].

ADRs cost-effectiveness analysis should be conducted based on the following direction: (1) ADR selection, (2) dose modification, (3) ADR and quality of life, and (4) multiple ADR. However, literature approach is restricted to some of these aspects isolated, considered to only one type of cancer and restricted to a specific health-care institution. In this perspective, a wide range of treatment cost can be found. For instance, the cost of erythropoietin treatment to address anticancer drug-related anemia can vary from £ 190,000 to £ 9000 per QALY gained [7].

Albeit individual patient characteristics contribute to ADRs in addition to drugs, multiple drug-related factors are involved like drug formulation, dosage, administration route, drug interactions (drug-drug, drug-food), allergic reactions, and metabolism [12].

The physicochemical drug features are highly related to the onset of ADRs. These drug features are directly involved in key aspects of drug metabolism like absorption, distribution, efficacy, transformation, excretion and drug promiscuity.

Ideally, candidate drug molecules should comply to a roll of principles initially established by Lipinski and cols. in 2001. [12].

Albeit designed to oral-administrated drugs, the "rule of five" of Lipinski (R05) can, in certain extension, be applied to intravenous drugs as well: R01, drug should not exceed a molecular weight of 500 g/mol; R02, the hydrophobicity, represented by log P value, of less than 5; R03 do not exceed 5 hydrogen bond donors and 10 hydrogen bond acceptor sites; R04 do not exceed a polar surface area of 140 Å; and R05 do not exceed 10 rotatable bonds [12].

Intravenous drugs tend to have more ADRs due to its faster and broadly systemic effect than oral-administrated drugs.

Notably, most anticancer drugs do not comply to R05 simply because they were developed before 2001.

High molecular weight and log P values are related to off target binding (drug promiscuity), and highly lipophilic compounds (high P log) are more likely to promote cell toxicity due to its high affinity to proteins [12].

The traditional approach to access ADRs is patients' spontaneous report. Prompt identification of drug safety problems enforces regulatory measures from health authorities to preclude further damage to patients [8, 11].

However, this approach is not so successful in oncology pharmacology due to different reasons:

1. Usually, cancer patients are severely ill, the anticancer drugs used are frequently very toxic, and consequently, ADR reports fairly high. The treatment risk/benefit evaluation by physicians is related to clinical course/severity of the disease as well as the prognostic. In this regard, anticancer ADRs are considered a low-priority secondary problem to clinicians.
2. The new developed drugs (first in class) targeting molecular cell receptors never tried before that have limited support from the literature. A selected study evaluated 12 anticancer target agents approved to access ADRs identification in the post-

marketing period. Seventy-six serious ADRs were included in the updated labels, 50% of them were potentially fatal, and 58% were unpredicted in the initial label. In addition, 42% received one or more boxed warnings.

3. Fatal ADRs can take longer times to be identified. For example, genetically susceptible patients may have bone marrow depression due to thioguanine after 36 years of the therapy.
4. It is worth mentioning that the population tested in premarketing studies is fairly different to that receiving the drug in the post-marketing phase [4, 8, 11].

In general terms, anticancer drugs are directed to completely eradicate the malignancy or, alternatively, to reduce disease severity in a palliation effect [6, 12].

This goal is achieved through drug lethal cytotoxic induction and, consequently, tumor regression. Classically selected targets to drug actions are centered in the different steps of metabolic DNA and RNA pathways, direct attack to DNA and cell division apparatus. These strategies are perfectly achievable but not restricted to cancer cells. Irrespective of various types of metabolic imbalances and defections in cancer cells, they are alike to normal (nonmalignant) cells, and consequently, anticancer drugs have a broad action through the whole organism. The off-target binding related to lack of drug specificity is termed drug promiscuity [6, 11, 12].

Anticancer drugs partial selectivity is achieved due to some characteristics of tumor mass: (1) higher demand of metabolites, (2) higher demand of blood supply, (3) higher mitosis index, and (4) higher cell death index [11, 12].

It is important to take into account that most of these characteristics are shared to normal tissues, especially hematopoietic and epithelial. In this perspective, some ADR can be predicted. A high epithelial cells turnover can anticipate hair loss (alopecia), gastrointestinal disturbance (vomiting, diarrhea, mucositis), and hematopoietic disturbance (reducing numbers of white blood cells, leukopenia; reducing numbers of red blood cells, anemia; reducing of platelets numbers, thrombocytopenia) [11, 12, 14].

Transient or not, these ADR suggests an additional (adjunct) drug therapy is frequent. Adjunct drug therapy aims to improve patient's quality of life in the case of vomiting, diarrhea, mucositis, or anemia, for example, but sometimes, it is absolutely mandatory. Leukopenia is related to an increased incidence of body infection (mainly in skin and guts) and the incidence of other types of tumors in addition to the primary target of the cancer therapy. Thrombocytopenia and its potential to compromise blood clot formation is a life-threatening condition that must be addressed with adjunct therapy as well [4, 11].

Additional concerns related to anticancer drugs include resistance and adaptation. In both situations, using two different types of drugs in combination or intercalated is the main strategy to address the problem. Drug combined therapy usually is short termed due to its markedly high incidence and intensity of ADRs [4].

In fact, dose, dose schedule, administration route, and the type of cancer contribute to toxicity of the drug prescribed to the patient; however, cancer drugs have a narrow limit of safety [4, 8, 12].

### 11.1.1 Most Common ADRs

**Hepatotoxicity** In considering drug dose set and possible drug adaptation, the access to patient's liver status is fundamental. Hydrophobic, high-molecular-weight drugs are fairly aggressive to the liver, particularly if used for long-lasting scheduled therapies. Hepatic cirrhosis or steatosis are frequent ADRs in long-term anticancer drug therapy. Therapeutic dose set may be even more difficult in patients exhibiting liver metastasis [9].

Anticancer drugs elimination from the cell and the entire organism involves cell membrane transporters in addition to liver and kidney.

The P-glycoprotein is a cell membrane transporter dedicated to remove drugs from the cells. It is expressed in a wide variety of cell types and is able to transport different types of drugs irrespective of hydrophobicity and molecular weight. Due to capacity to disturb drug absorption and metabolism, it influences drug bioavailability and toxicity, enhancing ADRs frequency [9].

P-glycoprotein activity modulation frequently occurs in anticancer drugs combination (multidrug) therapy.

Drug excretion is mainly directed through the liver and kidney. A fraction of the unchanged drug can be eliminated directly through biliary system and renal tubules. However, the most part of the ingested/injected drug is metabolized in the liver in two types of reactions. In type I reactions, reduction, oxidation, and hydrolysis are conducted to make the drug compound more hydrophilic. The type II reactions have the same goal, but it is achieved through conjugation of some compounds (glucuronic acid, glycine, sulfate). The type II reactions may, in addition to direct excretion, activate the drug compound and potentiate ADRs, enhancing off-target binding (drug promiscuity).

Drug metabolites are much more prone to off-target protein binding and are implicated in ADRs like nausea, cardiotoxicity, and neurotoxicity in addition to idiosyncratic events [9].

**Kidney Toxicity** Drugs used in malignant disease can induce a variety of renal failures. The kidneys are the main route to eliminate drugs and their metabolites. Excretion may take two routes: (1) tubular secretion and (2) glomerular filtration. Glomerular filtration is only possible if the drug is not bound to proteins. In the case of protein-bound drugs, proximal tubules secretion is the route to excretion.

Anticancer drugs can affect glomerulus, tubules, interstitium, and microvasculature. Clinical manifestations range from asymptomatic serum creatinine elevation to acute renal failure, and they are categorized as acute kidney injury (AKI) due to thrombotic microangiopathy (TMA), toxic acute tubular necrosis, and crystal nephropathy; proteinuria/nephrotic syndrome due to TMA, focal segmental glomerulosclerosis (FSGS), minimal change disease, and membranous nephropathy; tubulopathies due to electrolyte, acid-base, and divalent disorders; and chronic kidney disease (CKD) due to glomerulopathies or interstitial nephritis [2, 10].

**Cardiovascular Toxicity**
Cardiovascular system is affected by anticancer drug as well, and cardiotoxicity is considered the most critical ADR and the primary cause of mortality of cancer survivors. A wide range of cardiovascular compromise was recorded: thromboembolic and vasospastic ischemia, dysrhythmia, arterial hypertension, and heart failure due to left ventricle dysfunction. Anticancer drugs cardiotoxic effects are related to reactive oxygen species (ROS) and reactive nitrogen species (RNS) production in cardiomyocytes.

Low levels of ROS/RNS are required to normal cardiomyocyte physiological function. The $H_2O_2$ produced is considered an endothelium-derived hyperpolarizing stimulus and a coronary circulation vasodilator in addition to chemical attack to many cell biomolecules.

Intracellular signaling inhibitor anticancer drugs induce imbalances in metabolic cascades that are critically related to myocardial function, especially in conditions of stress (hypertension/hypertrophy) [3, 13].

**Neurotoxicity** Most anticancer drugs induce neurotoxic ADRs. The more frequently described neurotoxic effects are related to peripheral nervous system. Dorsal root ganglions are frequently disturbed by anticancer drugs with consequent manifestations in altered sensitivity, including states of spontaneous pain. Motor and sensitive myelin nerves experience different grades of demyelination with loss of sensibility, weakness, neuropathy, loss of equilibrium, and defective sensory-motor reflexes. Cranial nerves are less frequently affected by anticancer drug ADRs. Central nervous system ADRs are rare due to blood-brain barrier; however, mood disturbances were recorded [5].

**Nausea and Vomiting** The vomiting reflex is a preserved behavior through different species and is considered as a protective mechanism against ingested toxins.

Anticancer drugs may cause emesis through different mechanisms. The best supported is related to the effect on the upper small intestine. After anticancer drug administration, free radicals are produced, leading to a local release of 5-hydroxytryptamine (5-HT). 5-HT then, through its receptors, acts on vagal afferent terminals in the bowel wall. Efferent fibers project from the dorsal vagal complex to the final effector of the emetic reflex. Diverse neuronal groups of the temporal lobe may be sources of efferent fibers that stimulate emesis, such as the amygdala [6, 8, 12].

**Diarrhea** The diarrhea is a common ADR reported in several anticancer drug regimens that cause a debilitated state and can potentially be life-threatening.

The triggering mechanism is not completely understood, but it is most likely a process that induces an imbalance between absorption and secretion in the small bowel segment. Some types of anticancer drugs induce acute damage to the intestinal mucosa that is evidenced by intestinal epithelium loss, inflammation of the bowel wall, and focal necrosis. Drug-induced mitotic arrest of intestinal epithelial crypt cells results in an increase in immature secretory crypt cell numbers in relation to absorptive cells, leading to an abnormal absorption and secretion of fluids and electrolytes. Additionally, brush border disruption compromises the enzymes involved in terminal digestion of carbohydrates and proteins. Opportunistic bacterial colonization collaborates to disturb the secretion of intestinal fluids and electrolytes [6, 8].

**Alopecia** Alopecia represents one of the most conspicuously reported ADR and a major unmet challenge in clinical oncology.

The main target of anticancer drug ADRs are the rapidly proliferating and vulnerable hair follicle and its associated pigmentary system. These systems undergo a rapidly apoptotic process after chemotherapeutic inoculation. The P-53 proapoptotic pathway is importantly involved in the process. Additionally, anticancer drugs disturb hair follicle vasculature and the sebaceous gland of the region, negatively affecting the hair follicle health and function [6, 8].

**Anorexia** Anorexia can be defined as the loss of desire to ingest food, consequently disturbing nutrients ingestion, prompting body weight loss.

Anorexia-induced chemotherapy is possibly related to a systemic or local activation of the hypothalamus through inflammatory mediators secondary to intestinal mucositis or the direct action of the drug in the brain. The increased levels of proinflammatory cytokines, notably interleukin-1β, may be related to the process.

In addition, anorexia due to chemotherapy has a strong relationship with dehydration states that are secondary to diarrhea, which may be induced by a wide variety of different types of anticancer drugs. Systemic dehydration is a well-described cause of anorexia that is triggered by the activation of osmosensitive nucleus in hypothalamus and vasopressinergic neurons. It is presently known that chemotherapeutic drugs can induce enough dehydration to activate the neuronal brain pathways involved in anorexia [6, 8, 12].

**Rheumatic Manifestations** Reports have been collected about rheumatoid arthritis (RA), Reiter's syndrome, and vasculitis in patients submitted to anticancer immunotherapy. Anticancer drugs exacerbate previous RA states and frequently induce post-chemotherapy rheumatism. Arthralgia, stiffness, and arthritis ADRs were reported after chemotherapy and frequently involve joints of the upper and lower extremity after a few months of chemotherapy begin. These reports were considered self-limited, noninflammatory, and temporary. In addition, the phenomenon had no relationship with metastasis occurrence.

The mechanisms underlying chemotherapy-related rheumatic manifestations are poorly understood; however, it is supposed that anticancer drugs disrupt severally the immune system inducing an imbalance in cartilage matrix turnover, including the production of autoantibodies, resembling an autoimmune disease [6, 8, 12].

**Neutropenia** Chemotherapy-induced myelosuppression is among the earliest ADR reported of anticancer drugs and, commonly, the most important dose limiter of chemotherapy. Irrespective of the importance of all leukocyte types in body defense mechanisms, the neutrophil cell number reduction (neutropenia) has an immediate and profound effect in defense system [6].

Anticancer drug-induced neutrophil depletion severally impacts in inflammatory response. Neutrophil outnumbers the other leukocytes by a wide margin in "normal" blood, and it is a key component of innate immunity. Neutropenia reduces drastically antibacterial response, prompting infections due to unrestricted bacterial multiplication and invasion.

However, the most dangerous and life-threatening clinical feature is the reduction or the absence of the infection signs and symptoms. Basically, only fever remains present. Patients with this profile (febrile neutropenia) have a high risk of septicemia, so intravenous antibiotics and hospitalization are mandatory measures [6, 8, 12].

**Thrombocytopenia** Chemotherapy-induced myelosuppression, in addition to compromised leukocyte cell number (and function), reduces the platelet cell number as well (thrombocytopenia). The recent therapeutic use of myeloid growth factors and erythropoietic agents, have been reducing the incidence and severity of neutropenic fever and anemia, respectively. The same approach has not been so successfully applied to thrombocytopenia, so it remains an unsolved clinical problem.

Thrombocytopenic states are induced by intense anticancer drug administration, as in the setting of hematologic-origin malignancies and pediatric malignancies. In any case, hemorrhagic events and the necessity of platelet transfusion, as well as chemotherapeutic dose reduction and treatment delays, are commonly reported.

Thrombocytopenia may have different causes: (1) reduction of platelet production, (2) massive platelet destruction, and (3) spleen platelet sequestration.

It is worth to mention that in spite of platelet production reduction is the main cause of thrombocytopenia-related chemotherapeutic effects, different class of drugs act by different mechanisms:

1. The antimitotic effect on stem cells of busulfan and carboplatin leads to a reduction in platelet reduction that is long-lasting and refractory to treatments.
2. The antimitotic effect on progenitor precursors in later differentiation states of common cytotoxic drugs induces shorter periods of platelet reduction count.
3. Protease inhibitors (e.g., bortezomib), which act through nuclear factor K-ß inhibition, reduce the fully differentiated megakaryocyte capacity to shed platelets [6, 11].

### 11.1.2 Anticancer Drugs Classes and ADRs

Anticancer drugs can be classified according to their sites of action at specific points in the biosynthetic pathways of important biomolecules.

**Alkylating agents** This is a group of substances that react through electrophilic alkyl group or a substituted alkyl group that can bind covalently to nucleophilic site (including bases of DNA) bases of cytotoxic effect. Although it reacts to all cell in different cell-cycle phase, efficacy and toxicity are more evident in rapidly proliferating tissues. Common ADRs related to alkylating agents are nausea, vomiting, bone marrow atrophy, renal failure, interstitial pneumonitis, pulmonary fibrosis, gonadal toxicity, teratogenesis, alopecia, allergic reactions, immunosuppression, diarrhea, CNS disturbance, and induction of drug resistance.

As paradoxical as it seems be, new types of cancer may be induced along the treatment by anticancer drugs as they have a high mutagenic potential. For example, occurrence of acute non-lymphoblastic leukemia some 10 years after treatment to cure the original tumor has been observed. This is a particular problem related to the use of alkylating agent class [15].

**Cisplatin and Analogs** These compounds are based on platinum cell-killing potential. These compounds induce cell killing through the development of a covalent bifunctional bond to DNA. Common ADRs related to cisplatin and analogs are renal toxicity, cardiotoxicity, neurotoxicity, nausea, and myelosuppression [1, 16].

**Antimetabolites** Antimetabolites encompasses a group of substances that share structural resemblance to normal cell molecules, and they induce their predicted effect arresting or disturbing the metabolic pathways of nucleic acid synthesis. They fall into two main classes: the folate antagonists or antifolates, which interfere with nucleotide synthesis, and the purine and pyrimidine analogues, which are incorporated into DNA and affect the cell cycle.

Common ADRs related to antimetabolites are myelosuppression, mucositis, hepatotoxicity, interstitial pneumonitis, CNS disturbance, drug resistance induction, skin rash, chest pain, alopecia, neutropenic fever, anorexia, diarrhea, abdominal pain, and acute pancreatitis . Pediatric ADRs were reported: fever, myalgia, bone pain, conjunctivitis, malaise, peripheral neuropathy, and seizures.

Additionally, antimetabolites may induce other types of cancer: SCC, non-Hodgkin's sarcoma, and Kaposi's sarcoma [17].

**Topoisomerase Agents** DNA topoisomerase (Top) comprises a class of enzymes that alter the topology of the DNA and release torsional stress during replication and transcription. Top 1 and 2 isozymes are approved by the FDA. Common ADRs related to topoisomerase agents are mainly related to cardiotoxicity: tachycardia, hypotension, electrocardiogram changes, and arrhythmias [18].

**Antimicrotubular Agents** The mitotic spindle is part of a larger intracellular network of microtubules that is formed during prophase in the cell cycle. This larger network is a denominated cytoskeleton and participates in different cell functions, including the dislocation of organelles in the cell cytoplasm. The mitotic spindles comprise a group of different proteins, in addition to tubulins and centromere proteins, that are responsible on separating the newly duplicated cell DNA to the future daughter cells in the final phases of the cell division. Most microtubule inhibitor drugs are plant-derived compounds that have the ability to disturb tubulin polymerization, consequently disrupting mitotic spindles and cell division process.

**Taxanes** Neutropenia is the main toxicity effect, starting on day 8–10 and lasting 5–10 days.

Major hypersensitivity reactions were detected in 3% of the patients and starts 10 minutes after drug administration. High corticosteroid doses are, usually, effective in the recovery, and it is believed to be triggered by histamine-like substances.

Peripheral neuropathy was also detected. Sensory loss, including deep tendon reflexes, was observed, and demyelination was observed in physiologic studies.

Cardiac ADRs are mainly related to a transient sinus bradycardia in 30% of the patients. However, congestive heart failure can be observed in patients receiving drug combinations.

Severe hepatotoxicity and pancreatitis are rare ADRs. Drug-induced alopecia is reversible, and nail disorders were reported as well.

**Vinca Alkaloids** This group has a marked neurotoxicity characterized by a peripheral, symmetric, mixed sensory-motor and autonomic polyneuropathy. Neuritic pain and deep tendon reflex loss were recorded in extended treatments. Neurologic studies demonstrated axonal degeneration and reduced axonal transport related to axonal microtubule dysfunction. Cranial nerves are rarely affected, and central neurotoxicity is rare.

Neutropenia is the more frequent ADR, but thrombocytopenia and anemia were reported as well.

The more frequent gastrointestinal effects reported were bloating, constipation, abdominal pain, pancreatitis, and mucositis [19].

**Small-Molecule Tyrosine Kinase Inhibitors** Basic science research has propelled the development of new anticancer drugs. The rationale is to circumvent or reduce "classical" anticancer ADRs due to its lack of specificity to cancer cells. Tyrosine kinase is one of these candidate molecules that have been targeted in drug development. The phase I and II clinical tests have been conducted, and some drugs approved by FDA (imatinib mesylate, dasatinib, nilotinib, erlotinib, among others).

Irrespective of the research/clinical efforts, mild-to-moderate ADRs have been reported. The most frequent ADR reported is drug adaptation, followed by mild-to-moderate skin rash and diarrhea. Additionally, VEGFR TKI-directed drugs may induce hypertension, proteinuria, wound healing problems, bleeding, reversible leukoencephalopathy, thrombosis, and hypothyroidism ([20]).

**Antibodies to Signal Transduction Molecules** Different cell death mechanisms can be triggered using antibodies that are available to clinical use. Strategies vary from complexing with ligand, stimulation or blockade of receptor, toxic payload delivery, and interactions with the immune system or complement system to stromal components targeting. EGFR inhibitory antibodies are related to paronychia, digits fissures, and hypomagnesemia. Mild fever, hypotension, tremors, skin rash, nausea, abdominal pain, and vomiting were also reported.

In clinical tests using Anti-VEGFR antibodies, fatigue, pain, arthralgia, and constipation were reported.

On the other hand, TNF-related apoptosis-inducing ligand antibodies exhibited a mild fever, hypotension, myalgia, fatigue, nausea, and diarrhea [21].

**Histone Deacetylase Inhibitors and Demethylating Agents** The clinical strategy is based on (1) the inhibition of DNA methyltransferases that mediate abnormal promoter methylation and (2) the inhibition of histone deacetylases that catalyze key repressive biochemical steps related to transcriptional repression.

Histone deacetylase inhibitor compounds used in hematologic malignancies induced fatigue, nausea, diarrhea, and thrombocytopenia in 45% of the patients. In electrocardiographic T waves, 80% experienced asymptomatic changes [22].

**Proteasome Inhibitors** Proteasomes are macromolecular complexes that conduct intracellular protein degradation. However, recent research indicates that proteasome protein degradation is directly linked to cell cycle and apoptosis. Consequently, proteasome became a potential target to anticancer drugs. A phase II clinical study in multiple myeloma reported thrombocytopenia, neuropathic pain, nausea, vomiting, constipation, diarrhea, neutropenia, and anemia [23].

**Thalidomide and Derivatives** Thalidomide is a drug developed initially as antiemetic and sleeping aid; however, due to its implications in severe children malformations, it was abandoned. Irrespective of its ADRs, thalidomide continued to be studied and have sporadic used. A new drug potential was detected in this sporadic use: It was effective against erythema nodosum leprosum and multiple myeloma. Anticancer effects are related to (1) inhibition of NF-kß transcription, (2) adhesion of myeloma cells to bone marrow stromal cells, (3) inhibition of growth factors (VEGF, FGF) production and TNF-a, and (4) enhance natural killer cell-mediated cytotoxicity.

In 2005, thalidomide received FDA approval, and its ADRs arise specially with long-term therapy: drowsiness, constipation, orthostatic hypotension, nausea, peripheral neuropathy, venous thromboembolic events, mood changes, pulmonary embolus, hash, and bradycardia [24].

## 11.2 Tumor Lysis

Tumor lysis syndrome is characterized by massive disruption of the plasma membrane of cancer cells, which can be spontaneously or induced by treatment, mainly chemotherapy. The first description of this clinical situation was in 1929 by researchers Bedrna and Polcak in patients with chronic leukemia. At that time, there was no treatment for leukemia, and the finding was an abundant spontaneous cell lysis, changing laboratory biochemical parameters [25, 33].

In the seventies of the last century, the mass destruction of tumor cells was described in a patient with a gastrointestinal carcinoma, developing hyperuricemia and, later, renal failure. The imbalance between cell growth and death found in most tumors generates an abundant number of new cells originated from uncontrolled growth. The introduction of chemotherapy and radiotherapies leads to direct effects on the cell duplication cycle and, consequently, tissue death.

The acute effects of certain treatments or the inability to support the newly formed tissue can generate tumor lysis. The effect of this severe acute metabolic disorder is currently characterized by hyperuricemia, hyperphosphatemia, hyperkalemia, and hypocalcemia. This induces an emergency situation, if not recognized and dealt with quickly, and leads to the death of most affected people [26, 34].

When cancer cells are lysed, they release potassium, phosphorus, and nucleic acids (purines) which are metabolized to inosine, hypoxanthine, then xanthine, and uric acid in humans. Hyperkalemia can cause serious and occasionally fatal adverse events such as arrhythmias. Hyperphosphatemia is another common metabolite in these patients as tumor cells have about four times more phosphorus than normal cells. Hyperphosphatemia can cause secondary hypocalcemia, leading to neuromuscular irritability (tetany), arrhythmia, and increased muscle tone. There is the precipitation of calcium phosphate crystals in organs, which can cause kidney damage and nephritic colic [35–37].

### 11.2.1 Hyperuricemia

The increase in uric acid in tumor lysis syndrome begins 48 to 72 hours after cell mass degradation. Uric acid is a nitrogenous compound formed by two rings of nitrogen (N) and carbon (C) linked to hydrogen (H) and oxygen (O) atoms with general formula C5H4N4O3. In the body, it is a metabolic product that is eliminated in the urine.

Urates are the result of the degradation of purine nucleic acids (adenine and guanine). Currently, the blood concentration of uric acid considered normal cannot exceed 7.0 mg/dL for men and 6.0 mg/dL for women, and values above are called hyperuricemia.

High levels of uric acid in the blood cause deposition of sodium urate crystals in other tissues and can lead to skin irritation (erythema). As the urinary system is responsible for filtering the blood and eliminating uric acid, it is commonly affected when there is hyperuricemia, and it can be affected by infections. In the kidneys, there may be the formation of kidney stones and, in more advanced conditions, acute or chronic renal failure. In the case of tumor lysis syndrome, the effect is acute and immediate, and if left untreated, it leads to kidney failure [30].

### 11.2.2 Hyperphosphatemia

Hyperkalemia is characterized by a serum potassium concentration greater than 5.5 mEq/L, according to the European Resuscitation Council, and the normal range for potassium would be between 3.5 and 5.5 mEq/L.

Potassium is a mineral that carries an electrical charge when dissolved in body fluids such as blood and is one of the main electrolytes in the body. Potassium is essential for the functioning of nerve and muscle cells, and its excess directly interferes with their functions.

In tumor lysis syndrome, hyperkalemia also occurs after a large amount of potassium is released from tumor cells, prior to the disruption of the cell membrane, which is why the high levels of this electrolyte increase 24 to 48 hours after chemotherapy, radiotherapy, or spontaneous injury. The rapid shift of potassium from cells into the blood can overwhelm the kidneys and result in life-threatening hyperkalemia.

Mild hyperkalemia causes few, if any, symptoms. When hyperkalemia becomes more severe, it causes abnormal heart rhythms. If the levels are too high, the heart may stop beating.

Diagnosis is made by measuring circulating potassium levels or associated with certain changes in the electrocardiogram (ECG).

Hypocalcemia, the decrease in calcium levels, is directly related to hyperphosphatemia, with very low values in the circulation. The total calcium concentration is <8.8 mg/dL (< 2.20 mmol/L) in the presence of normal plasma protein concentrations or ionic calcium plasma concentration < 4.7 mg/dL (< 1.17 mmol/L).

Figure 11.1 summarizes the events that occur after massive cell death in the tumor microenvironment. The speed of tumor lysis generates a large number of metabolites and, consequently, acute kidney injury [29].

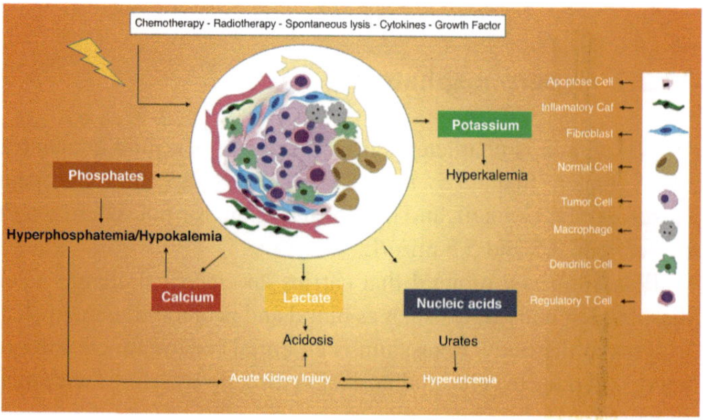


**Fig. 11.1** Diagram of tumor lysis syndrome pathophysiology. Massive cell death in the tumor microenvironment results in acute kidney injury

### 11.2.3 Malignancy and Tumor Lysis Syndrome Risk

After the conceptualization and characterization of TLS, numerous tumors have been observed with the ability to induce the picture of rapid cell damage and its consequences spontaneously or under treatment [38–40]. Currently, neoplasms that can lead to TLS are divided into three groups: (1) low risk, (2) moderate risk, and (3) high risk [32].

The main low-risk malignancies are medulloblastoma, breast carcinoma, gastrointestinal carcinoma, rhabdomyosarcoma, ovarian carcinoma, vulva carcinoma, thymoma, soft tissue sarcomas, metastatic seminoma, melanoma, prostate cancer, hepatocarcinoma, hepatoblastoma, and pheoblastoma of colon [28].

Tumors that present moderate risk, usually associated with treatment, are multiple myeloma, breast carcinoma under treatment with hormonal therapy or chemotherapy, small cell pulmonary carcinoma, and germ cells and neuroblastoma in ovaries. Here, it is worth noting that these are the most common at moderate risk and that both chemotherapy and radiotherapy treatments can lead other tumors that are not on this list to develop the syndrome [27, 41–44].

The neoplasms with high risk to develop TLS are high-grade non-Hodgkin's lymphoma, myeloid leukemia, acute lymphoid leukemias, Burkitt's lymphoma, and other high-grade hematologic tumors) [31, 45].

## 11.3 Extravasation

Anticancer chemotherapy extravasation refers to accidentally or inadvertently inoculation of fluid or drug that finds a way into the surrounding tissues. In the chemotherapy context, the surrounding tissues refer to perivascular connective tissue initially that may follow a spreading to the closer organs or tissues of the leaking site. Hence, clinical evidences are related to connective tissue responses to aggression, and they are related to (1) drug toxicity, (2) the amount of drug, and (3) how long it remained in the tissue [46, 49].

The clinical aspects of the consequences due to drug extravasation determines its classification: (1) vesicant, (2) nonvesicant, and (3) irritant.

Vesicants are usually related to pain, edema, and erythema that potentially induce a blister formation and are accompanied by ulceration and necrosis if not treated. Additionally, they can be divided according to the tissue damage mechanism: (1) DNA-binding drug, which induces apoptosis cell death and (2) non-DNA-binding drug, which induces cell death through drug's metabolization. Tissue damage is usually mild and improves over time [46, 49].

Irritants usually cause a transitory pain sensation and redness and are not related to necrosis; however, large volumes may cause ulceration.

Nonvesicants are usually related to mild reactions that are reported as mild inflammation and discomfort.

Estimative data indicates that extravasation occurs from 0.01% to 7% range in reported infusion procedures [46, 49, 51].

The main risk factors associated to extravasation are (1) blood vessels (veins) features (small, hardened/sclerotic, fragile, prominent but mobile), (2) diseases related to impaired circulation (Raynaud syndrome, advanced diabetes, severe peripheral vascular disease, lymphedema, or superior vena cava syndrome), (3) coagulation disturbance or related increase of vascular permeability, (4) vein access difficulties due to obesity, (5) sensorial deficits, (6) difficulties in communication (children, senile dementia/deficits, cerebral palsy), (7) prolonged infusion time, (8) inexperienced staff, (9) multiple attempts/difficulties at cannulation, (10) unfavorable regions to cannulation, (11) bolus injections, (11) high-flow pressure, (12) inadequate choice of the equipment (peripheral catheter choice, size, steel "butterfly" needle), and (12) inadequate dressings.

Obviously, prevention of drug extravasation relies on well-trained, experienced personnel aware of evidence-based protocols and able to implement preventive protocols [47, 51].

Extravasation identification is suspected if the following signs were present: burning, tingling, discomfort, pain, swelling, or redness in the site of the infusion. Blistering, ulceration, and necrosis may ensue, depending on the drug toxicity. The signs that usually indicate extravasation are resistance of the syringe's plunger, blood return absence, or interruption of the smooth delivery infusion [48, 55].

In the case of extravasation suspicion, a series of strict measures (protocol) should be followed: (1) Cannula should not be removed immediately, and (2) differential diagnostic should be conducted.

Differential diagnosis is mandatory because some anticancer drugs can cause local reactions similar to extravasation, even if correctly administered (skin erythema in the site around the cannula, in the accessed vein, local itching and urticaria) [51–55].

The chemical phlebitis (vein inflammation) may induce burning sensation in the cannula site, in addition to cramping, and it should be considered in differential diagnosis.

Immediate initiation of the treatment procedures is vital, and patient collaboration in symptoms identification is important.

Unspecific measures include the following: (1) Immediately halt and disconnect the infusion. The needle is maintained in place. (2) Identify extravasated agent. (3) Aspirate (if possible) extravasated agent, register the volume in patient record, and avoid manipulation of the region. (4) Mark the region with a pen. (5) Notify the physician and start specific measures.

Specific measures include an initial approach that is based in corticosteroids (hydrocortisone) injection site to avoid or ameliorate connective tissue defense response and reduce incidence of surgical debridement due to necrosis in the region.

Sodium thiosulfate is successfully used to inactivate extravasated DNA-binding drugs in subcutaneous administration route [51–55].

Dimethyl sulfoxide (DMSO) is an ordinary substance that has a potent solvent property and penetrates easily in tissues when topically applied. DMSO displays a free-radical scavenging property that enhances inactivation of the extravasated drugs from subcutaneous tissue.

Dexrazoxane is the antidote used to reduce cardiac toxicity in patients that received anthracycline-based chemotherapy. It is considered that the reduction of the cardiotoxic effects, induced by anthracyclines, is based on its capacity to chelate free and bound iron, reducing the formation of anthracycline-iron complexes, and consequently the generation of reactive oxygen species that are toxic to cardiac tissue.

Nonvesicant extravasated drugs are dealt very conservatively with local dry cold compresses.

Nevertheless, pain states that last more than 10 days and unresolved tissue necrosis are approached with surgical procedures. The surgical method consists of a three-dimensional removal of the necrotic tissue, a temporary coverage using biological dressings, accompanied by harvesting and storage of a split-thickness skin graft. Graft application is conducted only after the wound is clean, which usually is in 2 or 3 days. An alternative, and more recent, surgical procedure is subcutaneous washout. However, this surgical technique requires an experienced surgical unit [50].

In any event of extravasation, a detailed report must be done. Irrespective of different types of documentation used in diverse health centers, some items are obligatory for legal purposes and include (1) patient name and number (if applicable), (2) date and time of extravasation, (3) name of drug extravasated and diluent used, (4) signs and symptoms (also reported by patient), (5) description of the administration access, (6) extravasation area and the approximate amount of drug, (7) management steps with time and date, and (8) patient be informed about the event [51–55].

### 11.3.1 Others: Chemotherapy-Induced Emergencies

Anticancer drugs produce a not unconsidered amount of ADRs. Most of them can be predicted based on literature and clinical experience, and consequently, they can be prevented or, at least, diagnosed to avoid or reduce patient suffering. However, some types of predicted ADRs may occur in a disproportionally high intensity or an unpredicted ADR may occur. These types of occurrences are fewer than 1%, but they are potentially life-threatening and are defined as chemotherapy-induced emergencies. [57].

Emergency management is a challenging clinical situation that demands a prompt diagnostic and immediate institution of the treatment.

Life-threatening cardiac arrhythmias – Benign arrhythmias that are anthracycline induced are usual, but there are several reported cases of malignant arrhythmias with sudden death.

Acute pneumonitis – It is characterized by an acute-onset breathlessness accompanied by a diffuse infiltrate in the lungs. Acute pneumonitis is a potentially lethal complication induced by bleomycin, methotrexate, and cyclophosphamide.

Acute respiratory distress syndrome – It is characterized by a severe rapid-onset dyspnea with refractory hypoxia caused by gemcitabine, cytarabine, cyclophosphamide, methotrexate, and docetaxel. Mortality rate is high (40–65%).

Acute hemolytic anemia – Acute hemolytic anemia common symptoms are acute back pain, fever, and rigors. It has been related to cytotoxic compounds (fludarabine, cisplatin, carboplatin, oxaliplatin).

Acute pancreatitis – It can be caused by many chemotherapy drugs, but the phenomenon seems to be rare and poorly understood.

Cerebrovascular accidents – Some anticancer drugs (cisplatin, methotrexate, fluorouracil, L-asparaginase) increase the risk of stroke.

Reversible posterior leukoencephalopathy syndrome – It is a neurological disease characterized by headache, seizures, altered mental state, and visual disturbance. The syndrome has been associated with gemcitabine, cisplatin, cytarabine, cyclophosphamide, methotrexate, ifosfamide, and etoposide.

Drug-induced hepatotoxicity – Drug toxicity is related to different types of mechanisms (cholestasis, veno-occlusive disease, hepatic necrosis) that are related to the use of gemcitabine, docetaxel, and liposomal doxorubicin. Death due to fulminant hepatic failure has only been reported in a few cases.

Acute arterial occlusion – Acute limb ischemia due to large-vessel arterial occlusion is a rare event that is commonly related to cisplatin-based chemotherapy [56, 58].

# References

## Adverse Effects

1. Oun R, Moussa YE, Wheate NJ. The side effects of platinum-based chemotherapy drugs: a review for chemists. Dalton Trans. 2018;47(19):6645–53.
2. Malyszko J, Kozlowska K, Kozlowski L, Malyszko J. Nephrotoxicity of anticancer treatment. Nephrol Dial Transplant. 2017;32(6):924–36.
3. Zhang X, Zhu Y, Dong S, Zhang A, Lu Y, Li Y, Lv S, Zhang J. Role of oxidative stress in cardiotoxicity of antineoplastic drugs. Life Sci. 2019;232:116526.
4. Moreau-Bachelard C, Coquan E, LE Tourneau C. N. Imputability of adverse events to anticancer drugs. Engl J Med. 2019;380(19):1873–4.
5. Cavaletti G, Nicolini G, Marmiroli P. Neurotoxic effects of antineoplastic drugs: the lesson of pre-clinical studies. Front Biosci. 2008;3(1):3506–24.
6. Cridland MD. Antineoplastic and immunosuppressive drugs. Adverse effects and therapeutic problems. Drugs. 1972;3(5):352–65.
7. Pearce A, Haas M, Viney R. Are the true impacts of adverse events considered in economic models of antineoplastic drugs? A systematic review. Appl Health Econ Health Policy. 2013;11(6):619–37.
8. Wang Z, Yang X, Wang J, Wang S, Mao X, Li M, Zhao Y, Wang W, Qi X, Wu T. Risk of serious adverse event and fatal adverse event with molecular target anticancer drugs in cancer patients: A meta-analysis. J Cancer Res Ther. 2019;15(7):1435–49.
9. Tchambaz L, Schlatter C, Jakob M, Krähenbühl A, Wolf P, Krähenbühl S. Dose adaptation of antineoplastic drugs in patients with liver disease. Drug Saf. 2006;29(6):509–22.
10. Kintzel PE, Dorr RT. Anticancer drug renal toxicity and elimination: dosing guidelines for altered renal function. Cancer Treat Rev. 1995;21(1):33–64.
11. Tuccori M, Montagnani S, Capogrosso-Sansone A, Mantarro S, Antonioli L, Fornai M, Blandizzi C. Adverse reactions to oncologic drugs: spontaneous reporting and signal detection. Expert Rev Clin Pharmacol. 2015;8(1):61–75.
12. Chagas CM, Moss S, Alisaraie L. Drug metabolites and their effects on the development of adverse reactions: revisiting Lipinski's rule of five. Int J Pharm. 2018;549(1–2):133–49.
13. Tocchetti CG, Cadeddu C, di Lisi D, Femminò S, Madonna R, Mele D, Monte I, Novo G, Penna C, Pepe A, Spallarossa P, Varricchi G, Zito C, Pagliaro P, Mercuro G. From molecular mechanisms to clinical management of antineoplastic drug-induced cardiovascular toxicity: a translational overview. Antioxid Redox Signal. 2019;30(18):2110–53.

14. Hamnvik OPR. Thyroid dysfunction from antineoplastic agents. J Natl Cancer Inst. 2011;103(21):1572–87.
15. Tew KD. Alkylating agents. Chap. 25: Pharmacology of cancer chemotherapy. In: DeVita, Hellman and Rosenberg's Cancer: principles & practice of oncology. 8th ed. Philadelphia: Lippincott Williams & Wilkins; 2008. p. 407–19.
16. Reed E. Cisplatin and its analogs. Chap. 25: Pharmacology of cancer chemotherapy. In: DeVita, Hellman and Rosenberg's Cancer: principles & practice of oncology. 8th ed. Philadelphia: Lippincott Williams & Wilkins; 2008. p. 419–26.
17. Saif MW, Chu E. Antimetabolites. Chap. 25: Pharmacology of cancer chemotherapy. In: DeVita, Hellman and Rosenberg's Cancer: principles & practice of oncology. 8th ed. Philadelphia: Lippincott Williams & Wilkins; 2008. p. 427–37.
18. Rasheed ZA, Rubin EH. Topoisomerase-interacting agents. Chap. 25: Pharmacology of cancer chemotherapy. In: DeVita, Hellman and Rosenberg's Cancer: principles & practice of oncology. 8th ed. Philadelphia: Lippincott Williams & Wilkins; 2008. p. 437–47.
19. Lee JJ, Harris LN. Antimicrotubule agents. Chap. 25: Pharmacology of cancer chemotherapy. In: DeVita, Hellman and Rosenberg's Cancer: principles & practice of oncology. 8th ed. Philadelphia: Lippincott Williams & Wilkins; 2008. p. 447–56.
20. Lorusso PM, Ryan AJ, Boerner SA, HERBST RS. Small-molecule tyrosine kinase inhibitors. Chap. 25: Pharmacology of cancer chemotherapy. In: DeVita, Hellman and Rosenberg's Cancer: principles & practice of oncology. 8th ed. Philadelphia: Lippincott Williams & Wilkins; 2008. p. 457–68.
21. Cohen SJ, Cohen RB, Meropol NJ. Targeting signal transduction with antibodies. Chap. 25: Pharmacology of cancer chemotherapy. In: DeVita, Hellman and Rosenberg's Cancer: principles & practice of oncology. 8th ed. Philadelphia: Lippincott Williams & Wilkins; 2008. p. 469–77.
22. Gore SD, Baylin SB, Herman JG. Histone deacetylase inhibitors and demethylating agents. Chap. 25: Pharmacology of cancer chemotherapy. In: DeVita, Hellman and Rosenberg's Cancer: principles & practice of oncology. 8th ed. Philadelphia: Lippincott Williams & Wilkins; 2008. p. 477–85.
23. Molineaux CJ, Cews CM. Proteasome inhibitors. Chap. 25: Pharmacology of cancer chemotherapy. In: DeVita, Hellman and Rosenberg's Cancer: principles & practice of oncology. 8th ed. Philadelphia: Lippincott Williams & Wilkins; 2008. p. 486–90.
24. Copur MS, Rose M, Gettinger SN. Miscellaneous chemotherapeutics agents. Chap. 25: Pharmacology of cancer chemotherapy. In: DeVita, Hellman and Rosenberg's Cancer: principles & practice of oncology. 8th ed. Philadelphia: Lippincott Williams & Wilkins; 2008. p. 490–5.

## Tumor Lysis

25. Howard SC, Jones DP, Pui CH. The tumor lysis syndrome. N Engl J Med. 2011a;364(19):1844–54.
26. Coiffier B, Altman A, Pui CH, Younes A, Cairo MS. Guidelines for the management of pediatric and adult tumor lysis syndrome: an evidence-based review. J Clin Oncol. 2008a;26(16):2767–78.
27. Newton HB. Neurologic complications of systemic cancer. Am Fam Physician. 1999;59(4):878–86.
28. Azoulay E, Moreau D, Alberti C, Leleu G, Adrie C, Barboteu M, et al. Predictors of short-term mortality in critically ill patients with solid malignancies. Intensive Care Med. 2000;26(12):1817–23.
29. Benoit DD, Hoste EA, Depuydt PO, Offner FC, Lameire NH, Vandewoude KH, et al. Outcome in critically ill medical patients treated with renal replacement therapy for acute renal failure: comparison between patients with and those without haematological malignancies. Nephrol Dial Transplant. 2005;20(3):552–8.
30. Lanore JJ, Brunet F, Pochard F, Bellivier F, Dhainaut JF, Vaxelaire JF, et al. Hemodialysis for acute renal failure in patients with hematologic malignancies. Crit Care Med. 1991;19(3):346–51.
31. Tanvetyanon T, Choudhury AM. Fatal acute tumor lysis syndrome, hepatic encephalopathy and flare phenomenon following combined androgen blockade. J Urol. 2004;171(4):1627.
32. Vaisban E, Braester A, Mosenzon O, et al. Spontaneous tumor lysis syndrome in solid tumors: really a rare condition? Am J Med Sci. 2003;325(1):38–40.
33. Howard SC, Jones DP, Pui CHN. The tumor lysis syndrome. Engl J Med. 2011b;364(19):1844–54.
34. Coiffier B, Altman A, Pui CH, Younes A, Cairo MS. Guidelines for the management of pediatric and adult tumor lysis syndrome: an evidence-based review. J Clin Oncol. 2008b;26(16):2767–78.
35. Rahmani B, Patel S, Seyam O, Gandhi J, Reid I, Smith N, Khan SA. Current understanding of tumor lysis syndrome. Hematol Oncol. 2019;37(5):537–47.
36. Williams SM, Killeen AA. Tumor lysis syndrome. Arch Pathol Lab Med. 2019;143(3):386–93.
37. Criscuolo M, Fianchi L, Dragonetti G, Pagano L. Tumor lysis syndrome: review of pathogenesis, risk factors and management of a medical emergency. Expert Rev Hematol. 2016;9(2):197–208.
38. Russell TB, Kram DE. Tumor lysis syndrome. Pediatr Rev. 2020;41(1):20–6.
39. Mcbride A, Trifilio S, Baxter N, Gregory TK, Howard SC. Managing tumor lysis syndrome in the era of novel cancer therapies. J Adv Pract Oncol. 2017;8(7):705–20.
40. Greguska C. Managing tumor lysis syndrome. JAAPA. 2021;34(1):10–3.

41. Klemencic S, Perkins J. Diagnosis and Management of Oncologic Emergencies. West J Emerg Med. 2019;20(2):316–22.
42. Abu-Alfa AK, Younes A. Tumor lysis syndrome and acute kidney injury: evaluation, prevention, and management. Am J Kidney Dis. 2010;55(5 Suppl 3):S1–13; quiz S14–9.
43. Giammarco S, Chiusolo P, Piccirillo N, Di Giovanni A, Metafuni E, Laurenti L, Sica S, Pagano L. Hyperleukocytosis and leukostasis: management of a medical emergency. Expert Rev Hematol. 2017;10(2):147–54.
44. Findakly D, Luther RD III, Wang J. Tumor lysis syndrome in solid tumors: A comprehensive literature review, new insights, and novel strategies to improve outcomes. Cureus. 2020;12(5):e8355.
45. Durani U, Hogan WJ. Emergencies in haematology: tumour lysis syndrome. Br J Haematol. 2020;188(4):494–500.

## Tumor Extravasation

46. Strilic B, Offermanns S. Intravascular survival and extravasation of tumor cells. Cancer Cell. 2017;32(3):282–93.
47. Boulanger J, Ducharme A, Dufour A, Fortier S, Almanric K. Management of the extravasation of anti-neoplastic agents. Comité de l'évolution de la pratique des soins pharmaceutiques (CEPSP); Comité de l'évolution des pratiques en oncologie (CEPO). Support Care Cancer. 2015;23(5):1459–71.
48. Pérez Fidalgo JA, García Fabregat L, Cervantes A, Margulies A, Vidall C, Roila F. Management of chemotherapy extravasation: ESMO-EONS Clinical Practice Guidelines.; ESMO Guidelines Working Group. Ann Oncol. 2012;23(Suppl 7):vii167–73.
49. Jackson-Rose J, Del Monte J, Groman A, Dial LS, Atwell L, Graham J, O'neil SEMLERR, O'sullivan M, Truini-Pittman L, Cunningham TA, Roman-Fischetti L, Costantinou E, Rimkus C, Banavage AJ, Dietz B, Colussi CJ, Catania K, Wasko M, Schreffler KA, West C, Siefert ML, Rice RD. Chemotherapy extravasation: establishing a National Benchmark for incidence among cancer centers. Clin J Oncol Nurs. 2017;21(4):438–45.
50. Harrold K. Managing cytotoxic chemotherapy extravasation: use of saline washout. Br J Nurs. 2015;24(8):S36–7.
51. Yadavalli S, Jayaram S, Manda SS, Madugundu AK, Nayakanti DS, Tan TZ, Bhat R, Rangarajan A, Chatterjee A, Gowda H, Thiery JP, Kumar P. Data-driven discovery of extravasation pathway in circulating tumor cells. Sci Rep. 2017;7:43710.
52. Bahrami M, Karimi T, Yadegarfar G, Norouzi A. Assessing the quality of existing clinical practice guidelines for chemotherapy drug extravasation by appraisal of guidelines for research and evaluation II. Iran J Nurs Midwifery Res. 2019;24(6):410–6.

53. Zach L, Guez D, Last D, Daniels D, Grober Y, Nissim O, Hoffmann C, Nass D, Talianski A, Spiegelmann R, Cohen ZR, Mardor Y. Delayed contrast extravasation MRI for depicting tumor and non-tumoral tissues in primary and metastatic brain tumors. PLoS One. 2012;7(12):e52008.
54. De Wit M, Ortner P, Lipp HP, Sehouli J, Untch M, Ruhnke M, Mayer-Steinacker R, Bokemeyer C, Jordan K. Management of cytotoxic extravasation - ASORS expert opinion for diagnosis, prevention and treatment. Onkologie. 2013;36(3):127–35.
55. Harrold K, Gould D, Drey N. The management of cytotoxic chemotherapy extravasation: a systematic review of the literature to evaluate the evidence underpinning contemporary practice. Eur J Cancer Care (Engl). 2015;24(6):771–800.

## Others

56. Morgan C, Tillett T, Braybrooke J, Ajithkumar T. Management of uncommon chemotherapy-induced emergencies. Lancet Oncol. 2011;12(8):806–14.
57. Wagner J, Arora S. Oncologic metabolic emergencies. Hematol Oncol Clin North Am. 2017;31(6):941–57.
58. Mccurdy MT, Shanholtz CB. Oncologic emergencies. Crit Care Med. 2012;40(7):2212–22.

# Administration of an Oncology Pharmacy

# 12

Fred Soares dos Santos, Thais de Leles Balisa, Felipe de Souza Alves, and Wanessa Ferraz Neres

One of the biggest challenges of the health system is the search for a balance of financial resources and the quality of care provided. In this sense, the evolution and adequacy of programs to the health sector point to a historical process experienced in other sectors. In several countries, there is mobilization for quality programs in health organizations in order to develop management tools and improve the efficiency of these services. The sector's reform is based on the evaluation of a set of actions aimed at reducing health care costs within an administrative care policy.

---

F. S. dos Santos (✉)
Graduate Program in Pharmaceutical Sciences, Federal University of Golas, Goiânia, Brazil

T. de Leles Balisa
Graduate Program in Pharmaceutical Sciences, Faculdade Unida de Campinas, Goiânia, Golas, Brazil

F. de Souza Alves
Graduate Program in Pharmaceutical Sciences, Universidade Paulista, São Paulo, Brazil

W. F. Neres
Graduate Program in Pharmaceutical Sciences, Universidade Paulista de Brasilia, UNIP, Brasília, Brazil



C. W. P. Schmidt, K. M. Otoni (eds.), *The Golden Guide to Oncologic Pharmacy*, https://doi.org/10.1007/978-3-030-98596-7_12

The role of the pharmacist in oncology is relatively recent in Brazil. The activity with the multidisciplinary team is essential for the quality treatment offered to the patient. In addition, the performance of the pharmacist has a direct impact on reducing the employee's occupational risk, reducing costs for the company, improving the quality of service provided to the patient, and disposing of hazardous chemical waste. Service standards must be guided by quality standards and safety processes. The objective is to allow establishments to have positive results both in the quality of patient care and in the company's results. To start discussing planning and management, we first need to understand concepts. It is interesting to note that there are several schools, so the definitions may vary depending on the authors. The provocation that arises from this comment is that there is no right or wrong, but possibilities that need to be evaluated according to the peculiarities of each establishment. Based on these concepts, we have the following discussions: pharmaceutical care vs. pharmaceutical care, supply chain, scheduling and procurement, stock management techniques, storage and stock control, bag preparation, bag production safety, people management, and indicators in the oncology pharmacy.

## 12.1 Concepts and Definitions

1. Strategy: decisions that establish the organization or individual's position in the environment. This is the focus that must be expressed in behavior, either explicit or implicit.
2. Planning: is the translation of strategies and efforts to generate projected results.

The level of complexity of work relationships related to the health sector is increasing. We are facing even more participative consumers, healthcare operators acting in the revenue cycle, competition, and high costs. In this way, it is possible to insinuate that the strategy is the best path for the success of this type of undertaking. When designing the path, we must evaluate the following criteria:

- Long-term survival: operational continuity with quality patient/customer deliveries.
- Sustained growth: positive evolution over time and maintenance of the financial health of the business without reducing the level of service.
- Adequate profitability: compatible return on investment.
- Capacity for innovation: flexibility in the market and generation of new processes, products, and services.

In this way, we can say that the strategy consists of determining the steps of a company, often with assessments and perceptions that are not always accurate, which may be impacted by variations related to the complexity of the environment. Strategies must contain the following characteristics:

- Analysis of market and company results.
- Innovation.
- Compatible with company resources.
- Promote people's development and commitment.
- Follow company principles and values.

## 12.2 Pharmaceutical Assistance X Pharmaceutical Attention

Pharmaceutical assistance and pharmaceutical attention comprise concepts of health care in society. Both have their own concepts and different processes.

Resolution No. 388 of May 6, 2004 defines pharmaceutical assistance as a "set of actions aimed at the promotion, protection and recovery of health, both individual and collective, having the drug as an essential input and aiming at access and its rational use. This set involves the research, development and production of medicines and supplies, as well as their selection, programming, acquisition, distribution, dispensing, quality assurance of products and services, monitoring and evaluation of their use, with a view to obtaining concrete results and improvement of the population's quality of life."

Pharmaceutical attention is a concept defined for the first time in 1990 by Hepler and Strand as "the responsible provision of pharmacological treatment with the purpose of achieving concrete results that improve the quality of life of patients."

Pharmaceutical assistance and pharmaceutical attention are two definitions that sometimes get confused. It is noticed that both concepts place the pharmacist in the patient care process; that is, they seek to ensure the integrality of health actions.

## 12.3 Supply Chain

The supply activity of hospitals and clinics is no longer seen only as an operational activity of low relevance. When we talk about scheduling, acquisition, storage, and inventory control, we make clear the need for knowledge in management, business organization, and even pharmaceutical legislation and deontology.

The decision to keep stock or consignment and the operational condition of putting the logistics strategy into practice has a direct impact on the institutions' cash. If you buy more, you decrease the risk of stockouts, but you accumulate assets and stop stock devaluing on the shelves. If you buy less, it improves the cash flow and smoothes the volume of payments to be made, but puts the continuity of treatment at risk with the possibility of stockouts, for example, due to a lack of input in the market. Finally, what we are looking for is balance, how we can maintain inventories with a good safety margin, not negatively affecting the company's cash that is maintaining its financial competitiveness in the business.

For Chiavenato, administration is the vehicle through which organizations are aligned and guided to achieve excellence in their actions and operations to achieve results. The concept involves directing actions with certain resources to achieve the objective. In addition, a big question is to be able to use the resources within an oncology pharmacy in a context that guarantees the supply of medicines and/or materials within an optimized flow, because medicines and materials represent a large part of the logistical costs of an institution.

A complicating factor is that oncology pharmacies have a fluctuating demand and resupply cycle, which entails a degree of uncertainty in the availability of the products. In addition, we deal with a scenario of increasing costs, explained also by the technologies.

Given the context, the Pharmacist needs to seek tools that allow controls required for inventory management, including the involvement of information technology, which makes the use of software essential for decisions.

## 12.4 Programming and Acquisition

The first question is to understand what kind of institution the professional is inserted in. We need to assess whether it is a public or private company, accessibility to suppliers, public served, and financial resources.

The inventory management challenge is to maintain the need to invest as little as possible in inventory while at the same time meeting the patient's needs adequately [9].

Most pharmaceutical services use historical consumption as an acquisition criterion (partly by facilitating analysis and planning). However, the market already has software capable of generating a forecast of future consumption, based on protocols registered in hospital information systems (HIS). In this way, the consumption ratio for a given period analyzed, added to the delivery conditions (classification 123) and other points favorable to the analysis such as the ABC and XYZ classification, can generate direct impacts on inventory turnover and relief to institutional cash, given that we are talking most often about high-cost drugs, commonly used in oncology. In all programming methods, whether by epidemiological profile, service offer, historical or adjusted consumption, there are advantages and disadvantages. It is recommended that the adjustment be a combination of the various methods, for better programming adequacy [8].

## 12.5 Inventory Management Techniques

### 12.5.1 ABC Classification

The ABC classification allows the pharmacist to individualize attention by drug group. The ABC ranking is also known as the Pareto ranking (80% of your results depend on 20% of your effort) and aims to identify the product by a value reason. Items rated "A" are those that correspond to a small number of items and represent about 80% of the stock value. Items "C" are low value and high volume. Items "B" are of quantity or intermediate value; that is, they are those of average quantity and values in relation to items A and C. [8, 9]

### 12.5.2 XYZ Classification

The XYZ classification takes into account service levels such as service, local support, and others, always considering the criticality of the item for the activity. [9]

- X classification: low criticality, lack does not paralyze the activity, easy acquisition, and possibility of an equivalent to replace.
- Y classification: medium criticality, the fault can interrupt the activity and can be replaced by another material.
- Z classification: lack can interrupt activities and put people at risk, with no possibility of replacement by an equivalent product.

## 12.6 Storage and Inventory Control

Inventory control can be defined by the set of activities of registration, control, and analysis of movement that verify the amount needed to be purchased (how many) and the appropriate period for the purchase (when) in order to allow the company to continue operating. [9]

The storage of health products can be centralized (PSC – pharmaceutical supply center) or decentralized (satellite pharmacies). They involve receiving, storing, parameters for conservation, stock control, and security. Some of these activities can even be outsourced, depending on the size of the operation and if it is understood that it is not the institution's core business and that there may be improvement in the quality of delivery of the service provided. In any case, the institution's strategy will define the best path to be followed, being a good way to detail or define the storage and distribution strategy, making use of Portter's SWOT analysis.

The pharmacist must guide their actions by operating procedures for proper storage and handling of products. This action is necessary to ensure reproducibility and safety of processes. Definitions need to take into account current legislation and ongoing staff training.

Another relevant process is the systematic inventory process. The inventory can be an action that enables the identification of failures, in addition to directly affecting the replacement of inputs and possible stockouts. Accounting audits and transparency in inventory processes are extremely important to demonstrate financial efficiency and sustainability of institutions.

The pharmacist interested in working in the supply chain should seek to improve their knowledge of statistics, administration, and legislation. It should be noted that information technology plays an important role in sustaining the actions of the pharmacist. Finally, the entire process must be based on the effects of decision-making.

## 12.7 Bags Preparation

The advance of oncology was not limited only to new lines of treatment. Over the years, there was a need for progress in relation to the way in which medicines are cared for, understanding of current legislation and structural importance and processes, with the objective of optimizing resources, promoting pharmacoeconomic actions, and ensuring free production (bags) of risks to patients and professionals involved.

The understanding and use of a clean area are classified as essential in the production of manipulated bags and favored the creation of more robust and prepared environments for the development of activities safely. Therefore, there is a need to change processes. Before, the activity that was very close to the extension of patient care becomes more industrial, requiring the insertion of new concepts for better use of physical space and increasingly issues such as certification, validation, calibration, production line, volumetry, production peak, and many other concepts.

The service models of service will directly influence the way of operation of the compounding pharmacy. Understanding the business model in which the institution is inserted will determine the design of the best processes and flows.

Institutions that work with anticipation of manipulations (possible practice due to consultations and prescription releases on the day and/or period prior to the infusion) need to establish agreements with nursing regarding request times. Thus, there is a large volume of orders within the same period, but with a longer period for preparation, and the pharmacy team is responsible for evaluating the physical-chemical stability that will determine when the item can be prepared and sent to the infusion unit. As an advantage, there is a reduction in headcount for the demand and the main risk involved is the loss of the drug, due to the absence of the patient.

The model based on simultaneous releases after the patient's arrival reduces the risk of drug losses, but it requires a greater number of employees involved in the production line, as the "urgent" queues increase considerably. It is necessary to establish the delivery time of the prepared bags, in addition to being able to signal the quick application drugs, for example, those that do not require pre-chemotherapeutic drugs, to prevent these patients from spending too much time waiting. This signaling becomes useful for the team and allows for greater turnover in infusion stations, increasing the service capacity and improving the patient's experience, an important point to be considered, since the criterion for choosing which oncology center the patient is will perform the treatment is multifactorial.

The understanding that the pharmacy is strategically linked to the patient's experience increases the responsibility for managing processes and routines, cooperating with the satisfaction and the result of the NPS (net promoter score). It is a methodology created in 2003 by Brain & Company. The objective is to verify, through a rating from 0 to 10, how companies deal with their customers, where from 0 to 6 they are classified as detractors, potential complainants and customers who will poorly evaluate the service. The evaluation from 7 to 8 are neutrals and 9 from 10 are promoters, potential customers who will be loyal.

Therefore, questions like "What does the customer want?", "What is value to them?", "What is your expectation?" are important to define pharmacy strategies. Imagine a client with active life and disease under control visiting the oncology clinic for administration of medication with a 30-minute infusion. Many benefits and advantages can be offered to this patient, but a delay in the delivery of the drug that causes a very long stay will certainly affect their experience and relationship with the institution [10].

There is no better or worse model, work options that need to be carefully evaluated and check what is most suitable for the institution. Indicators of scholarship losses and their reasons, rescheduling rate, unit occupancy rate, and average hours of occupation of management posts can support decisions in an assertive manner. Services with large volumes of preparations benefit from the first model, being able to optimize the use of medications, reduce the queue, and make the service faster. Services that do not have large volumes, as well as have no problems with occupancy, benefit from the second model. Therefore, the study of workflow and processes is essential for this decision.

Understanding the preparation pharmacy as a business unit and assistance as a client of this service favors the administrative professionalization of the pharmacy management, not only as the guardian of medicines, but also as a generator of resources and one of the pillars for the patient experience, resulting in better institutional performance in terms of resources for materials and medicines, as well as service capacity. It presents, therefore, a new scenario for pharmacists within this context.

## 12.8 Safety in Bags Production

Combined with the productive importance, we have the safety of preparation. Neglecting the need to establish standards favors the possibility of errors, which can be fatal especially when dealing with drugs with a narrow therapeutic window and with many particularities.

Studies from 2014 show that hospitalized patients are subject to at least one medication error per day, estimating that per year in the United States, there are 7000 deaths due to these errors. It's like a large plane crashing every 18 days, which would draw a lot of attention. Faced with such a dangerous scenario, we have the production of medicine bags, and bringing with them their own brands, learning, and challenges to be increasingly safe for patients and professionals [11].

Currently, post-handling check methods, precision balance, light exposure check etc., are not common in most countries and pharmacy services. In addition, the subsequent check is more like redundancy and registration than process security, since the bag will already be ready and it will be necessary to repeat the activity. Therefore, what must be done for the process to end correctly, without variation from what was expected, is to develop robust, clear, feasible processes to ensure that all steps are adequate and assertive. As a result, there will be well-finished products.

### 12.8.1 Separation

Inventory organization and visualization act as barriers to failure. Commonly, drug makers leave their brands as marketing on their boxes, and as a result, they have many drugs that look similar and have similar names. Identifying these similarities and working so that very similar items are far away is necessary and are present as a mandatory error mitigation point in important national and international accreditation seals. The use of cabinets that allow the visualization of all items is also beneficial for reading before picking up the item, being able to use technology in its favor such as RFID (radio frequency identification) for controls, traceability, and even billing. Having computerized systems that block items that are not in the requests is also very important. For this, we can make use of bar code, qrcode, and data matrix readings that favor the identification of the drug by the system and constitute an important barrier to avoid continuity of the failed process.

Even so, training is essential, as is the resolution of failures in the day-to-day operation so that the employee does not bypass the barriers created for safety in the process, since they are used to performing manual operation as a contingency process. It is important to understand and put into practice that contingency is an exception, clearly defining when it can be used.

### 12.8.2 Sanitation

Activity that until recently was presented as a microbiological control point has been shown to be an important barrier in a failure situation for the continuity of the process. The presence of a properly trained professional, as well as the availability of technology that allows viewing the request, becomes a double-checking point. At this time, the verification of the quantity of bottles, diluents, and materials that will be used in the preparation can be verified.

### 12.8.3 Preparation

The preparation itself is easy to explain; however, it involves many nuances that highlight the latent need for professionals with knowledge of the process, but also of medicines. It is necessary to break the barrier of the professional who goes on autopilot. Peter Drucker, great master of management as a discipline, said: "It is common that when we do something for years on end, we go into automatic mode of operation, one in which we are aware and attentive, just repeating a very familiar pattern, being precisely it is at this time that we have lost sight of our great goal." The pharmacist needs to be a cooperator and check barrier in the process: check dilution, prescription information with the system, label to be stuck on the bag, infusion line chosen according to the route to be carried out, respect for the characteristics of the drug. Knowing all this will greatly enhance security. This moment is crucial, since an activity performed incorrectly can lead to an underdose, overdose, and change of medication that will not be easily evidenced by the care team.

### 12.8.4 Dispensation/Shipping

During this step, checks related to the equipment used, diluent, dilution, identifications, label information, coloring for specific drugs (doxorubicin, mitomycin, mitoxantrone, methotrexate, among others), if the infusion line is properly closed, use of all devices for safety, storage conditions (protection from light when necessary, refrigerated or at room temperature) are fundamental as safety barriers. When necessary, identify the destination unit and ensure adequate conditions during transport. It is worth highlighting the importance of recording the dispensing to ensure that the drug was delivered in ideal conditions, which will be important for the smoothness of the process and for event investigations, if necessary.

We could categorize anticancer drugs in different ways: injectable, oral, dermatological, synthetic, or biological. Perhaps biologicals need more attention due to their structural characteristics, as well as synthetic ones, due to their occupational risk. During transport, precautions are needed regarding the proper storage temperature, as in the case of biologicals, protein denaturations may expose epitopes in their amino acid chain, increasing the risk of immunogenicity reactions. Likewise, in the case of possible rupture of the bag for a cytotoxic product (most often synthetic), there is a need for barriers such as rigid transport boxes, spill, and registration kits, for future improvements.

In these steps, it is important to introduce some concepts to facilitate the execution of the processes. Visual communication, standardized work, demand study, and bulletin boards are some examples.

Visual communication concerns the information needed to carry out the process. The view of the workbench, the places where the equipment should be and the best layout of the room are small details that help to resolve doubts quickly.

One can see the importance of visual communication in how city traffic is organized with the idea of reducing accidents. Health services need this understanding in the processes. During the execution, questions arise that interfere with the result: "Where to start? What is the best way? Where should the manipulated bags be? What is the identification pattern? How to identify that something is not adequate?" The absence of these communications favors that information is restricted to an individual; when this is done, it impedes the individual's growth, and worse when he is not present, the pattern is lost. The reduction of professional variability is directly linked to the financial results of an institution.

Performing tasks in multiple ways is common. The lack of repetition and reproducibility favors the opportunity for mistakes, as each achievement resembles a new process. The ideal is equal execution, so that you can assess process flaws, timing, and performance. Standardized work differs from work instruction; it is a simple document with process images, directive phrases to ensure quick reference to the standard, avoiding unstudied variations in the process. However, individualized treatment creates some challenges, as the balance between the adjusted and standardized process with the individual's needs is necessary, and it cannot bureaucratize the final outcome, which is to ensure quality of care with sustainable processes.

Studying previous work demand, as well as monitoring to identify whether there is delay or potential delays, is important. Operational capacity calculations need to be part of compounding pharmacy management. Data collection as a time cycle (time required from separation to completion of preparation), relating this data to demand, understanding narrowing, and understanding the minimum number of employees needed to perform the task favor the establishment of plans for contingencies, displacement of demands and employees, before failures occur due to inadequate assessment or more commonly due to lack of assessment. [12]

Process narrowing is defined by the most stressful steps in the workflow, so speed and throughput will be limited for that specific period. Identifying and resolving narrowing is the first step to improve fluidity and eliminate unnecessary steps.

In the oncology production line, there are many possibilities of narrowing. Separation of materials and medicines, observation of physical space, number of employees and computers, and the variability of items separated at this stage may reveal the presence of queues. Queues make the pharmacist stop handling the kit to wait for a new kit, sanitization working at a slower pace than possible, and delays are generated.

Example: a pharmacy has a 15-minute time cycle for preparing a bag, that is, from the beginning of the separation of items until the bag is ready, it takes 15 minutes. Therefore, under the same conditions, in 1 hour it is possible to handle 4 bags. Mapping the process, we have the following situation:

- Separation = 8 minutes.
- Sanitization = 2 minutes.
- Preparation = 3 minutes.
- Dispensation = 2 minutes.

It is verified that the separation takes a long time, so it is necessary to understand which variables are involved to be worked on. Knowing that on any given day there will be a demand for 20 bags of patients who will be seen between 9 am and 11 am, we have:

Required demand/operational capacity = 20/8 (2 hours of work) = 2.5. So the need will be 2.5 times above the production capacity, with potential delays and, therefore, prior actions are necessary.

Anticipating demand, eliminating the separation queue, including another professional in the preparation, and reducing the waiting list are some valid options to avoid the accumulation of demand that favors conference failures.

In continuation: of the 20 bags, 8 were anticipated. Thus, when requested, they will not undergo separation and cleaning (reduction of 10 minutes per bag and 80 minutes in total). That leaves:

12 (demand) / 8 (operational capacity) = 1.5 and becomes less uncomfortable, with 1.5 times over capacity.

The example is simple but demonstrates the importance of knowledge of workflow and runtimes. Studies on value stream mapping are needed to reduce unnecessary steps, takt time (work rate time), and lead-time (waiting time). For the proper management of these points, these concepts must be present in the daily life of the pharmacist.

In the industry, there is the concept of Andon (Japanese word for lamp) which advocates light and sound signals to inform if the procedure is adequate (green) or if there is a problem (red), as well as traffic lights (the important thing here is the concept behind it). In the face of a failure, the process needs to stop, even in the health area; unfortunately, continuity is common, finding some ways to skip steps. Developing a quick intervention procedure in case of failures is important to avoid the continuity of the error, already illustrated by James Reason in the Swiss Cheese Theory. Errors are the result of several previous failures and eliminating one by one is the way [12, 13].

## 12.9 People Management

In the health area, it is common to form leaders by the group of healthcare professionals who have stood out in their previous careers. The good side of leadership is knowing the work process and the difficulties inherent in it. However, the disadvantage is that generally this professional has not been prepared for activities of a management and administration nature, whether of people and processes. Such professionals are shaped over time, but in a world of great transformations, this period can be exhausting for the institution, for employees, and for leadership.

Corporate saying goes that people are hired for their skills and fired for their behavior. It's a big reality, but there are some unanswered questions within that context. How are health environments prepared for development, to shape some behaviors? What is the management culture developed by the institution and what is the real culture? How clear are the values and how are they followed? Is the culture of safety and respect present? Are processes improved? Is there a continuing education program aimed at technical development and social skills? Is the environment harmonious, does it allow for new ideas, or is it a hostile and oppressive place?

There are many points that interfere in people management. The professional who leads needs to be attentive and engaged, as well as dealing with these and many other daily variables. Knowing how to control and balance these nuances will lead the reduction of turnover and, therefore, will maintain an expert team, reducing the need to prepare new employees.

It is important to emphasize that although a leader does not have some ideal characteristic for the development of his team, the leader's mindset (and also of his team) can be developed, trained, and stimulated. It is necessary to develop the leader within administrative and management nuances for full training and consequent evolution within the services [14].

Among the various tasks required, selection, development, monitoring, feedback, and promotions stand out – all within a respectful, transparent and fair strategy. A great challenge.

### 12.9.1 Selection

Many conflicts are created by misalignment of expectations that start with the selection of professionals. This step must be conducted with the greatest possible transparency, avoiding key information (pay, hours, workload, benefits, responsibilities, workplaces) without any surprises after a choice has been made. These points need to be subsides for decision-making. Frustrations are common within the work environment, arising from failures in communication and understanding at this stage.

It is essential to establish criteria for team selection, look for profiles that add potential communication skills, group interaction, leadership development, responsibility, and awareness, and rely on the human resources sector to create a script of questions that evidence these qualities and call for selection by competences. However, it is necessary to mix with technical knowledge to develop evidence of knowledge in the area and situations through problems that can demonstrate the ability of that candidate's immediate performance. In addition, understanding the profile of the institution's vacancy and culture is vital to getting it right at this time.

### 12.9.2 Development and Monitoring

The existence of a development plan, sometimes in manual form and a checklist, favors the direction of what must be learned first, establishing who will carry out the training and what this employee needs to achieve to meet the expectations of the function.

Balancing technical and behavioral development training supports the development of a work culture. Inserting this employee in the full context of the institution and promoting lessons on how macro-processes and policies work are important supports.

The continuing education program must be established at least annually and, for that, the main flows can be considered, as well as the recurrent problems and events in the last period. In general, the repetition of errors comes from poorly designed processes.

Understanding the monitoring and improvement of routines must be present in management: these are essential actions for initial training, however of equal importance for older employees. It avoids the execution of processes that for years are not elucidated in relation to the purpose, an action that invariably impedes innovation and, therefore, including employees in the construction of standards and understanding the difficulties allows better performance and use of the workforce.

### 12.9.3 Feedback

To paraphrase Charles Kettering, finding a problem is half the solution and feedback should be seen as leadership and team alignment. The hardened and tragic concept surrounding this action must be in the past. Using the right tools and making the procedure natural favors frank and constructive conversations [15].

Having a feedback routine, whether good or bad, is important for aligning the direction you want to follow. In building processes and a team, conflicts and mismatches are and will be common. Allowing them to take a larger proportion than necessary is optional.

Leaders need to be trained for the most varied situations, from the most ordinary to difficult and personal conversations, which in many situations permeate processes, but impact work relationships. Knowing your team and tracing the behavioral profile will help you handle the most varied themes. Choosing a place and time are crucial for the success of this action. Having emotional skills and using appropriate words make a big difference. Conflicts are much more related to the way of speaking than to what was said. The choice of reserved and uninterrupted places preserves the collaborator.

Some situations require special interventions, senior leadership, human resources, and health issues. It is important to evaluate and not centralize the solutions themselves. Dividing the problematic issues is beneficial for the institution and the employee. Remember that success is an option, not an obligation. Understand the limits of the employment relationship.

### 12.9.4 Promotions

Recognition of a job well done needs to be part of the institution's culture, linked to real gains for employees in the form of remuneration, benefits, or privileges. The development of a culture of reward for merit/effort promotes individual motivation and the possibility of not losing professionals, avoiding becoming just a recruiter and developer of professionals for the market.

Establishing clear and fair criteria for participation in internal processes favors the maintenance of the work environment in the institution, avoiding the feeling of undue favoritism.

Despite being a benefit, promotions should be well studied, as they can generate many conflicts, as well as exposure of the promoted employee. It takes discernment not to lose important pieces at the operational level and place them in certain situations without the proper training and skills.

### 12.9.5 Task Distributions

Identifying the skills of employees allows distribution of tasks and development in multiple activities. Defining whether it will have more specialists than generalists, or the opposite, is a challenge to the leadership, which has to analyze not only the individuals, but also the volume of tasks and headcount available to them. It is common to find individuals who do not know or do not manifest their abilities. Leadership has to pay attention to performance and encourage job changes.

Forgetting can be avoided through the scales, which contribute a lot to this stage: planning the tasks, which person will do it, and when the person will do it. The overload of an employee stimulates the development of knowledge / improvement about new processes. The need to get the job done may seem very clear, but responsibility and direction remain paramount to getting it right.

## 12.10 Drug Management

The management of medications is increasingly important for the financial health of institutions. In oncology, this theme is highlighted, given the high cost of drugs used in treatments.

Failures in this management, from entry to exit, are common and often compromise the entire service chain.

### 12.10.1 Acquisition

For institutions that are just beginning their activity, this stage is a challenge since without a history of consumption, incorrect purchases can occur, which generates inventories and high operating costs. To this end, some measures can be taken to minimize this impact: establishing the treatment profile that will be carried out, for example. Still, it will involve many variables that can lead to drug shortages, affecting and influencing the experience of patients.

Initially, agreements with distributors are a favorable path. As a disadvantage (usually there is a higher cost in the purchase of items, but there are partnerships for quick availability), it can be a less traumatic path to maintain the stock, until the history and possibility of studying the variables are established. In general, this model has greater availability and variety of items; however, it requires greater control, especially because it is third-party stock.

Purchases of medication for oncology units must be linked to the institution's business model. As they are high-cost treatments, they generally require authorization from health plan operators and/or the patient to perform them. Health plan operators rely on the need for scientific basis to endorse the medical decision and this will determine the permitted dose, drug brands, and presentations for use, as well as what material was used.

Organizing this flow is vital to establish a margin of days for drug acquisition within the expected specifications. Participating in decision-making groups and agreements with health plan operators, standardizing presentations, requested brands, and criteria established by the pharmacy can ensure better use of medicines and reduction of waste and glosses.

To facilitate this account in an oncological scenario, the use of A, B, and C classifications is very interesting. In addition to this classification, it is important to assess what the drug is indicated for, which line of treatment, whether there is a possibility of waiting, etc. These factors will change the view of some ranking points.

A second classification with a difference between consumption and demand becomes important. Some institutions classify it as standard and non-standard. Consumable items are those with a consistent history of exit that generally have an indication for various types of tumors or for a tumor with high prevalence. They are the first line of treatment and are provided for in worldwide care protocols. Even if it is of high value, there may be days of stock, as the chance of loss is minimal. This action even allows for better negotiations, based on closed contracts and purchases of larger quantities. Likewise, there are medications from the three classifications that are specific to some health conditions. Irregular consumption considerably increases the risk of these drugs being in stock and expired. It must be classified as demand and a fast acquisition flow must be created to avoid delays in starting/continuing treatment. So, regardless of the value, care must be taken when purchasing. Outdated therapies are a great example.

All of this is counterbalanced by the level of service that the institution wishes to offer its market segment. As an example, we can ask: "Do I always want to have a box of all drug options for a particular patient?" It seems to be interesting from the patient experience point of view, but it is certainly inefficient from the point of view of the resources allocated to this action. See the chart below:

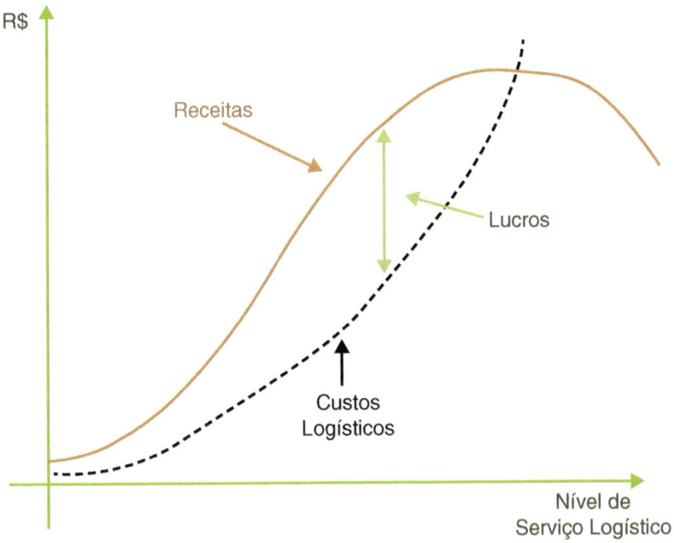


In addition, it is important to highlight medications used in hematological emergencies. Some diagnoses require immediate drug intervention, so there is no waiting time. This group of drugs should be available regardless of the financial risk, considering that the service has possible care in this specialty.

By providing the purchasing process with this information, decision-making tends to become simpler. Definition and monitoring of indicators for monitoring this process make management more adequate. Information such as inventory turnover, days of coverage, supply lead-time, and comparison of purchases with consumption should be part of the daily life of an oncology pharmacy.

It is important to highlight that services inserted within the hospital context need different treatment for oncological drugs. Despite being similar, small differences promote large process disruptions.

The service includes the existence of medication (which may even expire), especially in the case of emergencies. This is the operating cost of the service and is different from having all the drugs at all times, even if it was a possible service offer or a choice. It is recommended that there be a balance between attending to emergencies without disruptions and quality losses and avoiding unnecessary waste of assets in stock. This is the opportunity cost defined by Peter Drucker: the company provides resources to carry out another activity. We must always start from the premise that the opportunity cost represents the second best alternative for what the company could do with its resources. For example: a hospital group chooses to invest in a new unit and not in renewing ICU equipment. Or when we define between two protocols for the same disease, making it just a standard for the institution. So your opportunity cost was not having the protocol that was the second choice. Finally, what we want with this strategy is efficiency in processes, extracting the highest levels of benefits possible for our company.

A great truth is that resources are finite, whether in the private or public area. Everything costs time and money and you have to manage resources in the best way to make more profit or serve more patients.

### 12.10.2 Storage and Control

Purchases need to be matched with available storage space. In oncology, many medications are sensitive to temperature variations. Site evaluation and maintenance cost are essential to the process. Many institutions define processes based solely on current legislation and good practice manuals. It is noteworthy that these documents establish the minimum for the operation of a particular service. The assessment of the risks involved that will determine the degree of control must be established for those items.

There is legislation determining the verification of the temperature of medicine storage environments (closet, refrigerators, and rooms) at least three times a day. Since the 24 hours were due equally at three times, there will be a check every 8 hours. If a temperature deviation is found, some questions should be considered: "How long did this variation last? What were the temperatures recorded? What medications were in place?" The lack of these responses increases the risk of losses from inadequate storage. Online monitoring technologies show themselves as an opportunity to reduce these breakdowns. Minute-by-minute checks with alerts across multiple platforms allow for faster actions, ensuring the quality and use of medications.

The place must address humidity issues, in addition to keeping an eye on the external environment. There must be pest and dirt control, and assurance that the temperature is adequate throughout the environment. All details must guarantee the best conditions for the drug, even if it remains for considerable time on the shelf/refrigerator.

Controls through daily counts allow tracking of item usage, as well as tracking of breakdowns and deviations. It is important to consider that access controls and the use of cameras make it possible to detect situations and malfunctions more quickly, so that investigations can take place as soon as possible, whether due to procedural failure or effectively extra-institutional issue.

### 12.10.3 Losses

The drug preparation process generates considerable losses, even with all the relevant controls. Dose individualization, which considers body weight and surface area, has been characteristic of oncological treatments for many decades. This dose unitization, despite being beneficial to the patient, promotes a lot of wastage of medications. See below.

Medicine in the presentation of 50 mg with a unit cost of $ 20,000.00 with a dosage of 1.2 mg/kg, prescribed for a patient weighing 62.5 kg with application every 15 days: 75 mg and 2 vials will be needed (one whole and one half). Considering the stability of 24 hours after opening and having no patient to use, 25 mg will be discarded, equivalent to $ 10,000.00.

This cycle is repeated several times a month and with other medications of varying amounts. At the end of the period, there is considerable discarded value. Many systems do not allow tracking of this waste, leading to a misunderstanding of waste. The first action is to measure this value, either manually or through available system adequacy.

With data available, evaluation tools are used to define the drugs with the greatest history of waste. The Pareto diagram is useful for defining the most impactful items by sorting the values down and comparing them to the total. The study proposed in the Pareto diagram establishes that 20% of the items studied represent 80% of the impact on a process.

Line graphs show the evolution of the results achieved. They are ideal for use in monthly comparison views.

Example: counting of 20 medicines that generate waste during the month with the values available in the table.

| Medicine | Waste value |
|---|---|
| Med. 01 | $ 1,24 |
| Med. 02 | $ 6.000,00 |
| Med. 03 | $ 514,00 |
| Med. 04 | $ 24,00 |
| Med. 05 | $ 17.542,00 |

| Medicine | Waste value |
|---|---|
| Med. 06 | $ 10.000,00 |
| Med. 07 | $ 241,00 |
| Med. 08 | $ 124,00 |
| Med. 09 | $ 54,00 |
| Med. 10 | $ 900,00 |
| Med. 11 | $ 5.000,00 |
| Med. 12 | $ 57,00 |
| Med. 13 | $ 21,00 |
| Med. 14 | $ 47,00 |
| Med. 15 | $ 12,00 |
| Med. 16 | $ 34,00 |
| Med. 17 | $ 97,00 |
| Med. 18 | $ 21,00 |
| Med. 19 | $ 0,50 |
| Med. 20 | $ 20.000,00 |

Sort in descending order and add up all items.

| Medicine | Waste value |
|---|---|
| Med. 20 | $ 20.000,00 |
| Med. 05 | $ 17.542,00 |
| Med. 06 | $ 10.000,00 |
| Med. 02 | $ 6.000,00 |
| Med. 11 | $ 5.000,00 |
| Med. 10 | $ 900,00 |
| Med. 03 | $ 514,00 |
| Med. 07 | $ 241,00 |
| Med. 08 | $ 124,00 |
| Med. 17 | $ 97,00 |
| Med. 12 | $ 57,00 |
| Med. 09 | $ 54,00 |
| Med. 14 | $ 47,00 |
| Med. 16 | $ 34,00 |
| Med. 04 | $ 24,00 |
| Med. 13 | $ 21,00 |
| Med. 18 | $ 21,00 |

| Medicine | Waste value |
|---|---|
| Med. 15 | $ 12,00 |
| Med. 01 | $ 1,24 |
| Med. 19 | $ 0,50 |
| Total | **$ 60.689,74** |

Define the magnitude of each drug in relation to the total. **Waste value of each drug/total ×100**. In this way, there is a visualization of the items with the greatest impact.

| Medicine | Waste value | % |
|---|---|---|
| Med. 20 | $ 20.000,00 | 33% |
| Med. 05 | $ 17.542,00 | 29% |
| Med. 06 | $ 10.000,00 | 16% |
| Med. 02 | $ 6.000,00 | 10% |
| Med. 11 | $ 5.000,00 | 8% |
| Med. 10 | $ 900,00 | 1% |
| Med. 03 | $ 514,00 | 1% |
| Med. 07 | $ 241,00 | 0% |
| Med. 08 | $ 124,00 | 0% |
| Med. 17 | $ 97,00 | 0% |
| Med. 12 | $ 57,00 | 0% |
| Med. 09 | $ 54,00 | 0% |
| Med. 14 | $ 47,00 | 0% |
| Med. 16 | $ 34,00 | 0% |
| Med. 04 | $ 24,00 | 0% |
| Med. 13 | $ 21,00 | 0% |
| Med. 18 | $ 21,00 | 0% |
| Med. 15 | $ 12,00 | 0% |
| Med. 01 | $ 1,24 | 0% |
| Med. 19 | $ 0,50 | 0% |
| Total | **$ 60.689,74** | |

To define the most impactful items, add the percentage frequency with previous accumulated. Thus, it will be available for analysis based on the Pareto study.

| Medicine | Waste value | % | % Accum |
|---|---|---|---|
| Med. 20 | $ 20.000,00 | 33% | 33% |
| Med. 05 | $ 17.542,00 | 29% | 62% |
| Med. 06 | $ 10.000,00 | 16% | 78% |
| Med. 02 | $ 6.000,00 | 10% | 88% |
| Med. 11 | $ 5.000,00 | 8% | 96% |
| Med. 10 | $ 900,00 | 1% | 98% |
| Med. 03 | $ 514,00 | 1% | 99% |
| Med. 07 | $ 241,00 | 0% | 99% |
| Med. 08 | $ 124,00 | 0% | 99% |
| Med. 17 | $ 97,00 | 0% | 100% |
| Med. 12 | $ 57,00 | 0% | 100% |
| Med. 09 | $ 54,00 | 0% | 100% |
| Med. 14 | $ 47,00 | 0% | 100% |
| Med. 16 | $ 34,00 | 0% | 100% |
| Med. 04 | $ 24,00 | 0% | 100% |
| Med. 13 | $ 21,00 | 0% | 100% |
| Med. 18 | $ 21,00 | 0% | 100% |
| Med. 15 | $ 12,00 | 0% | 100% |
| Med. 01 | $ 1,24 | 0% | 100% |
| Med. 19 | $ 0,50 | 0% | 100% |
| Total | **$ 60.689,74** | | |

In the example, four medicines (20, 05, 06, and 02) represent 88% ($ 53,542.00) of the total waste. Therefore, the main actions for reduction need to be connected with these drugs.

The pharmacist has the technical knowledge to evaluate ways to reduce these discards. They are: physical-chemical stability assessment, scientific literature on extended stabilities, dose variation studies, and use of smart scheduler.

The study of physicochemical stability must consider the manufacturer's information and extended stability studies, in order to define the criteria for the level of evidence, weight, and place of publication. Currently, drug information consultation platforms have this information.

Once the drug has physicochemical stability, studies of microbiological conditions must be verified. Drug manufacturers tend to limit stability in the package insert, as it is not possible to guarantee the aseptic technique of each institution, and each organization is responsible for managing this important parameter.

The media fill test is a simulation of aseptic operations, replacing the product (medicament) with validated culture media, which are capable of demonstrating whether the designed process produces sterile products or not. The weekly control of areas and preparers complement the procedure's safety screening measures, with regard to microbiological control. Tests are established by regulatory agencies in each country.

With the guarantee of the parameters, one can choose to use the leftover drug for other preparations as long as there is a guarantee that the drug will be under adequate storage conditions, free from contamination and under control after opening. In this way, it is possible to carry out the so-called reuse, which will minimize losses, generate more resources, and reduce the production of chemical waste.

Using that example, considering that the first medicine (Med. 20) and the fourth (Med. 02) are in conditions of reuse, the expected reduction will be $ 26.000,00, which represents 43% of the total. This amount represents $ 312.000,00 in 12 months: important savings in resources.

When evaluating the step, it is necessary to adjust processes and structure that require investments to adapt the pharmacy and promote conscious and safe reuse. For this, it is necessary to assess the potential for reducing losses and waste, which will be the counterbalancing indicator for this process. Currently, the market has tested and validated devices that allow manipulations in a closed system and guarantee safety for the preparer. In addition to promoting care, studies demonstrate the guarantee of product sterility for up to 14 days. It may be a faster and less costly alternative for the institution; however, the use of these devices does not exclude the need to follow up on mandatory tests and follow-ups.

In the impossibility of using the mentioned stabilities, making use of intelligent scheduling is a possibility of reducing losses.

The objective is to insert, on pre-established days, patients undergoing treatments with the same drug. Thus, leftovers from one preparation can be used in another without compromising the quality of the medicine. The challenges for performing this task lie in the multiple agreements that must be made with the medical, nursing, scheduling, and authorization teams.

Studying the real gain for such a movement cooperates for decision making, considering the cost-benefit of such changes.

Considering the initial example: on the same day of application in the 75 mg patient, patient Y will be scheduled with a dose of 70 mg. It is possible to proceed as follows for the second patient: 1 bottle of 50 mg and 20 mg of the first preparation. Therefore, a supposed loss of 25 mg ($ 10.000,00) will become 5 mg ($ 2.000,00): a reduction of 80%

Another possibility of having many patients on the same day is taking advantage of overfill. It refers to the surplus present in the ready-to-use medicine bottles. There are manufacturers whose drugs have about 10% more than the nominal volume.

In a certain drug, it is described that it has 100 mg/4 ml. Consider 25 mg/ml for manipulations. However, in that same bottle, it is possible to obtain 4.4 ml, that is, 110 mg. Thus, in a prescription with a dose of 420 mg, 16.85 ml (5 vials) will be needed. If each vial has 4.4 ml, it is possible to determine 17.6 ml with 4 vials (440 mg) and 0.75 ml (18.75 mg) will be left over for new preparation.

In a scenario of large volumes, it is possible to prepare doses with a smaller number of bottles in order to use the surplus. With the data from the previous example and considering a day with the use of 20 bottles, at the end of the day it would be 8 ml (200 mg) of use and, therefore, 2 bottles would not have been used. It is up to the institution to define how this process will be handled. Some institutions call it an economy; others call it overfill. The important thing is to define flow for these items and establish adequate controls.

This method is of great importance in reducing disallowances by health plan operators because it can mean disagreement in the payment of the dose used/charged in the account. With the above method, it is possible to round up the volume of vials without reducing doses, contemplating better use of the available resource and successive cost reduction chain, from handling to payment for the service provided.

Dose reduction should also be evaluated. There are guidelines published in respected worldwide databases in which reductions of up to 10% in the patient's final dose do not alter the clinical outcome. In cases of drug administration (such as the example already mentioned) of a bag of a certain drug containing 440 mg (17.6 ml) in a final volume of 100 ml (e.g., saline solution), the final residue (prime) that remains in the gravitational equipment, which is discarded due to the impossibility of infusing the entire volume, can reach up to 10 ml of the final solution. The representativeness of these 10 ml, at a final solution concentration of 4.4 mg/ml, reaches 44 mg, that is, 10% of the final dose. The above case is common to be observed in anticancer therapy services that do not provide a specialist pharmacist. Even in this case, if we add a closed system device, added a 20 ml syringe with saline solution to wash the route in the equipment and with the objective of not generating the losses of the doses described above, we could easily conclude that 40 mg of the drug would be infused the most. It should also be added: the same that is usually done on a daily basis with 5 vials of that particular drug could be done with only 4 vials and the addition of the devices mentioned above.

The work described so far is fundamental for the development of the processes. Considering the context, we need to assess whether the parameters are in line with the company's needs. For this, it is necessary to "measure" and "qualify" the work developed. We need to define indicators capable of measuring the quality and efficiency of our processes.

## 12.11 Indicators in the Oncology Pharmacy

Monitoring the quality and efficiency of health services in their entire context is essential and has proven to be increasingly important for decision-making within these services [16].

The concern of health institutions in relation to the experience of customers, who are increasingly demanding with the services offered, quality certifications, and financial results that guarantee the sustainability and perpetuity of institutions, focusing on quality and safety, increases the need for constant improvements [17]. Given this new scenario, indicators or KPIs (key performace indicators) are one of the most used tools to measure improvements and show them [17]. In health-related aspects, there are essential criteria for evaluating, monitoring, and validating the service offered. Among them are safety, quality, and the outcome of various situations, in order to ensure that you have adequate assistance that goes beyond the use of processes. To measure this care, there are indicators that can assess or monitor quality, with the main function of ensuring patient safety.

KPIs are valuable tools for measuring the performance of oncology pharmacy strategic activities and are already embedded in many sectors [22]. However, there are specific challenges associated with implementation such as: having relevance to all stakeholders; difficulty in measuring activities; lack of resources for data collection; limited understanding of indicators by pharmacists and what impacts they may have on the future of pharmaceutical practice [19, 20].

Thus, there are some points that must be considered for the development of a KPI, including relevance and measurability [21]. Linked to this, the indicators have their great importance demonstrated by the ability to compare the levels of quality of health care offered by the clinical service [22]; elucidate the performance of actions performed based on their organizational objectives, comparing the results achieved with their projection; financial impacts on the perspective of attention and care; degree of patient orientation and medication adherence that can influence their clinical outcomes; opportunity for weaknesses and points for improvement [23].

The information needed to measure quality can be obtained at any time during the process and is related to service satisfaction. The data collected communicates performance, strategy, results, control, and improvement, in addition to allowing benchmarking between organizations [24]. To better understand and apply, we can divide it into four broad categories [25]:

- Strategic: analyze whether the goals are being achieved as planned, comparing the current scenario with the previous one and how it plans to be (e.g., inventory accuracy and losses).
- Productivity: aims to measure the level of efficiency of resources and inputs used from the assessment of deliveries (e.g., the number of bags produced and pharmaceutical intervention).
- Quality: measuring the level at which activities are being carried out, helping to understand any deviation or non-conformity that occurred during a process (e.g., guidance in patients on the beginning of treatment and contamination in the clean area).
- Capability: measure the response potential of a process in a given parameter (e.g., percentage of problems with suppliers and therapeutic failures) [25].

By monitoring the institution's practices, opportunities for improvement are identified. These points are important and necessary to support the management with regard to both administrative/production issues and clinical pharmacy services, being essential for decision-making and prevention of complications, and thus provide adequate care for cancer patients.

### 12.11.1 The Application

The choice of KPIs must be planned and well defined by the pharmacy management and, with this, develop an adequate and safe instrument for data collection. The lack of a precise instrument or mistaken data collection generates false results that may compromise the reliability of the information, bringing negative results.

Given the scarcity of resources in health, given the increasingly expensive needs in cancer treatment, measuring the quantity and quality of services provided to the patient provides the manager with control over the productivity and efficiency of the activities performed, as an evaluation correct results in proper management and better allocation of available resources [26]. According to Kaplan and Norton (1997), what is not measured is not managed and therefore cannot be improved [27]; the application of this concept in oncology pharmacy management becomes vital for the sustainability of the business. The biggest revenue and the biggest cost of oncology still come from the use of anticancer drugs and with the development of new drugs, with increasingly higher costs, it is necessary to measure and manage them.

### 12.11.2 Management in Practice

Through the indicators, it is possible to operationalize care, assess whether the process is really meeting the institution's needs, and analyze points that need to be modified so that the defined goal can be achieved [28]. The monitoring of a single indicator does not translate faithfully to reality, requiring the association of several for possible intervention [29].

The application of indicators in the management of oncology pharmacy aims to monitor the performance of the operation through the analysis of results and thus manage processes that make sense in the institution. Among these possibilities, we can check some applicability according to Table 12.1:

**Table 12.1** Indicators applicable in oncology pharmacy management

| Indicators |
|---|
| Number of chemotherapy bags handled in a given period of time |
| Manipulated drug delivery time |
| Loss rate during chemotherapy preparation |
| Cost for loss or diversion of chemotherapy drugs in a given period of time |
| Savings on manipulated drugs (accounting for leftovers and overfill); |
| Inventory accuracy |
| Purchase orders for urgent anticancer drugs |
| Request for purchase of non-standard medicines at the institution |
| Types and percentages of errors in the separation of drugs from the chemotherapy protocol |

Logistics and production activities (handling of chemotherapeutic/antineoplastic drugs), ranging from drug acquisition to dispensing, are important processes so that they are available at the right time for the patient and, together with the clinical pharmacy, act to ensure rational use and thus prevent drug-related problems.

Clinical pharmacy is defined by the American College of Clinical Pharmacy (ACCP) as "the science of health in which pharmacists provide patient care, optimize drug therapy and promote health and well-being centered on patient safety." [30] The pharmacist performs this function through patient assessment; identification of drug therapy problems, such as necessity, safety, and effectiveness; carrying out follow-up evaluations and monitoring of medications and other activities [32].

Thus, the importance of clinical pharmaceutical services has gained great prominence in the hospital scenario and demonstrating that pharmaceutical monitoring of cancer patients is necessary for the detection and resolution of problems related to chemotherapy drugs is essential. For this, indicators are used as shown in Table 12.2:

**Table 12.2** Indicators applicable to clinical pharmacy in oncology

| **Indicators** |
|---|
| Pharmaceutical guidance for patients beginning venous or oral chemotherapy treatment (including hormone therapy) |
| Pharmaceutical guidance for patients changing their intravenous or oral chemotherapy protocol (including hormone therapy) |
| Adverse events related to chemotherapy infusion |
| Pharmaceutical interventions in the medical prescription analysis process (dose, dilution, interval of chemotherapy cycles, incompatibilities, dilution, infusion time, and others) |
| Pharmaceutical interventions in chemotherapy extravasation |
| Waiting time of patients when dispensing oral chemotherapy/patient satisfaction |
| Pharmacotherapeutic monitoring |
| Rate of notification of occurrences in the process of validation of prescription, separation, and handling of chemotherapy |
| Index of therapeutic failures (interrupted treatments) |
| Monitoring of patients using new active principles |
| Number of pharmaceutical interventions accepted by the care team |

Crucial point for the success of the indicators in the institution is to consider critical points and implement what is most necessary and urgent to be monitored. It should be started with caution, always taking into account the issues of quality versus quantity. Remember that KPIs are quantifiable measures that will be used to track the institution's performance and allow tracking of results over time [33]. Therefore, a correct analysis ensures the implementation of improvements in clinical practice and improves the quality of care, which is always a priority in the healthcare area, including safety, efficacy, and patient experience.

As presented, we are faced with concepts that need to be evaluated according to the needs of each institution. What we want to bring in this chapter is that there is no right or wrong, but concepts and practices that need to be evaluated. For this, it is necessary to know in depth the processes and objectives to be achieved. We cannot fail to mention that processes are not static and that the pharmacist must always keep up to date.

We try to bring, in an objective and practical way, routines of the dilution center with regard to the management of processes and people, presenting minimum management criteria for the sustainability of an oncology pharmacy.

## Bibliography

1. Júnior GDG, Vieira MMF. Qualidade total e administração hospitalar: explorando disjunções conceituais. Ciênc. Saúde coletiva. 2002;7(2):325–34. Available in: https://doi.org/10.1590/S1413-81232002000200012.
2. Gomes HMS, Nascimento JCHB, Sousa ARC e Almeida ANM. Gastos do sistema público em saúde com tratamento em oncologia. Revista de Administração Hospitalar e Inovação em Saúde. 2021;18(2):74–89. Available in: https://doi.org/10.21450/rahis.v18i2.6877
3. Medici AC. Aspectos teóricos e conceituais do financiamento das políticas de saúde. In SF Piola, SM Vianna (orgs.). *Economia da saúde: conceito e contribuição para a gestão da Saúde* IPEA, Brasília. 1995. pp. 23–68.
4. Chiavenato A. Administração, teoria, processo e prática. 4th ed. São Paulo: Elsevier; 2007.
5. Brasil, Ministério da Saúde. Resolução RDC n.50, de 21 de fevereiro de 2002. Dispõe sobre o Regulamento Técnico para planejamento, program-

ação, elaboração e avaliação de projetos físicos de estabelecimentos assistenciais de saúde.
6. Brasil. Ministério da saúde. Resolução n°338 de maio 2004. Available in: https://bvsms.saude.gov.br/bvs/saudelegis/cns/2004/res0338_06_05_2004.html.
7. Hepler CD, Strand ML. Opportunities and responsibilities in pharmaceutical care. Am J Hosp Pharm. 1990;47(3):533–43.
8. Brasil. Ministério da saúde. Secretaria de Ciência, Tecnologia e Insumos Estratégicos. Departamento de Assistência Farmacêutica e Insumos Estratégicos. Aquisição de medicamentos para a assistência farmacêutica no SUS. Available in: https://bvsms.saude.gov.br/bvs/publicacoes/aquisicao_medicamentos_assistencia_orientacoes_basicas.pdf. Acessado em: 01/20/201.
9. André AM. Gestão estratégica de clínicas e hospitais. 2nd ed. Atheneu: São Paulo; 2014.
10. Endeavor. NPS: como as maiores empresas do mundo medem a satisfação de seus clientes. Available in: https://endeavor.org.br/estrategia-e-gestao/nps/. Access 12/10/2021.
11. Programa Nacional de Segurança do Paciente. Anexo 03: Protocolo de segurança na prescrição, uso e administração de medicamentos.
12. Kaizen express: Fundamentos para a suajornada lean = Kaizen express: fundamentals for your lean journey/TshikoNarusawa& John Shook. São Paulo: LeanInsitute Brasil, 2009.
13. Aperfeiçoando a Jornada do Paciente: Melhorando a segurança do paciente a qualidade e a satisfação, entanto desenvolvemos habilidades para resolver problemas. Keyte, Beau et al. São Paulo: LeanInsitute Brasil, 2013.
14. Mindset: a nova psicologia do sucesso/Carol Dweck: 1ª Edição. São Paulo: Objetiva. 2017.
15. LaHote. Dave. Por que uma solução de problemas efetiva começa com uma boa definição do problema? LeanInsitute Brasil.
16. Hronec SM. Sinais vitais: usando medidas do desempenho da qualidade, tempo e custo para traçar a rota para o futuro de sua empresa. São Paulo: Makron Books; 1994. p. 256.
17. Malik AM, Schiesari LMC. Qualidade na gestão local de serviços e ações de saúde. Revista Qualidade na gestão local de serviços e ações de saúde, p. 227–227, 1998.
18. Fenandes O, Le Piane F, Ahmed H, Toombs K. Should key performance indicators be a component of performance assessment for individual clinical pharmacists? The "con" side. Can J Hosp Pharm. 2014;67(2):166–8.
19. Doucette D, Millin B. Should key performance indicators for clinical services be mandatory. Can J Hosp Pharm. 2011;64:55–7.
20. Lloyd GF, Bajorek B, Barclay P, Goh S. Narrative review: status of key performance indicators in contemporary hospital pharmacy practice. J Pharm Pract Res. 2015;45(4):396–403.

21. Minard LV, Deal H, Harrison ME, Toombs K, Neville H, Meade A. Pharmacists' perceptions of the barriers and facilitators to the implementation of clinical pharmacy key performance indicators. PLoS One. 2016;11(4):e0152903.
22. Fernandes O, Le Piane F, Ahmed H, Toombs K. Should key performance indicators be a component of performance assessment for individual clinical pharmacists? The "con" side. Can J Hosp Pharm. 2014;67(2):166–8.
23. Ibrahim N, Altwoijri A, Alabdulkarim H, Alnajjar F, Alsaqa-aby M. Challenges in applying pharmacoeconomics at the hospital level: experts based approach. Glob J Med Therap. 2019;1(1):1–4.
24. Lo E, Rainkie D, Semchuk WM, Gordman SK, Toombs K, Slavik RS. Measurement of clinical pharmacy key performance indicators to focus and improve your hospital pharmacy practice. Can J Hosp Pharm. 2016;69(2):149.
25. Modelos de KPIs: os 4 principais para acompanhar o desempenho da empresa e orientar melhor as tomadas de decisão. Siteware, 2020. Available in: https://www.siteware.com.br/gestao-estrategica/modelos-de-kpis/. Access on 13 de Out. de 2021.
26. Hursman A. Measure what matters-seven strategies of selecting relevant key performance indicators. Inform Manage Mag. 2010;20:1–2.
27. Kaplan RS, Norton DP. A estratégia em ação: balancedscorecard. 4th ed. Rio de Janeiro: Gulf Professional Publishing; 1997.
28. Yin S, Wang G, Yang X. Robust PLS approach for KPI-related prediction and diagnosis against outliers and missing data. Int J Syst Sci. 2014;45(7):1375–82.
29. Bisbe J, Malagueno R. Using strategic performance measurement systems for strategy formulation: does it work in dynamic environments? Manag Account Res. 2012;23(4):296–311.
30. American College of Clinical Pharmacy. The definition of clinical pharmacy. 2012.
31. Available in: http://www.accp.com/docs/positions/commentaries/Clinpharmdefnfinal.pdf. Access on 10 de out. de 2021.
32. Harrison JJ. Key performance indicators for clinical pharmacy services in New Zealand public hospitals: stakeholder perspectives. J Pharm Health Serv Res. 2010;1(2):75–84.
33. Carvalho DCMF, et al. Manual de Farmácia Clínica e Cuidado ao Paciente. Rio de Janeiro: Atheneu; 2017.

# Stem Cell Transplantation 13

Fumiko Takahashi Ito, Cintia Vecchies Morassi,
Gabriela Sandoval da Silva,
Larissa Zuppardi Lacerda Sabino,
and Mariana Perez Esteves Silva Motta

## 13.1 Pre-transplant Evaluation

### 13.1.1 Stem Cell Transplantation

Stem cell transplantation (SCT) is a treatment modality for some diseases that mainly affect blood cells, such as lymphoproliferative and myeloproliferative diseases, hemoglobinopathies and other malignant and benign diseases. SCT's purpose is to replace the diseased bone marrow with normal cells, which may be from the patient himself (autologous) or from the donor (related or unrelated allogeneic) [1].

F. T. Ito (✉)
Brazilian Society of Pharmacists in Oncology, São Paulo, Brazil

C. V. Morassi · G. S. da Silva · M. P. E. S. Motta
Department of Oncology Pharmacy, Albert Einstein Hospital, São Paulo, Brazil

L. Z. L. Sabino
Oncology and Hematology Center, Albert Einstein Hospital, São Paulo, Brazil



C. W. P. Schmidt, K. M. Otoni (eds.), *The Golden Guide to Oncologic Pharmacy*, https://doi.org/10.1007/978-3-030-98596-7_13

**Table 13.1** Commonindications for STC

| | | |
|---|---|---|
| Autologous transplantation | Neoplastic diseases | Multiple myeloma<br>Hodgkin's lymphoma<br>Non-Hodgkin's lymphoma<br>Acute myeloid leukemia<br>Neuroblastoma<br>Ovarian cancer<br>Germ cell tumors |
| | Other diseases | Autoimmune diseases |
| Allogeneic transplantation | Neoplastic diseases | Acute myeloid leukemia<br>Acute lymphoblastic leukemia<br>Chronic myeloid leukemia<br>Myelodysplastic syndrome<br>Myeloproliferative disease<br>Hodgkin's lymphoma<br>Non-Hodgkin's lymphoma<br>Chronic lymphocytic leukemia<br>Multiple myeloma |
| | Other diseases | Anemias (aplastic, Fanconi, and sickle cell)<br>Thalassemia major<br>Epidermolysis bullosa<br>Blackfan diamond syndrome<br>Severe combined immunodeficiency syndrome<br>Osteopetrosis<br>Mucopolysaccharidosis<br>Granulomatous disease |

### 13.1.2 Stem Cell Transplantation Indication

SCT is an increasingly used modality in the treatment of hematological diseases, whether hereditary or acquired. Table 13.1 shows the main indications of SCT [2, 3].

### 13.1.3 Pre-transplant Phase

SCT is a complex procedure that involves a long and complicated path for the patient. Transplantation carries a significant risk of morbidity and mortality in which the relationship between the need for transplantation and the disease risk versus the transplantation risk should be considered [4].

In the pre-transplant phase, previous meetings should take place with patients, family members and caregivers to clarify each stage of SCT, and also all procedures to be performed. At this stage, the multidisciplinary SCT team should be presented and the patient should receive the necessary guidance before hospitalization.

The results of this pre-transplant evaluation help to adapt the transplant modality, such as conditioning regimen, graft type, stem cell source, post-transplant strategy, and detection of any abnormalities that may lead to post-transplant complications. This complete review serves as a reference and facilitates the comparison of results from the tests performed before, during, and after the transplantation [4].

### 13.1.4 Multidisciplinary Team in Stem Cell Transplantation

The multidisciplinary team is composed of different specialized professionals, who, in cooperation, play an important role in the management and care of hospitalized patients, providing support to patients and family members and supporting them to adapt to the treatment plan.

Professionals should be involved in decision-making during multidisciplinary meetings, provide education to patients and family members, and plan patient discharge and post-hospital discharge care [5].

The SCT clinical pharmacist is an integral member of the multidisciplinary SCT team that provides a variety of educational services, optimizes the adherence to the proposed drug treatment, and assists in the care based on patient safety [6]. The evaluation of pre-transplant patients, pharmacotherapeutic follow-up during hospitalization and post-discharge, allows the pharmacist to develop a care plan based on the safe and effective drug therapy management [7].

According to this active role in the multidisciplinary team, the pharmacist is responsible for the correct use of the drug and should develop guidelines and standard procedures regarding the drug therapy used by patients in SCT [8].

### 13.1.5 Pre-transplant Pharmaceutical Evaluation

When the patient begins the hospitalization process for SCT, the pharmacist performs a complete review of the patient medication profile and drug reconciliation, in order to provide the drug therapy management to multiple chronic diseases such as diabetes, hypertension, dyslipidemia, etc. He should manage the recommended anti-infectious prophylactic therapies for SCT, such as antifungals, antivirals, and antibacterials. He should intervene on self-medication, mainly regarding the use of herbal medicines or medicinal plants, and use of supplements and alternative medicines. This allows monitoring all diseases that the patient treats, avoiding iatrogenic cascade, and prevents prescriptions duplication by different members of the multidisciplinary team and also assesses untreated conditions or diseases [6, 9].

In the pre-transplant pharmaceutical evaluation, it is possible to identify drug allergies, drug interactions, need for adequacy of pharmaceutical formulations according to the patient preference and need, especially in elderly or pediatric patients, and need for adjustments when changes in laboratory parameters occur [6]. Drug-related problems (DRPs) should be identified, such as adverse drug reactions (ADRs), and medication errors or any errors during the prescription and use process of the drug [6, 9–11]. A medication error may arise in the medication choice, dose, administration route, and frequency or duration of treatment. Inadequate prescription may also be related to individual characteristics or co-existing treatments of the patient [10, 11].

At the time of hospital admission, unintentional omission or changes in the treatment regimen may occur. Inaccurately obtaining the medications history may result in potential damage to the patient. The pharmacotherapeutic follow-up, when the pharmacist monitors the individual clinical needs of the patient, allows the detection, prevention, and resolution of possible DRPs [11].

For any identified problem, the pharmacist should intervene with the multidisciplinary team suggesting dose adjustments, suspensions, or substitutions to avoid toxicities and inefficacy to treatment [10].

### 13.1.6 Drug Therapy Management

During hospitalization in the SCT, the pharmacist should be responsible for the daily analysis of the medical prescription. In the context of SCT, where high-risk drugs are prescribed and administered, the pharmacist plays an important role in providing specific information for the correct use and administration of these medicinal products [12].

The pharmacist must manage [12]:

- Chemotherapy drugs used in the SCT conditioning. After the technical evaluation of the medical prescription, he should be responsible for the handling, technical evaluation of the drug, dilution choice, storage, and guidance regarding the administration time.
- Drugs with narrow therapeutic margin such as immunosuppressants, anti-infectious, anticoagulants, and chemotherapy agents. Monitoring should be performed through laboratory test results and/or signs and symptoms.
- Selection of antimicrobials for prophylaxis of viruses, fungi, and bacteria infections due to risk factors for transplant patients, such as febrile neutropenia, taking into account institutional protocols, treatment cost, and institutional microbial resistance parameters.
- Medications in the treatment of pre-existing comorbidities or those associated with the therapy applied to the transplanted patient, in which the combination of various therapies may cause drug interactions and/or exacerbate pre-existing conditions, such as graft-versus-host disease (GvHD) treatment that can worsen conditions in patients with diabetes.

- Nutritional support that occurs after SCT due to factors such as: insufficient oral intake induced by chemotherapy (nausea, vomiting, mucositis), anorexia, and GvHD. The pharmacist may assume responsibility for the introduction and discontinuation of prolonged parenteral nutrition, blood glucose monitoring, and electrolyte disorders.
- GvHD therapy options, based on the signs and symptoms shown by the patient concomitant with complications, risks of infectious complications, such as cytomegalovirus reactivation, nephrotoxicity, and steroid-refractory treatment.
- Maintenance therapy after SCT, where some drugs of choice are of high cost and the pharmacist should guide the patient and family member about the access to these drugs available through local care programs.
- Toxicities to post-transplant therapy, when patients have transplant-related toxicities that can become chronic problems and require long-term monitoring, such as chronic pain management, anticoagulation for venous thromboembolism, post-transplant bone health, steroid-induced hyperglycemia, and chronic GvHD. The pharmacist role in the long-term management of these complications is an opportunity to improve the patient quality of life.

## 13.2 Pre-hematopoietic Stem Cell Transplantation Conditionings

Preparatory or conditioning regimens are administered to patients with malignant diseases and eligible for SCT and have two main objectives: promote medullary aplasia with the purpose of preventing graft rejection and reducing the tumor burden of the disease before transplantation. To achieve these objectives, doses of total body irradiation (TBI) and chemotherapy agents are used, with no overlapping toxicity [13].

Conditionings have been classified into three categories, according to their intensity: myeloablative conditioning (MAC), reduced intensity conditioning (RIC), and non-myeloablative conditioning (NMA) [14].

### 13.2.1 Conditioning Types

#### 13.2.1.1 Myeloablative Conditioning (MAC)

It consists of a single agent, or a combination of chemotherapy agents, obtaining deep pancytopenia, which is caused by the destruction of hematopoietic cells in the bone marrow and, in this case, this is the most expected side effect of this type of conditioning [13].

Such effect begins within 1–3 weeks of the conditioning onset and its duration is prolonged and irreversible. In this case, the SCT is responsible for the hematopoiesis restoration and reversal of the pancytopeniccondition [15].

MACs cause adverse effects, in addition to medullary toxicity, such as: mucositis, nausea, vomiting, diarrhea, skin rash, peripheral neuropathy, pulmonary and hepatic toxicities, among others [13].

Some examples of MACs are Cy/TBI, Bu4/Cy, Flu/Bu4, BEAM, CBV protocols, and Melphalan protocols [16].

#### 13.2.1.2 Reduced Intensity Conditioning (RIC)

They do not meet the criteria for myeloablative conditioning, nor for non-myeloablative conditionings. This type of conditioning causes cytopenia with varied duration that often is not reversible. Patients eligible for this type of conditioning should undergo a stem cell support [14]. In general, what differentiates a MAC from a RIC is that in RIC, the chemotherapy or TBI dose is usually reduced by approximately 30% of the doses applied in MACs [13].

Examples of reduced intensity conditioning: Flu/Mel, Flu/Bu2, Flu/Cy, Flu/Bu/Tiothepa [16].

#### 13.2.1.3 Non-myeloablative Conditioning (NMA)

In some diseases indicated for SCT, greater action of the immunological effects promoted by donor cells and less need for cytotoxic effects on pre-transplant conditioning is required. In these cases, non-myeloablative conditionings have been studied as a better option, since they cause minimal cytopenia, with no need for stem cell support for recovery [14].

Although GvHD is a condition avoided to the maximum in SCT, it is necessary to consider that not all diseases indicated for the procedure have a high risk of GvHD. Follicular lymphoma, chronic lymphocytic leukemia, mantle cell lymphoma, and chronic myeloid leukemia are diseases where GvHD is most recurrent. Acute lymphocytic leukemia and Hodgkin's lymphoma are relatively resistant to GvHD complications. This can also be a factor of choice for non-NMAs conditionings [13].

NMAs also allow transplantation in elderly, high-risk patients or previously treated patients of any age, because they have lower toxicity and are associated with lower mortality from treatment.

Examples of NMAs: Flu/TBI, TLI/ATG.

Drugs involved in pre-SCT conditioning can cause medullary toxicity; however, they also affect other organs, as shown in Table 13.2 [17]:

The choice of a regimen is based on some principles such as age and patient performance status, comorbidities, availability of a donor, and also factors related to the disease, such as the remission risk and status of the disease at the time of transplantation [13, 14]. Regarding the patient comorbidities, it is necessary to know that patients with advanced age or comorbidities of great relevance end up not being candidates to receive MAC, but are eligible for RIC or NMA [13, 14].

The status of the disease prior to transplant can also be an eligibility criterion to choose the type of conditioning. For example,

**Table 13.2** Agents commonly used in STC and the organs most affected by its toxicity

| Agent used in the STC | Organ most affected by toxicity |
|---|---|
| Irradiation | Lung, heart |
| Cyclophosphamide | Heart |
| Busulfan | Lung |
| Etoposide | Liver |
| Carmustine | Lung |
| Cytarabine | Central nervous system |
| Melphalan | Lung, gastrointestinal |

Adapted from Robert S Negrin. Preparative regimens for hematopoietic cell transplantation. In: UpToDate.

in malignant hematological diseases, there is a need to eradicate as many hematopoietic cells as possible in order to prevent the disease from relapsing. For this, a MAC would be the one indicated. When bone marrow transplantation is indicated for patients with immunodeficiencies or aplastic anemias, the main objective of conditioning is immunosuppression. For this purpose, a less intensive regimen may be a more indicated alternative. Fanconi anemia, for example, is particularly sensitive to toxicities from chemotherapy and radiotherapy. Patients with this diagnosis should undergo less intense conditioning [13, 18].

The current status of the disease can also define the type of conditioning intensity; for example, when the disease is not in complete remission, a MAC is necessary.

Generally, MACs are the choice for young patients with good performance status or difficult-to-control diseases. The choice between the different types of conditioning also depends on institutional preferences, medications availability, transplant center experience, and the factors mentioned above [18].

### 13.2.2 Irradiation

Total body irradiation (TBI) has been included in many pre-bone marrow transplant conditionings, both autologous and allogeneic, due to its immunosuppressive property and penetration capacity at hard-to-reach sites (sanctuary sites). Currently, TBI-based conditionings have the total dose of fractional radiation usually in 4 days in a row, which helps to decrease toxicity and increase tolerability to conditioning. Conditionings generally combine doses between 12 and 16-Gy with chemotherapy agents with antineoplastic and immunomodulatory properties, such as Cyclophosphamide. Higher doses of TBI can produce non-hematological toxic effects, and also hinder the grafting of hematopoietic cells and success in the bone marrow transplantation procedure [13].

Major limitations of this modality include mucositis, lung toxicity, and infertility [14].

## 13.2.3 Pharmacotherapeutic Follow-Up

### 13.2.3.1 Busulfan

#### Pharmacokinetics of Busulfan

Busulfan is a chemotherapy agent constantly used in allogeneic pre-transplant conditioning regimens. This is a drug with high pharmacokinetic variability, where, for example, the area under the curve (AUC), concentration versus time, can range between 3 and 7 times in patients receiving high doses of this drug, calculated based on the patient weight, or his body surface. Busulfan AUC has been related to toxic effects, modifications in bone marrow grafting time, and relapse in patients undergoing conditioning with Busulfan and Cyclophosphamide; but these losses can be extrapolated to other conditionings than Busulfan. Factors such as age and obesity have been identified as predictors of Busulfan clearance [19].

Due to the heterogeneous pharmacokinetics of Busulfan, transplant centers have been seeking drug plasma monitoring as an alternative to avoid unfavorable endpoints with the use of this medication, minimizing toxicities and preventing graft rejection. Busulfan drug level plasma monitoring consists of a series of blood samples collected for up to 6 hours after the beginning of the first and second infusion of the drug. Busulfan plasma concentrations are quantified to calculate the AUC. Taking into account the target AUC of the chosen conditioning, it is possible to guide yourself to define the AUC that the patient should still receive [19].

#### Prophylaxis of Seizures

Because it is a drug with highly easy penetration into the blood-brain barrier, reaching identical proportions in plasma and central nervous system, Busulfan can cause convulsive seizures due to these high concentrations in the CNS. To avoid this adverse effect, drugs are used to prevent this condition. Studies indicate that convulsive conditions may occur at a frequency from 1% to 40% in patients who have not received anticonvulsant prophylaxis [20,

21]. Some drugs may be used in seizure prophylaxis, such as Levetiracetam, Phenytoin, and Clonazepam. The drug of choice should have rapid action and should not increase the toxicity or pharmacokinetics of the agents used in conditioning. In addition, it should cause as little hematological toxicity as possible, so that it does not interfere with the bone marrow engraftment. Also, one should choose a drug that does not cause dermatological toxicity that can be confused with GvHD, and that does not increase nausea, emesis, diarrhea, or mucositis, which are common symptoms to pre-transplant conditioning [21, 22].

Neurotoxicity, including seizures, can occur during the administration of Busulfan and within 24 hours after the last dose of this drug, so prophylaxis drugs should be indicated at least during this period of bone marrow transplantation [23].

#### 13.2.3.2 Drug Interactions

Busulfan pharmacokinetics, besides being heterogeneous, may suffer interferences due to the concomitant use of other medications. This is a critical situation where low plasma levels of Busulfan can lead to undesirable effects such as disease relapse, graft failure, and shortened survival. On the other hand, high plasma levels of Busulfan may increase side effects, such as mucositis, pulmonary toxicity, sinusoidal obstructive syndrome, and neurotoxicity, among others [23].

Table 13.3 shows the drugs that commonly interact with Busulfan, either by the action on cytochrome P450, interference in glutathione S-transferase, glutathione, or other transporters.

#### 13.2.3.3 Cyclophosphamide and Uroprotection

One of the adverse effects that should be monitored in patients undergoing pre-SCT conditioning composed of Cyclophosphamide or Pelvic Irradiation is hemorrhagic cystitis, which is characterized by hematuria. Hemorrhagic cystitis is an inflammatory process induced by acrolein, a toxic metabolite of Cyclophosphamide, and can be aggravated by the immune system subsequent activation by producing a greater number of pro-inflammatory agents. Acrolein is derived from the hepatic metabolism process of alkylating agents, filtered by

**Table 13.3** Drugs that interact with Busulfan

| Drug | Interaction result | Recommendation |
|---|---|---|
| Acetaminophen | Increased serum levels of Busulfan | Do not use the drug 72 h before and 72 h after the administration of Busulfan |
| Itraconazole, voriconazole | Increased serum levels of Busulfan | Use with caution and monitor the toxic effects of Busulfan; consider fluconazole as an alternative |
| Metronidazole | Increased serum levels of Busulfan | Do not use the drug 72 h before and 72 h after the administration of Busulfan |
| Phenytoin | Decreased serum levels of Busulfan | Consider the administration of another anticonvulsant; if the option is phenytoin, monitor Busulfan AUC wisely |
| Deferasirox | Increased Busulfan AUC | Consider another drug option for iron quelation |
| Ethacrynic acid | Inhibition of Busulfan-GSH conjugation | Consider a change in diuretic therapy |
| Ketobemidone | Increased serum levels of Busulfan | Consider the use of another opioid agent, such as morphine, for example |

Adapted from Myers AL, et al. and Glotzbecker et al. [24]

the kidneys and concentrated in the bladder. From 10% to 40% of patients are affected by hemorrhagic cystitis and patients undergoing SCT have a high risk of developing this condition, which is more common after a MAC than in RIC [25].

The most effective treatment for hemorrhagic cystitis and certainly the safest for the patient is prevention, where the strict intravenous hydration of the patient is recommended, and also the use of Mesna. In addition, monitoring and attention to initial symptoms of cystitis are important for the prevention of more severe forms of this condition [25].

Mesna is a drug that inactivates acrolein in the urine and reduces the risk of cystic toxicity. This should be given before Cyclophosphamide; i.e., Mesna should already be present in the bladder by the time the alkylating agent starts. Because the half-life of Mesna is approximately 90 minutes and that of alkylating agents ranges between 6 and 7 hours, additional doses of Mesna are required, usually 4 and 8 hours after cyclophosphamide administration. Generally the final dose of Mesnato be fully administered represents 60% of the total dose of Cyclophosphamide [25].

#### 13.2.3.4 Melphalan and Mucositis

Mucositis is one of the most common adverse effects of SCT, especially when due to radiotherapy or high doses of Melphalan. This effect is often mentioned by patients as one of the most debilitating of all onco-hematological treatment, which can cause dehydration, malnutrition, potential opportunistic infections, and reduced disease-free survival time [26].

Studies indicate that after high doses of Melphalan, 20–45% of patients develop severe mucositis. When we analyze the incidence of mucositis in all grades, this number is between 70% and 90% [27].

Prophylactic and curative measures can significantly reduce these values. Some of them are: cryotherapy, antiviral, antifungal and antimicrobial prophylaxis, total parenteral nutrition, topical anesthetics, and mouthwashing solutions, among others [28].

Pharmacist may carry out interventions with the medical and dental service in cases of patients undergoing bone marrow transplantation, who use radiotherapy or high doses of Melphalan.

#### 13.2.3.5 Cytarabine and Conjunctivitis

Cytarabine is part of some pre-SCT conditioning protocols, especially those associated with radiotherapy and/or cyclophosphamide. High doses of Cytarabine are used, and some characteristic adverse effects are eye disorders such as conjunctivitis, eye pain, blurred vision, photophobia and sensation of foreign bodies in the eyes. These symptoms develop in 40–100% of patients receiving doses of Cytarabine 2 $g/m^2$/day. Such disorders result from the transport of Cytarabine from plasma into the tear fluid, inhibiting the division of the cornea epithelial cells. Although the concentration of Cytarabine in the tear fluid is ten times lower than in the bloodstream, it is enough to cause such eye disorders [29].

For the prevention and control of this adverse effect, the use of corticosteroid-based eye drops has been reported. The choice of eye drops is not standardized in the conducted studies, and either the use frequency, but the use of betamethasone eye drops at 1%, prednilosone 1% or prednisolone 0.5% is pointed out. The association of corticosteroid eye drops with artificial tear has shown good results and improvement in the patient quality of life. Regarding the frequency, some centers start the eye drops administration 48 h before the first dose of Cytarabine and maintain it for up to 28 days after treatment. Other centers start the prophylaxis for conjunctivitis on the day of Cytarabine administration and maintain it for 5 days after the last administration of Cytarabine [29, 30].

The pharmacist plays an important role in the follow-up of these cases, since prophylaxis can reduce the incidence of conjunctivitis caused by Cytarabine at high doses from 85% and 92% to 8% and 16% [31].

In patients undergoing SCT, the occurrence of conjunctivitis may be aggravated due to the association with TBI, which may cause synergistic toxicity to that of Cytarabine [31].

## 13.3 Care Before Engraftment

### 13.3.1 Introduction

Communication and coordination of the SCT team, including a multidisciplinary team, are important for establishing and maintaining a successful care plan [32].

At this stage of SCT, after bone marrow infusion and before engraftment, care is intended to manage toxicities to conditioning chemotherapy. Preventive managements should be carried out for infections and graft-versus-host disease (GvHD), and engraftment syndrome. But there are other risks during this phase due to individual characteristics [32].

Common factors that may contribute to complications during SCT [32]:

- Previous treatments
- Status of the disease at the time of SCT
- Existence of comorbidities
- Conditioning regimes developed
- Type of SCT
- Organic dysfunction
- Infections prior to SCT
- Age of donor and recipient

### 13.3.2 Drug Toxicity

During conditioning, high doses of chemotherapy are usually used associated or not with radiotherapy, which will be administered in the days prior to the infusion of hematopoietic progenitor cells (CPH).

The conditioning stage aims to eradicate residual disease or reduce tumor load, create space in the bone marrow that will be filled by donor cells, and induce immunosuppression to prevent graft rejection in allogeneic SCT [33].

The high dose of chemotherapy results in predictable toxicity, but in individualized intensity.

The commontoxicities of conditioning chemotherapy are:

- Gastrointestinal complications: nausea, vomiting, mucositis, and diarrhea
- Liver complications: sinusoidal obstructive syndrome (SOS)
- Hematologicalcomplications: Cytopenias (neutropenia, anemia, and thrombocytopenia)
- Kidney and lung complications

#### 13.3.2.1 Nausea and Vomiting

Chemotherapy causes damage to gastrointestinal tissue that results in the release of neuroactivating agents and vagal stimulation, located in the brain stem, which activates the center of vomiting. Later nausea and vomiting have a cause that differs from toxicity to conditioning. Prevention is the key to success in the management of nausea and vomiting in the peri-transplant period.

The choice of drugs like antiemetic should be according to the emetogenic potential of the drugs used in conditioning and corticosteroids for some types of SCT. Therapy and prevention should be managed according to the type of transplantation and drug interaction, especially in allogeneic transplantation [34]. In the 2020 American Society Clinical Oncology (ASCO) guideline update, the use of integrative medicine as non-pharmacological measures to complement treatment for nausea and vomiting is endorsed.

#### 13.3.2.2 Oral Mucositis

The pathophysiology of mucositis is complex and involves direct damage to mucosal tissue, generation of inflammatory cytokines, and microbiome changes.

Acute oral mucositis is one of the common sources of morbidities in patients undergoing SCT and affects more than 80% of patients undergoing transplantation [34].The pain and dysphagia caused by this reaction leads to a consequence such as a drastic reduction in food and liquid intake and affects quality of life throughout the affected period [32]. The mucosal barrier is predisposed to bacterial, fungal, and viral infections and may remain locally or spread, especially if the patient is in a period of medullary aplasia, and the most common is candidiasis.

Prevention can be performed with laser therapy – photobiomodulation (before the start of chemotherapy and until recovery time), cryotherapy (before and during chemotherapy), and oral hygiene (before the start of chemotherapy and until recovery time). The initial clinical manifestation is erythema of soft tissues of oral mucosa or palate with burning sensation. After the mucositis onset, pain management with opioid analgesics may help in the intake of food and liquids [32].

#### 13.3.2.3 Diarrhea

There are numerous possible causes of diarrhea during SCT. Approximately 80% of patients will have at least one event of diarrhea during the SCT process. The most common cause soon after the bone marrow conditioning and infusion regimen is the toxicity of high doses of chemotherapy, called non-oral gastrointestinal mucositis, which in addition to diarrhea can include nausea, vomiting, and abdominal pain. This occurs between 7 and 14 days after chemotherapy. Reaction should be taken into account by non-chemotherapy drugs such as antibiotics and immunosuppressive drugs, and it may be treated with medication or excluding medicinal products suspected of causing diarrhea. During cytopenia, the cause may also be infection or GvHD [32].

#### 13.3.2.4 Liver Complications

Liver dysfunction is a common complication in SCT that can be identified in increased bilirubin and liver enzymes, asymptomatic, sinusoidal obstructive syndrome (SOS), hepatic GvHD, and fulminant death from liver failure. Early detection and treatment results in its prognosis.

### 13.3.3 Infections

SCT patients are at increased risk of a variety of infections based on their degree of immunosuppression and exposure to the infectious agent. Infection in these patients is associated with high morbidity and mortality. Patients may develop a variety of bacterial, fungal, viral, and/or parasitic infections after SCT. Antimicrobial prevention should be according to the history of symptomatic and asymptomatic infections of both the donor and the recipient.

The management of prophylactic antibiotics should consider the rate of quinolone strain resistant and multi-resistant to various drugs [35]. Prevalence rate of bloodstream infection should also be evaluated.

For the antifungal use, the patient risk for fungal infection should be known according to pre-transplant evaluation.

The pharmacist has a fundamental role for the management of prophylactic and preemptive antimicrobials, which should be according the individualized risk of the patient, and monitored by laboratory tests and signs and symptoms of the patient.

### 13.3.4 Immunosuppression

Due to the intensive pre-transplant conditioning regimen, both cellular and humoral responses are severely impaired. Immune reconstitution is an important component for a successful transplantation, not only because immune defects are related to post-transplant morbidity, but also because they can influence the risk of relapse and development of secondary malignancies after transplantation [36].

Soon after allogeneic stem cell transplantation (SCT), the circulating lymphocyte in the recipient is from the donor that has a small impact on residual cells with effective immune effect. After this period, there is an immunological reconstitution of the receptor through the dependent T-pathway that performs the rearrangement of T-cell receptor genes. T cells generated by this pathway maintain recognition and immunocompetence to various antigens. Another reconstitution pathway of T-cells may be the peripheral expansion pathway, i.e., the proliferation of mature T-cells present in the graft [36].

The reconstitution of the receptor immune system requires the formation of new antigen-specific T-lymphocytes, derived from the hematopoietic progenitor cells of the donor. The production of these new lymphocytes is dependent on the thymic function of the receptor, which decreases depending on the age [36].

When the peripheral blood of the receptor begins to be restored, the first granulocytes appear, followed by lymphocytes, and also red blood cells and platelets.

The lymphoid system reconstitution may also be impaired by the manifestations of GvHD [36]. In the prophylaxis of GvHD, the patient is placed subjected to a clinical protocol with immunosuppressants to control the action of residual T cells from the donor blood, avoiding rejection. A standard combination of immunosuppressants has been established for GvHD prophylaxis, in which the use of calcineurin inhibitor such as tacrolimin or cyclosporine is usually used in combination with or without methotrexate. Other combinations such as calcineurin inhibitor with mycophenolate (MMF) are also used and depend on the conditioning regimen and type of SCT [37].

These drugs have high toxicity associated with the narrow therapeutic range and should have plasma level control and high vigilance regarding toxicity and effectiveness. In addition, they have numerous drug interactions, leading to an increase or decrease in plasma levels, resulting in toxicity or therapeutic failure. The pharmacist should monitor and manage plasma levels of these drugs frequently and make the necessary adjustments for safety and efficacy [37].

In general, GvHD is caused by the reaction of mature T-cells grafted into the inoculum against host alloantigens. Acute GvHD (aGvHD), after histocompatible hematopoietic progenitor cell transplantation, has a small effect on lymphoid reconstitution time. The thymus can be selected as a target organ, and also the skin, liver, and intestine [37].

Immunological reconstitution is the key to successful transplantation, which includes the choice of conditioning and maintenance of post-transplant monitoring even after spinal grafting.

### 13.3.5 Laboratory Tests

After SCT, there is a need to monitor the patient clinical conditions through constant multidisciplinary medical and multidisciplinary visits and through laboratory tests.

Blood test is a daily control routine to identify the need for transfusion support, for white and differential cell count, and engraftment can be followed as the first step towards the SCT success. The detection of viral infections reactivation is of paramount importance for early therapy. Due to the use of several medications, drug interaction is inevitable in the SCT process. Liver functions and kidney functions should be monitored to avoid and treat complications. Serum electrolyte and immunosuppressive plasma levels should be monitored and managed early.

Other tests will be requested according to the patient clinical status and should be considered in the pharmacotherapeutic follow-up.

## 13.4 Complication in Progenitor Cell Transplantation

After stem cell transplantation, the patient undergoes a period of neutropenia and immunodeficiency and, therefore, complications are more susceptible. Several factors contribute to these complications, such as conditioning regimen, age, transplantation type, comorbidities, and underlying disease. Below are the main complications involved.

### 13.4.1 Febrile Neutropenia and Bacterial, Fungal, and Viral Infections

Fever during neutropenia is common in post-stem cell transplantation (SCT) patients and is a non-specific symptom that may be associated with several causes, such as: bacterial infections, fungal infections, viral infections, drug reactions, transfusion reactions, mucositis, engraftment syndrome, GvHD, cytokine release syndrome, immune rejection of donor cells mediated by host cells and hemophagocytosis. Since infection by gram-negative bacteria, including *Pseudomonas aeruginosa*, can result in a rapid deterioration of the patient clinical condition, empirical antibiotic therapy should be considered until the cause or pathogen identification and the best treatment are defined [38].

Febrile neutropenia is defined as a single measurement of oral temperature greater than 38.3 °C, or a sustained measurement for more than 1 hour above 38 °C in patients with neutrophil count below 500 cells/μL [39]. Infectious complications can occur at different stages of SCT (stem cell transplantation) [40]:

- *Phase I or pre-graft phase:* up to 45 days after hematopoietic stem cells infusion. Febrile neutropenia and skin barrier rupture result in increased risk of bacteremia and fungal infections by *Candida species* and *Aspergillus species*, and reactivation of herpes simplex virus type I and II.

- *Phase II or post-graft phase*: from 30 to 100 days after hematopoietic stem cells infusion. At this stage, infections are related to cell-mediated immunity impairment. The scope and impact of this defect are determined by the extent of GvHD and immunosuppressive therapy for it. Herpes viruses, such as cytomegalovirus (CMV), are the most common infectious agents in this period, besides *Pneumocystis jiroveci* and *Aspergillus species*.
- *Phase III or late phase*: 100 days after hematopoietic stem cells infusion. At this stage, patients with chronic GvHD (cGvHD) and unrelated donor transplanted patients have a higher risk of infection and its severity is proportional to the severity of GvHD during phases II and III. Major pathogens include cytomegalovirus (CMV), varicella-zoster virus (VZV), and infections by encapsulated bacteria such as *Streptococcus pneumoniae* [40].

### 13.4.2 Toxoplasmosis (*Toxoplasma gondii*)

Toxoplasmosis is a rare infection in a patient after hematopoietic stem cell transplantation. Although there are reports in patients undergoing autologous transplantation, its prevalence is higher in patients undergoing allogeneic transplantation. This occurs mostly by latent reactivation; however, it can also be transmitted by the donor and for this reason it is important to determine the patient serology before transplantation. The main risk factors are associated with acute GvHD and its treatment and incidence of *Toxoplasma gondii* disease varies according to geographic prevalence [38].

### 13.4.3 Complications of Bleeding, Thrombosis, and Endothelial Origin

Complications related to bleeding and thrombosis are an important cause of SCT-related morbidity and mortality. Approximately one quarter of patients have a hemorrhagic event in the first year after transplantation. The main thrombotic complications are:

venous thromboembolism such as catheter-related thrombosis, sinusoidal obstructive syndrome (SOS), and thrombotic micro angiopathy associated with transplantation. Bleeding is related to the gastrointestinal or respiratory tract and is more common in thrombocytopenic patients or with GvHD [38].

Sinusoidal obstructive syndrome is a systemic endothelial disease with onset occurring days or weeks after the stem cell transplantation (SCT) with refractory thrombocytopenia, hepatomegaly, ascites, and jaundice, and can progress rapidly to multiple organ dysfunction and death. For this reason, effective management is essential to reduce associated morbidity and mortality.

Thrombotic microangiopathy associated with transplantation is a potentially fatal complication of transplantation caused by endothelial injury that appears through renal dysfunction and/or unexplained neurological dysfunction, with evidence of intravascular hemolysis [41].

### 13.4.4 Graft-Versus-Host Disease (GvHD)

GvHD is a common complication in allogeneic hematopoietic stem cell transplantation and one of the main causes of morbidity and mortality. This complication occurs when donor T lymphocytes recognize host antigens as foreign [42]. Initially the GvHD was classified taking into account the time of symptoms onset and, therefore, when they appeared up to 100 days after transplantation they were classified as acute and after 100 days they were classified as chronic. Based on clinical manifestations, the National Institutes of Health (NIH) accept the following subclassification [42]:

- Acute classic GvHD: appears within 100 days after transplantation with classic clinical characteristics of acute graft-versus-host disease (aGvHD)
- Persistent, recurrent or late-onset of acute GvHD: appears with clinical characteristics of classic acute GvHD, but after 100 days of transplantation

- Classic chronic GvHD: appears after 100 days of transplantation with classic clinical characteristics of chronic GvHD
- Overlap syndrome: can appear at any time after transplantation with acute and chronic GvHD characteristics

Risk factors for acute GvHD manifestation [42]:

- HLA incompatibility degree
- Gender difference between donor/recipient
- Intensity of the transplant conditioning regimen
- GvHD prophylactic regimen
- Graft source

Main organs affected in acute GvHD [42]:

- Skin
- Gastrointestinal tract
- Liver

Risk factors for the manifestation of chronic GvHD [42]:

- HLA incompatibility degree
- Advanced age (donor or recipient)
- Gender difference between donor/recipient
- Graft source
- Previous manifestation of acute GvHD
- Lymphocyte infusions
- Cytomegalovirus-positive serology in the donor and/or recipient
- Donor with positive serology for Epstein-Barr virus

Main organs affected in chronic GvHD [42]:

- Mucocutaneous manifestations – changes in skin, nails, scalp and body hair, mouth, eyes, and genitalia
- Liver
- Gastrointestinal tract
- Lung
- Musculoskeletal: fasciitis and myositis

### 13.4.5 Lymphoproliferative Syndrome

Post-transplant lymphoproliferative diseases (PTLD) are potentially fatal and occur due to the proliferation of B cells previously infected with Epstein-Barr virus (EBV) in the absence of normal T cells. The main risk factors related to its development are the degree of immunosuppression, age, race, and time after transplantation. The most common symptoms are fever, weight loss, and fatigue in addition to symptoms related to viral infection, lymphadenopathy, and dysfunction of the involved organs and extranodal masses [43].

## 13.5 Hospital Discharge and Outpatient Follow-Up

Hospital discharge can be defined as a care transition process, in which it is transacted from the health team to the patient and their relevant caregivers. It is considered a delicate phase, in which patients are more susceptible to the occurrence of adverse events related to the use of drugs and opportunistic infections, which justifies the increase in the demand for urgent and emergency care and in new hospitalizations [44]. As a strategy to prevent problems related to the use of medications, the pharmacist at discharge advices the patient regarding the home use of medications such as dosage, storage and administration, contributing to the safe use of medications, in addition to the treatment adherence monitoring and follow-up [45].

The criticality of discharge is not only due to the constant changes in the patient pharmacotherapy, but also because of the large amount of information that the patient can receive. The pharmacotherapy instructions should begin during hospitalization to establish a link with the patient and caregivers to evaluate their degree of understanding, so that the patient can assume, at hospital discharge, the use of his medications safely. During this period, patients and their caregivers will have the opportunity to clarify their doubts [46].

On the day of the patient discharge, the information should not be given only orally. The pharmacist can offer the therapeutic plan in writing or printed, which can be in the form of a table, which facilitates the patient understanding. All educational material should be adapted to the understanding of the patient and his family member or caregiver. If possible, a contact channel should be offered so that they can clarify any questions that may arise [45].

After hospital discharge, the pharmacist should follow up the patient on an outpatient basis, either in face-to-face appointments, telemedicine, or by telephone contact. The role of the pharmacist in outpatient follow-up can prevent the occurrence of adverse effects and identify therapeutic failures and problems related to therapy through drug conciliation.

### 13.5.1 Chronic Graft-Versus-Host Disease (cGVHD)

Chronic graft-versus-host disease is the most important cause of long-term morbidity and mortality among patients who have undergone SCT. It usually occurs between 3 months and 2 years after SCT, and with 2/3 of cases in the first 12 months. It is estimated that about 80% of patients who developed cGvHD had already developed aGvHD.

The pharmacist should periodically monitor plasma immunosuppressive levels through laboratory tests and immunosuppression regimens, such as GvHD prophylaxis, assist the patient in accessing immunosuppressive therapies [47], monitor the serum level of electrolytes, because calcineurin inhibitors can lead to electrolyte imbalance [48], and intervene with therapeutic alternatives in relapse to immunosuppressants. In the use of corticosteroids, such as cGvHD treatment, the follow-up of de-escalation is of paramount importance for patient safety [47].

Regarding corticosteroid withdrawal, the SCT team may find difficulty during patient follow-up. Some patients may not tolerate the withdrawal of these drugs, in the absence of the disease reagudization, and this condition is called steroid withdrawal syndrome. This syndrome is characterized by the appearance of physical symptoms, such as vomiting, asthenia, cephalalgia, among others and psychological, such as mood change and emotional lability, and delirium and psychotic states. The syndrome may occur in all patients, including children and adolescents who do not tolerate the withdrawal of these drugs [49].

### 13.5.2 Other Late Complications

Other late complications after SCT are described in Table 13.4, and the conduct suggestions to the pharmacist during outpatient follow-up [47, 50].

### 13.5.3 Vaccination

Patients undergoing SCT, due to treatment, lose acquired immune memory through exposure to infectious agents during life and through prior vaccination [51]. Therefore, the reexposure of patients undergoing SCT to vaccines is advocated by several medical groups that have developed several guidelines for the immunization program after SCT. This mobilization is justified by the fact that the immunological recovery of these patients takes up to 2 years after transplantation, especially in individuals who keep the chronic graft-versus-host disease active. Post-transplant patients should be vaccinated according to the vaccination schedule of choice of the transplant team.

However, the decision to include the patient into an immunization program should be made by an expert, especially in cases where the patient should continue with post-transplant maintenance treatment [52]. Vaccination protocols may vary depending on the SCT center [51]. Table 13.5 describes one of the recommendations on adult patient vaccination after SCT.

In the group of patients after SCT, the incidence rate of children has been increasing greatly in recent decades. This population also benefits from reimmunization, but after a rigorous evaluation of a specialist professional. This is because there is a high risk of developing infections and serious adverse events. In addition, no large-scale vaccine study has evaluated the clinical outcome in disease prevention in this population [53].

Basic principles regarding the vaccination of children subjected to SCT [53]:

**Table 13.4** Monitoring of late effects in patients after SCT

| Late effects | Incidence | Mortality | Monitoring | Pharmaceutical monitoring |
|---|---|---|---|---|
| Cardiovascular toxicity | + | + | Cardiovascular risk and cardiac function with echocardiogram to evaluate ventricular ejection fraction and electrocardiogram | Follow-up drug interactions that increase QT interval |
| Endocrine toxicity: Thyroid dysfunction | ++ | – | Thyroid function | Instruct the patient about the drug dosage and monitor treatment adherence |
| Diabetes | ++ | + | Serum glycemia and glycated hemoglobin | |
| Dyslipidemia | ++ | – | Cholesterol: Total cholesterol, HDL, LDL, and triglycerides | |
| Liver toxicity | + | – | Liver function and viral load for hepatitis B and C | Adjust the drugs dose according to liver function |
| Renal toxicity | + | + | Renal function: Creatinine and urea | Adjust the drugs dose according to renal function |

Adapted from Late effects of blood and marrow Transplantation (Inamoto Y, Lee SJ); Long Term Complications After Hematopoietic Cell Transplantation (Majhail NS)

Abbreviations: *HDL* high density lipoproteins, *LDL* low density lipoprotein

**Table 13.5** Recommendation on patient immunization after SCT

| Immunization agent type | Schedule |
|---|---|
| Influenza A and B | 1 dose annually, throughout life, before the start of the influenza season. Data suggest that response rates are better 4–6 months after SCT. |
| Diphtheria/Tetanus/Pertussis/ Inactivated Polio/Haemophilus Influenzae type b/Hepatitis B | Starting 6 months after transplantation, 3 doses at 1-month interval. |
| Meningococcal Group B (Men B) | Starting 6 months after transplantation, 2 doses, 2-month interval. |
| Meningococcal Groups A, C, W and Y (ACWY Men) | From 6 months after transplantation, a single dose. |
| Pneumococcal (*Streptococcus pneumoniae*) | Starting 6 months after the transplant. |
| Measles / mumps / rubella | Starting 24 months after transplantation, 2 doses with 1-month interval. |

Adapted from Immunization Schedule for Autologous and Allogeneic Blood and Marrow Transplant Recipients (Oxford University Hospitals)

- The use of vaccines with inactivated viruses is generally safer than vaccines with attenuated viruses. If attenuated virus vaccine is required, look for safety and efficacy data in the literature.
- Healthcare professionals and caregiver/family members around the patient should also be vaccinated.
- Follow the most recent recommendations regarding vaccination in this population.
- Consider antibody testing to evaluate vaccine response.

The pharmacist should follow up the patient regarding the vaccination schedule adopted by the transplant center, guiding the patient regarding doubts in the reimmunization process, assist the multidisciplinary team in the calendar follow-up, and, in case of children, can assist the medical team, when necessary, in seeking information on vaccines available in the local market.

### 13.5.4 Withdrawal of Prophylactic Infectious Therapies and Immunosuppressants

After conditioning, patients undergo a phase known as the pre-graft phase. An aplastic phase characterized by deep neutropenia [54]. One of the consequences of this aplastic period is the chance of infections by bacteria, fungi, and viruses, making the use of antibiotic prophylaxis necessary [55]. The engraftment time may vary depending on the source of donor cells [54]. Even after the patient medullary recovery, he still remains immunosuppressed by the use of immunosuppressants and the fact that the humoral immune response is only recovered at the end of 2 years of allogeneic transplantation [55, 56]. In the first 100 days after SCT, the patient is still susceptible to gram-positive and negative bacterial infections, fungi and viral reactivations including cytomegalovirus (CMV), and Epstein-Barr virus (EBV) [54].

After 100 days of SCT, there may be an important decline in the possibility of the patient acquiring an infection, because he may have already recovered the amount and functioning of neutrophils, and lymphocytes already have some functionality. At this time antibiotic prophylaxis withdrawal may begin and the patient is redirected to seek medical care in the presence of febrile peak, chills, diarrhea, and any other symptoms that may be indicative of an infection [55].

The same occurs with immunosuppressants, after immunological reconstitution with allogeneic transplants, but in general, patients may take longer to achieve this reconstitution due to GvHD, either by the pathophysiology itself, having a small effect on the lymphoid reconstitution time, and even by the use of immunosuppressants for GvHD prophylaxis that may contribute to a deficiency of the immune system [56].

The pharmacist should monitor the use of specific anti-infectious and C-reactive protein (CRP) tests. For immunosuppressants, strict follow-up of serum levels and dose adjustment is required when necessary. Therefore, long-term follow-up should be optimized and individualized to the specific needs of the patient and can last for years [47].

## References

1. Figueiredo MS, Kerbauy J, Lourenco DM. Guia de Hematologia – Unifesp. Editor Manole: São Paulo; 2021.
2. American Society for Blood and Marrow Transplantation. Beyond fundamentals of hematopoietic cell transplantation training course. Florida: ASBMT; 2017.
3. American Society of Health System Pharmacists, Inc., and American College of Clinical Pharmacy – BCOP, Hematopoietic Stem Cell Transplantation/Blood and Marrow Transplantation. 2013.
4. Bompoint C, Castagna A, Hutt DA, et al. The European Blood and Marrow Transplantation Textbook for Nurses: Under the Auspices of EBMT. Chapter 4: Transplant Preparation. Cham, Switzerland: Springer; 2017.
5. Taberna M, Moncayo FG, et al. The Multidisciplinary Team (MDT) approach and quality of care. Front Oncol. 10: 85. Published online March 2020.
6. Clemmons AB, Alexander M, DeGregory K, Kennedy LA. The hematopoietic cell transplant pharmacist: roles, responsibilities, and recommendations from the ASBMT Pharmacy Special Interest Group. Biol Blood Marrow Transplant. 2018;24:914–22.
7. Derman BA, Kordas K, Ridgeway J, Chow S, Dale W, Lee SM, Aguada E, Jakubowiak AJ, Jasielec J, Kline J, Kosuri S, Larson RA, Liu H, Mortel M, Odenike O, Pisano J, Riedell P, Stock W, Bishop MR, Artz AS. Results from a multidisciplinary clinic guided by geriatric assessment before stem cell transplantation in older adults. Blood Adv. 2019;3(22):3488–98.
8. Langebrake C, Admirral R, et al. Consensus recommendations for the role and competencies of the EBMT clinical pharmacist and clinical pharmacologist involved in hematopoietic stem cell transplantation. Bone Marrow Transplant. 2020;55:62–9.
9. Shah GL, Majhail N, Khera N, Giralt S. Value-based care in hematopoietic cell transplantation and cellular therapy: challenges and opportunities. Curr Hematol Malig. 2018;13(2):125–34.
10. Velo GP, Minuz P. Medication erros: prescribing faults and prescription errors. Br J Clin Pharmacol. 2009;67(6):624–8.
11. Panel de consenso ad hoc. Consenso de Granada sobre Problemas relacionados com Medicamentos. Pharm Care Esp. 1999;1:107–12.
12. Langebrake C, et al. On behalf of the EBMT Working Group. Consensus recommendations for the role and competencies of the EBMT clinical pharmacist and clinical pharmacologist involved in hematopoietic stem cell transplantation. Bone Marrow Transplant. 2020;55:62–9.
13. Gyurkocza B, Sandmaier B. M. Conditioning regimens for hematopoietic cell transplantation: one size does not fit all. Blood 2014;124(3):344–353.

https://doi.org/10.1182/blood-2014-02-514778. Available from: https://pubmed.ncbi.nlm.nih.gov/24914142/. Accessed 21 March 2021.
14. Jethava YS, et al. Conditioning regimens for allogeneic hematopoietic stem cell transplants in acute myeloid leukemia. Bone Marrow Transplant 2017 ;52(11):1504–1511. https://doi.org/10.1038/bmt.2017.83. Available from: https://www.nature.com/articles/bmt201783. Accessed 21 March 2021.
15. Caballero MD, et al. BEAM chemotherapy followed by autologous stem cell support in lymphoma patients: analysis of efficacy, toxicity and prognostic factors. Bone Marrow Transplant. 1997 ;20(6):451–458. https://doi.org/10.1038/sj.bmt.1700913. Available from: https://pubmed.ncbi.nlm.nih.gov/9313877/. Accessed 21 March 2021.
16. Gratwohl A, Carreras E. Principles of conditioning. In: Apperley J, Carreras E, Gluckman E, Masszi T, editors. ESH-EBMT handbook on haematopoietic stem cell transplantation 2012, vol. 2012. 6th ed. Paris: European School of Haematology.
17. Negrin RS. Preparative regimens for hematopoietic cell transplantation. In: Up-To-Date Available from: https://www.uptodate.com/contents/preparative-regimens-for-hematopoietic-cell-transplantation?search=preparative%20regimens%20for%20stemm&source=search_result&selectedTitle=2~150&usage_type=default&display_rank=2. Accessed 21 March 2021.
18. Bacigalupo A, et al. Defining the intensity of conditioning regimens: working definitions. Biol Blood Marrow Transplant. 2009 15(12):1628–1633. https://doi.org/10.1016/j.bbmt.2009.07.004. Available from: https://pubmed.ncbi.nlm.nih.gov/19896087/. Accessed 21 March 2021.
19. Lindley C, et al. Intraindividual variability in busulfan pharmacokinetics in patients undergoing a bone marrow transplant: assessment of a test dose and first dose strategy. Anticancer Drugs. 2004;15(5):453–9. https://doi.org/10.1097/01.cad.0000127145.50172.51. Available from: https://pubmed.ncbi.nlm.nih.gov/15166618/. Accessed 2 May 2021.
20. Chan KW, et al. Lorazepam for seizure prophylaxis during high dose busulfan administration. Bone Marrow Transplant. 2002; 29(12):963–965. https://doi.org/10.1038/sj.bmt.1703593. Available from: https://www.nature.com/articles/1703593. Accessed 2 May 2021.
21. Eberly AL, Anderson GD, Bubalo JS, McCune JS. Optimal prevention of seizures induced by high dose busulfan. Pharmacotherapy 2008;28(12):1502–1510. https://doi.org/10.1592/phco.28.12.1502. Available from: https://pubmed.ncbi.nlm.nih.gov/19025431/. Accessed 2 May 2021.
22. Akiyama K, et al. Comparison of levetiracetam with phenytoin for the prevention of intravenous busulfan-induced seizures in hematopoietic cell transplantation recipients. Cancer Chemother Pharmacol. 2018; 82(4):717–721. https://doi.org/10.1007/s00280-018-3659-8. Available

from: https://www.ncbi.nlm.nih.gov/pmc/articles/PMC6132870/. Accessed 2 May 2021.

23. Myers AL, et al. Clarifying busulfan metabolism and drug interactions to support new therapeutic drug monitoring strategies: a comprehensive review. Expert Opin Drug Metab Toxicol 2017; 13(9):901–923. https://doi.org/10.1080/17425255.2017.1360277. Available from: https://pubmed.ncbi.nlm.nih.gov/28766962/. Accessed 19 May 2021.
24. Glotzbecker B, Duncan C, Alyea E 3rd, Campbell B, Soiffer R. Important drug interactions in hematopoietic stem cell transplantation: what every physician should know. Biol Blood Marrow Transplant. 2012; 18(7):989–1006. https://doi.org/10.1016/j.bbmt.2011.11.029. Available from: https://pubmed.ncbi.nlm.nih.gov/22155504/. Accessed 19 May 2021.
25. Linder BJ, Chao NJ, Gounder MM. Chemotherapy and radiation-related hemorrhagic cystitis in cancer patients. In: UpToDate. Available from: https://www.uptodate.com/contents/chemotherapy-and-radiation-related-hemorrhagic-cystitis-in-cancer-patients?search=Chemotherapy%20and%20radiation-related%20hemorrhagic%20cystitis%20in%20cancer%20patients&source=search_result&selectedTitle=1~150&usage_type=default&display_rank=1. Accessed 2 May 2021.
26. Blijlevens N, et al. European Blood and Marrow Transplantation Mucositis Advisory Group. Prospective oral mucositis audit: oral mucositis in patients receiving high-dose melphalan or BEAM conditioning chemotherapy–European Blood and Marrow Transplantation Mucositis Advisory Group. J Clin Oncol. 2008; 26(9):1519–1525. https://doi.org/10.1200/JCO.2007.13.6028. Available from: https://pubmed.ncbi.nlm.nih.gov/18268357/. Accessed 19 May 2021.
27. Johansson JE, et al. Cryotherapy as prophylaxis against oral mucositis after high-dose melphalan and autologous stem cell transplantation for myeloma: a randomised, open-label, phase 3, non-inferiority trial. Bone Marrow Transplant 2019; 54(9):1482–1488. https://doi.org/10.1038/s41409-019-0468-6. Available from: https://pubmed.ncbi.nlm.nih.gov/30718802/. Accessed 19 May 2021.
28. Rodrigues GH, Jaguar GC, Alves FA, Guollo A, Camandoni VO, Damascena AS, Lima VCC. Variability of high dose melphalan exposure on oral mucositis in patients undergoing prophylactic low-level laser therapy. Lasers Med Sci 2017 ;32(5):1089–1095. https://doi.org/10.1007/s10103-017-2211-0. Available from: https://pubmed.ncbi.nlm.nih.gov/28512727/. Accessed 19 May 2021.
29. Patel AK, Sheehan W, Jenkins A, Lane C, Kell J. Prophylactic treatment for cytosine arabinoside-induced keratoconjunctivitis. Int Ophthalmol. 2011; 31(3):191–5. https://doi.org/10.1007/s10792-011-9435-y. Available from: https://pubmed.ncbi.nlm.nih.gov/21424238/. Accessed 4 June 2021.
30. Kume T, et al. The effect of corticosteroid eye drops on the prevention of eye disorders caused by high-dose cytarabine therapy. Clin Oncol. 2017;

2:1246. Available from: https://www.clinicsinoncology.com/full-text/cio-v2-id1246.php; Accessed 4 June 2021.
31. Mori T, et al. Prevention of cytarabine-induced kerato-conjunctivitis by eye rinse in patients receiving high-dose cytarabine and total body irradiation as a conditioning for hematopoietic stem cell transplantation. Int J Hematol. 2011 Sep; 94(3):261–5. https://doi.org/10.1007/s12185-011-0912-x. Available from: https://pubmed.ncbi.nlm.nih.gov/21853271/. Accessed 4 June 2021.
32. UP-To-Date https://uptodate.com/contents/early-complications-of-hematopoietic-cell-transplantation. Accessed 21 Apr 2021.
33. Gyurkocza B, Sandmaier B. Conditioning regimens for hematopoietic cell transplantation: one size does not fit all. Blood. 2014;124(3):344–53.
34. Tuncer HH, Rana N, Milani C, Darko A, Al-Homsi SA. Gastrointestinal and hepatic complications of hematopoietic stem cell transplantation. World J Gastroenterol. 2012;18(16):1851–60. https://doi.org/10.3748/wjg.v18.i16.1851.
35. Mikulska M, Cordonnier C. Fluoroquinolone prophylaxis during neutropenia: what can we expect nowadays? Clin Microbiol Infect. 2018;24(7):678–9. https://doi.org/10.1016/j.cmi.2018.02.031.
36. Maria A, Reis L, Jeane EL. Immunology reconstitution after allogeneic bone marrow transplantation. Visentainer Rev Bras Hematol Hemoter. 2004;26(3):212–7. ISSN: 1806-0870.
37. Silva LCF da, Martins CL, Tofani AA. Perfil de Utilização de Imunossupressores para Profilaxia de Doença Enxerto Versus Hospedeiro em Pacientes Submetidos ao Transplante de Células-Tronco Hematopoiéticas. Rev. Bras. Cancerol. [Internet]. 3° de setembro de 2019 [citado 25° de maio de 2021];65(2):e-06148. Available from: https://rbc.inca.gov.br/revista/index.php/revista/article/view/148.
38. The EBMT Handbook. https://doi.org/10.1007/978-3-030-02278-5_35.
39. Zimmer AJ, Freifeld AG. Optimal management of neutropenic fever in patients with cancer. J Oncol Pract. 2019;15(1):19–24. https://doi.org/10.1200/JOP.18.00269.
40. Tomblyn M, et al. Guidelines for preventing infectious complications among hematopoietic cell transplantation recipients: a global perspective. Biol Blood Marrow Transplant. 2009;15(10):1143–238. https://doi.org/10.1016/j.bbmt.2009.06.019.
41. Up-To-Data. Available from: https://www.uptodate.com/contents/hepatic-sinusoidal-obstruction-syndrome-veno-occlusive-disease-in-adults?search=sos%20hep%C3%A1tico&source=search_result&selectedTitle=1~144&usage_type=default&display_rank=1. Accessed 19 May 2021.

42. UP-To-Date. Available from: https://www.uptodate.com/contents/clinical-manifestations-diagnosis-and-grading-of-acute-graft-versus-host-disease?search=gvhd%20agudo&source=search_result&selectedTitle=1~150&usage_type=default&display_rank=1. Accessed 18 2021.
43. UP-To-Date. Available from: https://www.uptodate.com/contents/epidemiology-clinical-manifestations-and-diagnosis-of-post-transplant-lymphoproliferative-disorders?search=sindrome%20linfoproliferativa%20pos%20tmo&source=search_result&selectedTitle=2~150&usage_type=default&display_rank=2. Accessed 19 May 2021.
44. Kipralani S, Jackson AT, Schnipper JL, Coleman EA. Promoting effective transitions of care at hospital discharge: a review of key issues for hospitalists. J Hosp Med. 2007;2(5):314–23.
45. Gato MIR, Dos Reis NA, Tofani A, et al. Transplante de células-tronco hematopoéticas: introdução para farmacêuticos. São Paulo: SegmentoFarma; 2018. p. 67–9.
46. Anderson SL, Marrs JC, Vande JPG, Hanratty R. Implementation of a clinical pharmacy specialist-managed telephonic hospital discharge follow-up program in a patient-centered medical home. Popul Health Manag. 2013;16(4):235–41.
47. Majhail NS. Long term complications after hematopoietic cell transplantation. Hematol Oncol Stem Cell Ther. 2017;10(4):220–7.
48. Yu ASL, Goldfarb S, Lam AQ. Hypomagnesemia: causes of hypomagnesemia. Up To Date, 2021. Available from: https://www.uptodate.com/contents/hypomagnesemia-causes-of-hypomagnesemia?csi=44745fac-8bcc-4f01-b9d2-183c4e6658e3&source=contentShare. Accessed 06 June 2021.
49. Alves C, Robazzi TCV, Mendonça M. Withdrawal from glucocorticosteroid therapy: clinical practice recommendations. J de Pediatria. 2008;84(3). Disponível em: https://www.scielo.br/j/jped/a/vVftgBpWqnGZVztFk6cC8DD/?format=pdf&lang=pt.
50. Inamoto Y, Lee SJ. Late effects of blood and marrow transplantation. Haematologica. 2017;102(4):614–25.
51. Machado CM. Reimmunization after bone marrow transplantation – current recommendations and perspectives. Braz J Med Biol Res. 2004;37:151–8.
52. Wareham D, Jeffery K. Immunisation schedule auto/allo BMT recipients. Department of Clinical Haematology Oxford BMT Programme, 2021. Available from: http://www.nssg.oxford-haematology.org.uk/bmt/long-term/B-2-13-allograft-and-autograft-immunisation-schedule.pdf. Accessed 06 June 2021.
53. Shetty AK, Winter MA. Immunization of children receiving immunosuppressive therapy for cancer or hematopoietic stem cell transplantation. Ochsner J. 2012;12:228–43.

54. Ogonek J, Juric MK, Ghimire S, et al. Immune reconstitution after allogeneic hematopoietic stem cell transplantation. Front Immunol. 2016;17:1–15.
55. Hospital Inglês especializado em transplante de medulla óssea - Transplante de Medula Óssea Complicações pós-transplante de medula óssea. Available from: http://www.hospitalingles.com.br/transplante-medula-ossea/complicacoes-pos-transplante-de-medula-ossea. Accessed 06 June 2021.
56. Reis MAL, Visentainer JEL. Reconstituição imunológica após o transplante de medula óssea alogênico. Rev Bras Hematol Hemoter. 2004;26(3):212–7.

# Oncology and Hematology in the ICU

# 14

Renan Gomes do Nascimento,
Nataly Any Barros Garrido de Paula,
MérciaPatrícia Ferreira Conceição,
Daniel Rodrigues de Bastos,
and Danilo de Oliveira Cerqueira

R. G. do Nascimento (✉)
Department of Clinical Pharmacy and Oncology, HSC – Hospital São Camilo, São Paulo, Brazil

Department of Education in Pharmacy Oncology, SENAC – Serviço Nacional de AprendizagemComercial, São Paulo, Brazil

Department of Education in Pharmacy Oncology, IPESSP – Instituto de Pesquisa e Ensino em Saúde de São Paulo, São Paulo, Brazil

N. A. B. G. de Paula
Department of Clinical Pharmacy and Oncology, ICESP – Instituto do Câncer do Estado de São Paulo, São Paulo, Brazil

M. F. Conceição · D. R. de Bastos
Translational Research Center in Oncology, ICESP – Instituto do Câncer do Estado de São Paulo, São Paulo, Brazil

FMUSP – Faculdade de Medicina da Universidade de São Paulo, São Paulo, Brazil

D. de Oliveira Cerqueira
Department of Clinical Pharmacy and Oncology, HSC – Hospital São Camilo, São Paulo, Brazil

Department of Education in Pharmacy Oncology, IPESSP – Instituto de Pesquisa e Ensino em Saúde de São Paulo, São Paulo, Brazil



C. W. P. Schmidt, K. M. Otoni (eds.), *The Golden Guide to Oncologic Pharmacy*, https://doi.org/10.1007/978-3-030-98596-7_14

## 14.1 Introduction

Since the beginning of the 1950s, the field of intensive care medicine has made significant advances [1]. Among patients with oncological and hematological diseases, approximately 10% may develop some life-threatening condition, which requires admission to an intensive care unit (ICU) [2, 3]. In addition, it is estimated that patients with malignant neoplasms represent about 20% of all admissions to ICUs [4, 5].

Different studies have reported that critically ill patients with cancer can benefit from intensive treatments [6–8]. Until the turn of the twentieth century, the survival rates of critically ill oncology and hematologic patients did not exceed the 30% mark [9]. Currently, it is known that the survival rates of these patients who present recurrent complications of cancer in ICUs have been greater than 50% [10].

The survival rates of critically ill onco-hematologic patients have improved dramatically due to different factors [11–16]. Among them, we can include:

- Advances in the treatment of solid tumors and hematological malignancies.
- Changes in screening patterns and early admissions to ICUs.
- More accurate investigation of organic failures.
- New therapeutic strategies to avoid toxicity.
- Greater understanding of the pathophysiological, genetic, and molecular aspects of onco-hematological malignancies.
- Greater collaboration and interaction between oncologists, hematologists, intensive care, clinical pharmacists, and other members of the multidisciplinary team.

Unquestionably, the use of resources in ICUs needs to be carefully discussed and a limiting factor remains the availability of sufficient beds for the admission of critically ill oncology and hematological patients [17, 18]. In addition, late or unplanned admission to ICUs, lack of reliable, and specific and clinical evidence-based recommendations have resulted in increased mortality of onco-hematologic patients [19].

Acute respiratory failure (ARF) is the leading cause of admission among onco-hematologic patients [20]. In particular, neutropenic patients and patients undergoing allogeneic hematopoietic stem cell transplantation (HSCT) are at increased risk of developing ARF [21, 22]. Therefore, an accurate diagnosis is essential, taking into account types of respiratory symptoms, radiological findings, and associated organic dysfunctions [21].

Approximately 1/3 of critically ill oncology and hematologic patients have acute kidney injury (AKI), and many of these patients require renal replacement therapy [23]. Sepsis, hypoperfusion, and nephrotoxic agents are the main factors for AKI [24].

Data from several cohort studies indicate that the provision of cytotoxic drugs associated with life support therapy of clinically critical onco-hematologic patients is feasible and associated with an increased survival of these patients [25]. Patient preferences, performance status, appropriate choice of anticancer agents, personalized dosing, and close monitoring need to be rigorously analyzed [26, 27].

Serious infections and sepsis are among the main serious complications observed in critically ill onco-hematologic patients under chemotherapy regimens, mainly caused by neutropenia and immunosuppression [28]. Therefore, antibiotic and antifungal therapy are at the heart of care for patients with cancer [29].

Multidisciplinary and multiprofessional collaboration is essential for personalized care, greater care, and better survival rates for patients with onco-hematologic neoplasms who present clinical complications in ICUs [30]. Meetings between oncologists, hematologists, and intensivists for care planning and goal setting have impacted mortality reduction and resource optimization [31]. The clinical pharmacist in particular is a key player in the multidisciplinary team of intensive care for critically ill onco-hematologic patients [32, 33]. Different studies have highlighted that the presence of clinical pharmacists in ICUs is essential to identify inappropriate drug administration, under-dosing, lack of laboratory monitoring, drug interactions, drug-related side effects, and overdosing [34]. Additionally, pharmaceutical interventions can lead to suspension of inadequate treatment, dose adjustment, additions of supportive therapies, changes in administration routes, and optimization of treatment [35–37].

## 14.2 Insertion of the Pharmacist in Hospitals and Their Activities in This Service Location

According to the pharmaceutical practice guidelines made available by the World Health Organization (WHO), all pharmacists have an obligation to ensure that the service they provide to each patient is performed in an appropriate and quality manner. To ensure this vital commitment of the profession, the pharmacist must provide medicines and other health care for people, helping them to make the best use of the medicines intended for them, thus promoting good quality and preventing new health problems [38]. Among the requirements of good pharmacy practices, cited in the Good Pharmacy Practice: Guidelines in Community and Hospital Settings (WHO), we can mention: concern for the patient's well-being in all environments, promotion of rational and economical prescription, appropriate use medicines, supplying medicines and other health products, and monitoring the effects of their use. It is extremely important that the pharmacist be constantly updated with regard to therapeutic innovations and new drugs made available on the market [38].

Among the main interventions performed by pharmacists in the hospital environment, we can mention: inclusion of missing information, dose change, prescription cancellation, change in infusion time, change in diluent volume, change in administration route, start of new drug, change in administration frequency, drug replacement, diluent replacement, among other interventions [39]. Considering pharmaceutical interventions, there are, among the main problems related to drugs, incomplete prescription, underdose, pharmacokinetic problem that requires dose adjustment, overdose, incorrect infusion time, duplicate prescription, dose regimen with frequency higher than recommended, incorrect diluent volume, inappropriate administration route, dose regimen often lower than recommended, among others [39].

The information mentioned above will be discussed below, with the details that the study requires, and, with particular emphasis, on the reality experienced by the pharmacist who works in an Intensive Care Unit (ICU) for patients with oncological and hematological profiles.

## 14.3 Pharmacists in Intensive Care

The hospitalized patient, who for some reason presents complications, needs personalized and vigorous care. The aforementioned care sector, called the intensive care unit (ICU), is a hospital service aimed at users in serious clinical situations, or at clinical or surgical risk, who demand intensive care, uninterrupted medical, nursing, and physiotherapy assistance, monitoring continuous 24 hours a day, in addition to equipment and a specialized multidisciplinary team [40]. Several organizations recognize the dedicated patient care pharmacist as an essential component of the multidisciplinary team to provide quality care [41, 42].

Through critical care pharmacy services in U.S. hospitals, which aimed to characterize the level of pharmaceutical services provided to intensive care units, it was possible to identify that the pharmacists interviewed in these services were involved in activities that involved constant need, sometimes, changes in drug therapy, monitoring, prevention of adverse events, provision of information about drugs, cost savings, and educational activities [43]. In that publication, it was found that these pharmacists are predominantly involved in the provision of care to patients and administrative functions, leaving, in moderate status, their involvement with educational and academic activities [43].

## 14.4 Critical Oncohematologic Patient

In cancer and hematology hospitals, considering the high complexity of comorbidities of patients and ensuring an effective and safe treatment, an interdisciplinary approach that provides comprehensive care is needed, with the pharmacist's action being a fundamental part of this care [39]. Added to the profile of the complexity of the treatments required for these patients, in many of them, due to various complications and peculiar clinical and pathophysiological characteristics, admission to the ICU is necessary [44, 45].

According to the natural history of cancer, after the detection of the disease based on symptoms or signs that occur at the beginning of the clinical phase or, disease at an advanced stage, the patient, after evaluation, will be directed to treatment and follow-up that may lead him to cure, control, or death [3, 46]. Due to advances in the field of cancer therapy, which contribute to the improvement of pharmacological practice and safety in clinical management, the observation of adverse effects associated with these new therapies is frequent, thus making intensive care support necessary, which helps to restore the patient's organic function [45].

According to the studies by the authors Bos MMEM, et al., the types of malignancy with the highest frequency of admission to the ICU were malignant neoplasms of the breast, lung, colon, prostate, and esophagus, the latter being the one that most commonly leads to the admission of oncohematological patients in ICUs [47]. The study "Characteristics and outcomes of cancer patients in European ICUs" evaluated the characteristics of patients with critical cancer and their prognosis, and it was possible to verify that the mortality rates in the ICU and hospital were similar in patients with solid tumors and without cancer [48]. In addition, this study and that of the authors of the study "Outcomes of haematology/oncology patients admitted to intensive care unit at the Canberra Hospital" found greater survival of patients with hematologic neoplasia when compared to solid tumors [48, 49].

## 14.5 ICU Admission Criteria

The screening procedures for admission of oncological and hematological patients to intensive care units take into account some criteria, among them, the characteristics of the patient, scientific evidence, personal experience of the medical team, hospital guidelines, and verification of preferences deserve to be highlighted of patients [50].

It is of paramount importance to identify patients with potential benefit for intensive care. For this benefit to be achieved and, consequently, improvements in results to be achieved, the existence of effective communication between intensivists and oncol-

**Table 14.1** Situations and outcomes of ICU admission criteria – oncological and hematological patients

| Situation | Ending |
|---|---|
| Low status/bedridden performance or palliative care | Admission to the ICU is not recommended, your comfort and palliative care will be prioritized. |
| Denial of admission to the ICU | |
| First line of treatment | The patient will be able to be admitted to the ICU and be re-evaluated from time to time. |
| Newly diagnosed disease | |
| Potentially reversible acute complication | |

Source: Adapted from Silva (2017)

ogists is essential [50, 51]. To avoid conflicts between teams and family, when admission to the ICU of a cancer patient is requested, it will be necessary to evaluate 2 situations (Table 14.1):

In addition to the information mentioned above, the severity of organic dysfunctions, impairment of functional capacity, cancer staging, and the application of prognostic indices should also be evaluated [51]. Therefore, admission to the ICU should not be denied solely based on the fact that the patient has a neoplastic disease. The prognostic assessment tools and the assessment of the patient's functional capacity serve as support for decision-making [45].

## 14.6 Reasons for Hospitalization of Cancer and Hematological Patients

Regarding the specificity of oncological and hematological patients in intensive care, it is necessary to list the main reasons for hospitalization, which are: sepsis, septic shock, acute renal failure, acute chronic renal failure, liver failure, upper digestive hemorrhage, lower digestive hemorrhage, tumor lysis syndrome, lowered level of consciousness (which may or may not be associated with medications), difficult-to-control convulsive crises (often due to metastases in the central nervous system), hepatic encephalopathy, respiratory failure, electrolyte changes, thromboembolism, cardiovascular changes (superior vena cava syndrome, drug toxicity), and surgical procedures [31].

## 14.7 Importance of Pharmaceutical Follow-Up in the ICU

Given the increased incidence of cancer in recent decades, the quality and life expectancy of cancer patients may be impaired due to errors during treatment [52]. Pharmaceutical care is essential in the care of critical patients, as it is responsible for circumventing adverse reactions and reducing the aggressiveness of the treatment to the patient, thus avoiding possible indifference in the proposed oncological therapy and thus increasing the well-being of the patient individual [53].

It is essential to realize that clinical pharmacists working in the oncology ICU must have an understanding of conditions associated with cancer, such as: febrile neutropenia, tumor lysis syndrome, malignant hypercalcemia, posterior reversible encephalopathy syndrome, diffuse alveolar hemorrhage, veno-occlusive disease, anemia and chronic diseases such as spinal cord compression, and pathological fractures, among other complications [33]. One of the most important complications of this patient profile is the toxicities associated with poorly planned chemotherapy regimens [31].

When comparing a service specialized in intensive care and a non-specialized one, it is notorious that there is an increase in the number of pharmaceutical interventions [54]. However, to achieve these interventions that optimize therapy and simultaneously identify drug-related problems, a standardized and structured approach is needed [55]. One of the mnemonics used in the daily evaluation of pharmacotherapy is the FASTHUG-MAIDENS (Table 14.2).

These points function as a daily checklist for patient assessment. The daily use of this tool, in conjunction with pharmaceutical interventions, can increase ventilator-free time, decrease the time of empirical antibiotic therapy, decrease the duration of cen-

**Table 14.2** FASTHUG – MAIDENS Mnemonic

| Letter | Definition |
|---|---|
| F | Feeding |
| A | Analgesia |
| S | Sedation |
| T | Thromboprophylaxis |
| H | Hyperactive or hypoactive delirium |
| U | Stress ulcer phophylaxis |
| G | Glucose control |
| M | Medication reconciliation |
| A | Antibiotics or anti-infectives |
| I | Indications for medications drug dosing |
| D | Drug dosing |
| E | Electrolytes, hematology, and other laboratory results stop dates |
| N | No drug interactions, allergies, duplications, side effects |
| S | Stop dates |

Source: Adapted from Mabasa (2011)

tral venous catheter use, and increase rates of adherence to therapies to prevent venous thrombosis prophylaxis and stress ulcer prophylaxis [56].

All these parameters involved in this pharmaceutical assessment tool, FASTHUG-MAIDENS, aim to prevent events, stop or delay the disease process, prevent a disease or symptom, eliminate or reduce the symptomatology, and cure the disease. These goals demonstrate that healthcare institutions should use clinical pharmacists as a vital component in a process improvement strategy and in promoting optimal pharmacotherapy. The activities of this mnemonic are described in more detail below:

### 14.7.1 Feeding

Nutrition in ICU patients presents a variety of alternatives and situations, namely: oral ingestion, tube feeding, parenteral nutrition, and also diet as tolerated [55].

The pharmacist in these situations will be able to act both in changing the routes of medications and in optimizing drug therapy. In addition, you should check the best pharmaceutical form to be administered to the patient without harming the treatment. The verification of the concomitant use of a drug and a nutritional formulation is also important and necessary, as there may be changes in drug absorption [55]. Thinking about food, laboratory tests are considerable in this evaluation, because for patients receiving parenteral nutrition, for example, it is essential to check these tests and thus analyze the need or not to change the composition of the diet [56].

### 14.7.2 Analgesia

Cancer-related pain is one of the most common and uncomfortable symptoms that affect this patient profile. Articles show that it is reported by over 70% of patients [57]. It is considered one of the most commonly reported stressors in patients in ICUs, which can exert considerable negative effects on their recovery [58].

Appropriate management will only be possible with an appropriate diagnosis, based on a detailed clinical history, comprehensive physical examination, and correct interpretation of tests; and these activities are carried out by the intensive care team. In addition, the patient's psychosocial situation should also be taken into account [59]. Its inadequate management can lead to devastating consequences that directly affect the patient's quality of life, reduce functionality, and also affect the emotional level of both these and their families [60].

The ideal level is present when the patient receives an amount consistent with their clinical condition and their real need, in an adequate and not excessive way, from an adequate method. In the case of an unwanted amount, the hypothesis can be mentioned that the patient is inadequately sedated and presents respiratory depression and, consequently, an unsuccessful weaning from the ventilator [61]. Therefore, the pharmacist is responsible for evaluating and suggesting to the medical team the best therapy and the most assertive method to administer the medication for this patient profile [61].

### 14.7.3 Sedation

For cancer patients undergoing various procedures during their treatment, which are often painful due to various causes, such as the oncological and hematological disease itself causing pain, with the existence of marked functional decline, uncontrolled symptoms, it is necessary, in many cases, sedation. In this context, criteria for the desired depth of sedation, the patient's health status, fasting status, and medication property must be checked with extreme rigor [59].

The pharmacist in intensive care is responsible for ensuring that sedative drugs used by patients are appropriate. Among the most common sedatives used are: midazolam and lorazepam. However, it is imperative to highlight that other classes may be indicated depending on the critical situation in which the patient finds himself [32]. Depending on this clinical situation and the period of sedation (continuous infusion, intermittent dosage) that the patient needs, the pharmacist should be involved in the decision to start, stop, and adjust the doses of these medications. This assessment is performed daily and always discussed together with the intensivist team [59].

### 14.7.4 Thromboprophylaxis

Venous thromboembolism (VTE) is a term that covers two conditions: deep vein thrombosis and pulmonary thromboembolism. These conditions are usually asymptomatic or have non-specific symptoms, which contribute to negative outcomes [62, 63].

Hospitalized patients have at least one risk factor for the development of venous thromboembolism; therefore, thromboprophylaxis is the initial strategy to improve the safety of these patients [62, 63].

The eighth American College of Chest Physicians (ACCP) Consensus on VTE prevention highlights that the vast majority of hospitalized patients have at least one risk factor for developing VTE, and about 40% have three or more, and it is assured that thromboprophylaxis is the initial strategy to improve the safety of hospitalized patients [62].

### 14.7.5 Hyperactive or Hypoactive Delirium

Critically ill patients present in many situations pain, stress, anxiety, and an interrupted sleep-wake cycle. These conditions may increase the risk of UTI-related delirium. Delirium, the most common brain dysfunction in critically ill patients, affects not only short-term recovery, but can also lead to long-term cognitive impairment, post-traumatic stress disorder, and reduced quality of life [58].

To identify the presence of delirium, there are tools and methods that can help in the detection and, subsequently, in choosing the best treatment, which is both pharmacological and non-pharmacological [64]. In this context, the pharmacist, when using these strategies, in addition to seeking the cause and consequently the best approach to correct this clinical condition, must guide the medical team in choosing the best agent to be used. After the choice, it is necessary for the pharmacist to routinely assess whether the regimen and dose are optimal and should monitor the patient for efficacy and adverse reactions [55, 65].

### 14.7.6 Stress Ulcer Phophylaxis

Stress ulcers are defined as stress-induced gastritis or gastropathy in which the gastric and sometimes esophageal or duodenal mucosal barrier is disrupted secondary to severe acute illness [66, 67]. They are associated with extreme physiological stress such as sepsis, multiple dysfunction, multiple trauma, or severe burns. The most common sites for these ulcerations are the gastric body and fundus, as well as the antrum and duodenum [68].

In Intensive Care Units, patients who receive mechanical ventilation are at risk for this complication. An incidence of approximately 1.5% of clinically important gastrointestinal bleeding related to stress ulcers has been demonstrated [68]. In cancer patients in particular, this pathophysiology is not yet fully understood; it was hypothesized that splanchnic hypoperfusion, compromised microcirculation, and the pro-inflammatory state predispose patients to rupture of the gastric mucosal barrier and the occurrence of stress ulcers [68, 69].

Because of this risk, prophylactic medications must be administered; the pharmacist must ensure that the patient is receiving an appropriate and prophylactic agent, based on the patient's medical history. The drug should be discontinued when the pharmacist re-evaluates and realizes that the patient's condition is better and there is no more risk of stress ulcers [70]. Among the drugs used, include histamine receptor antagonists and proton pump inhibitors [55].

According to a study that evaluated 2000 physicians who were members of the Society of Critical Care Medicine, it was found that the implementation of a stress ulcer prophylaxis scheme, which may be related to possible bleeding of the mucosa, is necessary for patients in ICU, even though it is a relatively rare event. Therefore, the pharmacist should actively act in these situations together with the intensive care team and oncologists [70].

### 14.7.7 Glucose Control

Before starting a chemotherapy treatment, by the medical team, it will be necessary to be aware of the patient's blood glucose level, under penalty of affecting the successful completion of the treatment, generating, for example, an adverse event, development of an infection and/ or hospitalization during treatment and increased risk of reduction or discontinuation of chemotherapy [71].

In the case of a patient in intensive care, it is necessary to control the insulin in the blood, and consequently, the glycemic alterations: hyperglycemia and hypoglycemia. This monitoring should be followed according to the protocol of each institution [63].

In critically ill patients, hyperglycemia is common. This situation is characterized by significant morbidity and mortality in intensive care units and resulting from the existence of several facts: the release of stress hormones (epinephrine, glucagon, growth hormone and cortisol) and the use of medications such as corticosteroids (these drugs are often used in conjunction with chemotherapy) and catecholamines, in addition to the release of inflammatory cytokines, in cases of sepsis or surgical trauma [63]. These risk factors, which can trigger this change in blood sugar, are commonly found in cancer patients. In this regard, the pharmacist plays an important role, as he is able to advise, when necessary, the team on the properties of prescribed drugs and help in the best pharmaceutical approach for the situation in question [63, 71].

### 14.7.8 Medication Reconciliation

Due to the critical condition of oncologic and hematologic patients, upon admission to the ICU, continuous-use medications should be evaluated at the time of admission. Among these drugs are the chemotherapeutics themselves, which are often used orally at home or injectable chemotherapeutics (which coincide with the cycle at the time of hospitalization), in addition to antihypertensives, oral hypoglycemic agents, anxiolytics, antidepressants, and antipsychotics [36].

The evaluation consists of verifying the need or not for temporary suspension, dose adjustment, or continuity of treatment, even if it is due to a change in the pharmaceutical form, aiming at a better adequacy of the administration route to be used at the specific moment. In addition, post-ICU pharmaceutical care is also needed [72]. Among examples, the following situations stand out: during the transition period to hospitalization in the ICU, there may be unintentional continuation of medications and, in other cases, the unintentional continuation of medications prescribed in the ICU after the patient's clinical improvement [73]. Therefore, the medication reconciliation activity is among the interventions that reduce medication errors [74].

### 14.7.9 Antibiotics or Anti-infectives

Antimicrobials constitute a therapeutic class of paramount importance in critical oncology and hematological patients, given that their prescription positively impacts treatment: thus reducing failure rates and optimizing antimicrobial therapy. With these activities, it is also possible to verify improvement in clinical outcomes related to the treatment of infections, reduction of antimicrobial resistance, and promotion of rational use [55].

To achieve these improvements, it is necessary to verify, by the pharmacist, whether there is a need for adjustments in subtherapeutic and supratherapeutic doses, escalation or de-escalation, site of infection, antimicrobial sensitivity test, incorrect duration of treatment, adjustment of the infusion time, drug interactions and incompatibilities, dilution and reconstitution adjustments, and also the need or not to collect cultures [55, 63].

### 14.7.10 Indications for Medications

During the stay of an oncologic and hematologic patient in an intensive care unit, it is possible to verify that the amount of medication present in the prescription created by the doctor is vast. This situation happens with some frequency, since patients are complex and require medication to treat multiple changes. Due to this complexity in pharmacotherapeutic regimens, the pharmacist plays an essential role in this scenario [75].

Under these conditions, the pharmacist is responsible for daily reviewing all scheduled medications and checking the need or not of a certain medication for an appropriate indication [55, 75].

When a drug is detected that is no longer suitable for the patient's current situation, the pharmacist should discuss with the intensive care team about a possible withdrawal of the medication, providing guidance with justifications and also informing that this withdrawal, for example, can reduce the risk of events adverse effects, renal and liver overload, drug interactions, medication errors, and costs, among others [75]. In addition, the pharmacist must also be able to verify whether, in case of untreated dysfunction, it is possible to insert a medication for this purpose [55].

### 14.7.11 Drug Dosing

Due to the clinical state in which the patient is, even more in cancer patients where multiple organs can be affected, both due to chemotherapy treatment and the involvement of the disease itself, in many situations, the renal and hepatic functions can fluctuate [55]. On these occasions, the pharmacist must have knowledge and know how to verify information with a scientific basis in order to suggest dose adjustments to the medical team, if necessary, ensuring, in addition to the adequacy of doses, the prevention of drug accumulation in the body and, consequently, achieving outcomes desired [55, 63].

In addition, this analysis should be daily, with monitoring of both clinical examinations by the physician, and laboratory tests, so that the pharmacist, when necessary, adjusts the doses again according to the respective clinical evolution, thus avoiding under dosing, for example [55, 63].

It is also important to pay attention to the doses of oncological treatment drugs itself (during the stay in the critical sector), when continuation is suggested by oncologists and intensivists, as these may require periodic adjustments. Remember that this decision to continue chemotherapy, during the ICU stay, is analyzed on a case-by-case basis by the medical team and based on the risk/benefit binomial that the patient will present with this exposure [55].

### 14.7.12 Electrolytes, Hematology, and Other Laboratory Results

In critically ill patients, routine pharmaceutical evaluation requires laboratory tests. In the aforementioned analysis, it is necessary to check the complete blood count, electrolytes (potassium, magnesium, calcium, sodium, and phosphorus), biochemistry, and blood gases (gas exchange, oxygen saturation, oxygen partial pressure, carbon dioxide partial pressure, bicarbonate, and lactate). Furthermore, it is also necessary for the pharmacist to verify the information that the nursing team checks, such as temperature, heart and respiratory rate, blood pressure, blood glucose, diuresis, bowel movements, gastric residue, vomiting, fluid balance, and debts and drains [63]. From these controls, the pharmacist can intervene recommending the start or discontinuation of electrolytes, nutrients, minerals, blood, among others [55].

### 14.7.13 No Drug Interactions, Allergies, Duplications, Side Effects

The risk of drug interactions is a very routine situation in a hospital environment, especially when it comes to a critically ill patient who uses polypharmacy [55].

The pharmacist should identify possible interactions based on the prescription made by the physician and identify them as real and potential, in addition to verifying drug interactions between drug-food and drug-laboratory tests, and, when possible, it is plausible to recommend an alternative therapy [55].

Among the drug incompatibilities found, we can mention the physicochemical reactions that occur in vitro between two or more drugs, when the solutions are combined in the same syringe, equipment, or bottle [76]. Furthermore, physical reactions can cause visible changes such as precipitation, color change, consistency, opalescence, or gas production [33].

When admitting patients, it is essential to verify, both with them and with their families, the known and reported allergies. Based on these collected elements, the pharmacist must assess, for example, whether it is an actual allergy or a matter of intolerance. After this analysis, the pharmacist, when necessary, will talk to the medical team to make the relevant adjustments and monitor the patient with the use of medications [76].

In addition, as mentioned above, when checking the daily prescription of each patient admitted to the ICU, drugs that are duplicated or when more than one drug is used for the treatment of a given complication are also checked, and often this would not be necessary administration, which can lead to drug overload [33].

With the help of the multidisciplinary team, in conjunction with the intensive care team, it is important to pay attention to possible adverse reactions that the patient may have or has already had, and the pharmacist should make a careful assessment of these details [33].

### 14.7.14 Stop Dates

The prescription of medications needs to be guided by the establishment of a schedule, with a demarcation of the beginning and possible end. The pharmacist, in this context, will be responsible for monitoring the days of treatment and reassessing, together with the medical team, the best time for interruption [63].

Furthermore, it is important to highlight that the pharmacist is the specialized and reference professional on drug therapy, incumbent on him, therefore, with the duty to ensure that the drugs are not discontinued prematurely and, therefore, is prescribed observing the appropriate duration. In addition, it is their responsibility to advise on dose adjustments, timing guidelines, infusion rate, appropriateness of dilution, and reconstitution [55, 63].

## 14.8 Hematopoietic Stem Cell Transplantation

Stem cells are widely distributed throughout the human body. They consist of a population of cells that have not undergone differentiation, but which have the ability to become highly specialized, renewing the body's tissues. Stem cells can be found in greater abundance in bone marrow and umbilical cord. Its physical location is associated with different proliferative properties and functions [77]. Hematopoietic stem cells (HSC) comprise a particular group capable of self-renewal and differentiation into blood tissue and immune system cells [78].

Hematopoietic stem cell transplantation (HSCT), more popularly known as bone marrow transplantation, is a procedure where healthy hematopoietic stem cells are administered to patients who have bone marrow dysfunction. HSCT was proposed as a treatment strategy about 60 years ago and is the most widely used cellular immunotherapy to date. It has wide application, being performed for the treatment of hematological neoplasms and congenital and acquired diseases, including its application in some cases of solid tumors [79]. The number of diseases that affect the bone marrow is vast, leading to the pathological process. Thus, the types of malignancies for which HSCT has been indicated are increasing substantially, including neoplasms such as multiple myeloma, Hodgkin's and non-Hodgkin's lymphoma, acute myeloid leukemia, acute lymphocytic leukemia, myelodysplastic syndrome, myeloid leukemia. chronic/chronic lymphocytic leukemia, myelofibrosis, essential thrombocytosis, polycythemia Vera, and solid tumors; and non-malignant diseases such as: aplastic anemia, severe combined immunodeficiency syndrome (SCID), thalassemia, sickle cell anemia, among others.

It is important to understand that despite the indications, a compatible donor must be chosen. For this, the human leukocyte antigen (HLA) system is analyzed, the main histocompatibility complex (MHC). HLA is made up of proteins expressed on the surface of cells, and is considered a type of signature for each individual. Briefly, six types of HLA are evaluated: HLA-A, HLA-B, HLA-C, HLA-DP, HLA-DQ, and HLA-DR, which the first three are encoded by MHC class I and the others by MHC class II. Determining compatibility requires comparing the donor's HLA with that of the recipient in order to choose the one with the greatest genetic similarity to the recipient [80].

The HSCT is commonly divided into two groups: autologous and allogeneic, and less frequently, a third group appears, the syngeneic. In autologous transplantation, stem cells come from the patient and can be removed from the marrow or peripheral blood. The material receives a treatment and after purification methods the product is reinfused in the patient. The main advantage of this technique is the absence of graft-versus-host disease (GVHD). However, as disadvantages there may be relapses due to the limitations of purification techniques, allowing abnormal cells to remain and be administered to the patient. Another critical point is that its application doesn't cover all cases of bone marrow abnormalities, limiting the use of the technique [81].

Allogeneic transplant requires a donor. The donor may or may not be a family member as long as it is compatible with the recipient. To verify compatibility, HLA analysis is performed. Once compatibility is confirmed, the stem cells are collected, processed, and infused into the receptor [82, 83]. The syngeneic type HSCT is less widely discussed due to the low cases number of identical twins, which one of them requires a transplant. Interestingly, Gahrton et al. (1999) observed a significant association, which syngeneic transplants had better overall survival compared to allogeneic transplants [84]. Other works discussed syngeneic transplantation showing similar results. A summary of HSCT types can be found in Table 14.3.

**Table 14.3** Stem cell transplantation types

| Type | Origin | Donor | Advantage | Disadvantage |
|---|---|---|---|---|
| Autologous | Bone marrow, peripheral blood | The patient is his own donor | No GVHD | Relapses |
| Allogeneic | Bone marrow, peripheral blood, umbilical cord | *Family*: siblings or other compatible family member | | GVHD |
| | | *Non-family*: Any person in society who is compatible | | |
| Syngeniec | Bone marrow, peripheral blood | Identical twins | Low risk of relapse | Rare cases due to the low frequency of identical twins |

Source: Adapted from Gahrton (1999)
*GVHD* graft versus host disease

Complications such as respiratory failure, shock, organ failure, among others may arise after HSCT, and for this, intensive care is required, leading to the patient's admission to an intensive care unit (ICU). The type of HSCT, HLA incompatibility, graft disease, and conditioning intensity are risk factors associated with admission of these patients to the intensive care unit [85, 86].

The level of autologous or allogeneic post-HSCT complications is different. In the first case, mortality is estimated at less than 3% and the main cause of death is related to disease recurrence, which corresponds to 69% of the causes of death [87]. The admission rate of these patients to the ICU is 3.3%, which the mortality rate increases drastically, reaching 38% of these cases [88]. In allogeneic HSCT, the risk of GVHD directly influences the mortality rate due to chemotherapy side effects, with prolonged immunosuppression. The estimated ICU admission rate for allogeneic HSCT is 16% with a range from 9% to 30% in different studies [85, 89]. An index based on allogeneic HSCT patient comorbidities (HCT-IC) appears as a predictive tool that helps to select candidates for transplantation. The HCT-IC generates a score and it is categorized into low risk, intermediate risk, or high risk. In a cohort of 377 patients admitted in the ICU, it was observed that low-risk HCT-IC groups had a better overall survival (OS) than those classified as high-risk [90].

The mortality rate and OS of HSCT patients admitted to ICU has shown an improvement over time; however, the prognosis is still poor. In a systematic review, this progressive improvement was observed and between 2000 and 2015 the mortality ranged up to 75%, while OS was not higher than 30%. These data can be even worse compared to previous years [85].

As highlighted by Bayraktar (2016), medical decisions to admit the patient to ICU should be based on pre-transplant comorbidities, patient functional status, and GVHD grade [85]. These parameters were related to the patient's outcome; however, more comprehensive studies with specific objectives need to be conducted in order to identify the best criteria associated with the prognosis of the HSCT patient admitted in the ICU. It is also important to highlight that the development of reduced intensity conditioning regimens, an early admission to the ICU, and the use of non-invasive mechanical ventilation has contributed to better outcomes for these patients [91].

## 14.9 Toxicity Managment

### 14.9.1 Hypersensitivity Reactions

Hypersensitivity reactions (HR) has become increasingly common. With multiple causes, HR is an adverse effect in which an exaggerated or inadequate immune response occurs due to the exposure to an antigen or allergen [92]. HR can be divided into three distinct groups based on immediate responses: type I, type II, and type III; and the fourth as a late-response group, type IV. Types I to III occur within 24 hours, and type IV occurs after 12 and up to 72 hours of exposure to the allergen (Table 14.4) [93].

**Table 14.4** Types of hypersensitivity reactions and their clinical manifestations in patients admitted to ICU

| Type | Post-exposure reaction started | Mechanism of action | Clinical manifestations |
|---|---|---|---|
| I | Before 24 hours | Reaction mediated by IgE antibodies | Anaphylaxis, allergic bronchial asthma, allergic rhinitis, allergic conjunctivitis, food allergy, atopic eczema, drug allergy |
| II | | Cytotoxic reaction mediated by IgG or IgM antibodies | Immune thrombocytopenia, autoimmune hemolytic anemia, autoimmune neutropenia, hemolytic disease of the fetus and the newborn, good pasture syndrome, pemphigus |
| III | | Reaction mediated by immune complexes | Serum sickness, Arthus reaction |
| IV | After 12 hours | Reaction mediated by T cells | Contact dermatitis, tuberculin-type hypersensitivity, and granulomatous-type hypersensitivity |

Source: Adapted from Kanji (2010)

The evaluation of HR can include clinical and laboratory analysis, using the blood count, immunoglobulin dosages (IgE, IgG, IgM), skin test, and antibody dosage. In addition to these tests, differential analyses may be ordered depending on the patient's characteristics and general condition. The treatment corresponds to the diagnosed condition, which may include clinical management, drug administration, identification, and suspension of the allergen or even surgical procedures such as tracheotomy in the presence of severe laryngeal edema [94, 95].

### 14.9.2 Corticosteroid Treatment

Corticosteroids (CS), also known as corticosteroids or cortisone, constitute a group of steroid hormones that are produced by the adrenal glands. The synthetic form of CS was identified in 1935 and since then a series of studies have investigated its benefits, succeeding in wide use throughout the world and in almost all areas of medicine [96].

CS can be divided into glucocorticoids and mineralocorticoids. While the first is involved with the metabolism of carbohydrates, lipids, and proteins, resulting in immunosuppressive, anti-inflammatory and vasoconstrictor activities; mineralocorticoids affect the transport of ions from the epithelial cells of the renal tubules through electrolyte regulation and water balance [97].

Because they have anti-inflammatory and immunosuppressive properties, corticosteroids are commonly used in the treatment of asthma, allergic disorders, septic shock, rheumatoid arthritis, inflammatory bowel disease, multiple sclerosis, autoimmune conditions, post-transplantation, blood cancers, and other immune disorders. Despite the numerous beneficial effects, the use of corticosteroids is limited due to adverse effects caused by high dosage or long duration of use. Side effects include skin atrophy, osteoporosis, abdominal obesity, hypertension, diabetes, adrenal insufficiency, glaucoma, cataract, vascular necrosis, growth retardation, and infections [97–99]. Thus, long-term systemic corticosteroid therapy must precede a historical evaluation and complete physical examination in order to assess risk factors and potential drug complications, as well as the definition of frequency for monitoring the patient's general status.

Corticosteroids can still cause HR, although it is a rare event considering the general population. However, in high-risk groups, HR is not uncommon. CS-induced hypersensitivity reactions can be divided into two categories: immediate reactions, which occur within the first hour after drug administration; and not immediate, which can manifest after an hour of drug administration. The non-immediate is the most common [100]. Among the HR classifications, CS trigger IgE-mediated reactions, thus being type I. The incidence of hypersensitivity caused by CS varies depending on the study population, with allergic contact dermatitis being the most common non-immediate reaction. Immediate systemic reactions are rarer regardless of whether administration is oral, parenteral, or intra-articular [100, 101]. It is unquestionable that more comprehensive studies are needed to assess immediate reactions after CS administration.

The use of CS can lead to side effects even in patients who use a low dosage, although less frequently. In addition to the possibility of exacerbating the patient's pre-existing conditions or inducing new complications, medical knowledge about its clinical manifestations caused by the administration of CS is extremely necessary.

## 14.10 Transfusion of Blood Components

The blood components are obtained through physical or chemical procedures that results in albumin, globulin, and coagulation factor concentrate separation from blood. It also includes platelets, red blood cells, and plasma. Nevertheless, the use of these valuable components depends on a limited supply and viability [102, 103].

According to data from the year 2013 obtained from World Health Organization (WHO) Global Database on Blood Safety (GDBS) in the reported period there was a total of 112.5 million blood donations around the world. The majority of donations were observed in high-income countries wich corresponded to 47% of the global donation [104]. Approximately 85 million units are transfused per year globally [105, 106]. In the United States for the year 2013 the second largest number of red blood cells (RBC) units were allocated to hematology and oncology. In 2015, the largest number of RBC and platelet units were also used in hematology and oncology hospital units [107].

Transfusion of red blood cells is a critical care resource used in different clinical services including supportive care in cardiovascular and transplant surgery, massive trauma, and therapy for solid and hematological malignancies (WHO). Despite its beneficial role and potential to save lives, blood transfusion can threaten lives with the possibility of contamination with viruses and bacteria causing an infection [108]. In addition, blood products transfusion is associated with some adverse effects including transfusion-associated circulatory overload, hemolysis, acute lung injury, and immunomodulating effects [108–110].

Transfusions are common in patients with hematologic/oncologic disorders being blood loss and hemodilution the most common cause of RBC transfusions [105, 111]. Decrease in the count or function of platelets and/or coagulopathy is also a cause for transfusions in these patients [108]. Nevertheless, transfusion of blood products is an important procedure during cancer therapy because of myelosuppression caused by chemotherapy. Anemia, for example, commits 90% of patients during chemotherapy and transfusion is the procedure indicated to alleviate symptomatic anemia [102, 110, 112, 113]. In addition, transfusion can be used as a prophylactic treatment in that case physicians frequently use hemoglobin level as a transfusion need indicator [114].

In the intensive care unit, it is estimated that about 40% of critically ill patients receive at least one transfusion during ICU staying period [115]. Héber and colleagues demonstrated in their Transfusion Requirements in Critical Care trail study that implementation of a restrictive transfusion protocol reduced allogenic blood transfusion in 33% without affecting mortality between groups [106, 116]. Chantepie et al. studied the strategy of using a restrictive transfusion in patients who received intensive chemotherapy, for acute leukemia, or underwent autologous HSCT or allo-HSCT for hematologic malignancies. This group was designed to receive 1 unit of RBC per transfusion and was compared with a secondary cohort with similar inclusion criteria who received 2 units of RBC per transfusion. Despite 1RBC and 2RBC strategy, no difference was observed in RBC transfusion per patient and stay between groups. However, there was a significant reduction in RBC transfusions in the allo-HSCT subgroup [114]. The authors attribute their contrasting results compared to others in hematologic or nonhematologic diseases to the higher hemoglobin level threshold to transfusion indication used in their study [117–120]. Thus, several studies have shown that restrictive transfusion associated to a lower hemoglobin threshold may result in a reduction in RBC transfusion unit use. Therefore, applying a restrictive transfusion strategy, consequently, reduces hospitalization costs as a result of the reducing in number of RBC units transfused and represents a medical improvement.

## 14.11 Antimicrobial Therapy

In 1928 the physician and bacteriologist Alexander Fleming accidentally discovered penicillin and changed the infectious diseases perspective worldwide [121]. Since then, the administration of antimicrobial agents has significantly reduced the morbidity and mortality associated with infections. The term "antimicrobial" comprises pharmacological agents and include antibacterial, antifungal, antiviral, and antiparasitic drugs.

Due to the condition of immunosuppression caused by hematological diseases and treatment with chemotherapy, hematological and oncological patients are more susceptible to the acquisition of bacterial and fungal infections. This population most susceptible to infectious diseases includes patients with severe neutropenia, a condition of reduced number of neutrophils in the blood, and patients with hematopoietic stem cell transplantation [122]. The risk factors involved with infectious diseases acquisition include deficits in the immune system, associated comorbidities, and adverse effects of treatments [123, 124].

Thus, infection cases are frequent in these patients and, therefore, they undergo several cycles of antimicrobial therapy [125, 126]. In a significant portion of cases occur complications that contribute to the morbidity and mortality of this population, despite advances in the care offered to patients [127]. The high use of antimicrobials confers a selective pressure that favors resistant organisms, indirectly interfering, for example, in the prevalence of Clostridium difficile infection, associated with high mortality and prolonged hospitalization in this population [128, 129].

Fungal infection rates are increased in patients with prolonged neutropenia and/or deficit in immune system [122]. Cancer patients in the intensive care unit (ICU) are exposed to multiple factors that facilitate invasive fungal infections. The most frequent reponsable for fungal infections are Candida spp. but Aspergillus corresponds to an emerging cause of infection in ICU patients [130].

Gram-negative bacteria are the main infectious pathogen that affect these group of patients, but in recent decades infections by gram-positive bacteria increased [131, 132]. Infections with gram-negative bacteria resistant to multiple drugs (MDR) increased among cancer patients and are associated with high mortality rates from 36 to 58% due to limited treatment options [131].

Recently, a multicenter study carried out by Rello et al. (2020) investigated the challenges associated with the treatment of MDR bacteria infections in hematological patients in the ICU. According to the applied survey acute leukemia was the most common pathological condition found among the physicians responses (48.8%). In addition, pneumonia was the most frequent type of infection (53.7%) followed by bloodstream infection (31.7%) [131].

In addition, the study developed by the Spisas group identified that, among patients in treatment centers, the most frequent and high-risk infections in the ICU were caused by extended-spectrum B-lactamase (ESBL), Enterobacteriaceae spp. (57.5% of responses), Klebsiella pneumoniae resistant to Carbapenems and Pseudomonas aeruginosa resistant to Carbapenems, the latter being the most lethal according to 37.1% of participants [131].

According to this research in cases of febrile neutropenia, the initial treatment with anti-gram-negative and positive antibiotics was the regimen most indicated by the participants (41%) and monotherapy against gram-negatives represented only 23%. The most reported therapeutic strategies among the responses were the combination of antipseudomonal beta-lactams plus aminoglycosides (68.4%), carbapenem plus glycopeptides (20%), and carbapenem plus aminoglycosides (15%) [131].

There are different factors that guide the correct use of antimicrobial therapy and that must be considered for the definition of the therapeutic strategy that will be used. The diagnosis of the infectious disease, including identification of the infection site and, if possible, the etiologic agent, is an important step. The appropriate time to initiate therapy is determined by the severity of the situation; in patients in critical conditions such as febrile neutropenia, for example, empirical therapy should be started immediately after or during material collection for diagnosis [133].

It was reported that critically ill patients treated inadequately were more likely to die during hospitalization compared to those receiving adequate antimicrobial therapy [134]. Therefore, it is common to apply the strategy of using a broad spectrum of antimicrobials as an initial empirical therapy to ensure coverage of different pathogens with common clinical symptoms [133]. The factors to be considered when selecting the antimicrobial agent include renal and hepatic function, history of allergy or intolerance, and history of recent antimicrobial use [133].

The emergence of pathogens resistant to multiple drugs requires reduced antimicrobial inappropriate administration through correct selection, dosage, route, and duration of treatment [135]. The implementation of these strategies supports the minimization of ecological impacts caused by indiscriminate use, such as selection and dissemination of multi-resistant organisms.

The main objective of implementing and expanding the application of antimicrobial stewardship is to optimize clinical outcomes while minimizing the adverse effects of the use of antimicrobials such as toxicity, pathogen selection, and emergence of resistance [122, 135]. In addition, it has a secondary objective of reducing care costs without impacting its quality [135].

Based on different intervention studies on the use of antimicrobials in hospitalized adults the Infectious Diseases Society of America and the Society for Healthcare Epidemiology of America published a guideline about antimicrobial stewardship [135]. The development of multidisciplinary antimicrobial stewardship teams for the implementation of several strategies as prospective audit with intervention and feedback, formulary restriction and preauthorization requirements, educational efforts, and antimicrobial cycling among others is suggested t [122, 135].

Finally, the antimicrobial therapy use in ICU with hematological and oncologic patients is substantial due to the high rate of infections in these population. The antimicrobial use has several benefits including improvement in clinical outcomes and a positive impact on reducing mortality. However, it must be managed carefully and it is suggested to be assisted by an antimicrobial stewardship program.

## 14.12 Palliative Care

The palliation is an intervention method to alleviate a patient's suffering in a hospital or domiciliary environment. Its aim is to mitigate the consequences of severe diseases in the well-being of the diagnosed patient and members of their families [136, 137]. Palliative care (PC) is a multidisciplinary medical care modality specialized in symptom management, spiritual and psychosocial support, and assistance in treatment decision for patients diagnosed with severe diseases and their families. The professionals which compose this medical care modality include physicians, nurses, psychologist, social assistant, physiotherapists, and even dentists and nutritionists [135, 136].

The medical intervention realized by those professionals impacts positively in patients and their family's life, including improved psychosocial, physical, and spiritual symptom management, better prognostic comprehension and acceptance, and improved quality of life. An effective communication with the patients and their families helps for a better understanding and conduction of treatment during this complicated period. Also, patients' beliefs, choices, and history of life should be considered and respected, and the family members should be oriented and educated to understand how the disease is established, evolutes, and affects their relative [136, 138–140].

In the context of advanced Palliative care (PC) cancer palliative care are traditionally used more frequently with solid tumors, whereas just a few patients with hematologic malignancies received this specialized care. The possible reasons for this discrepancy include hematologist resistance due to fear of trigging anxiety and sadness on patients and the incorrect association of palliative care with end-of-life care [138, 139].

Palliative care professionals are trained in several areas useful in patients with serious illness care. The main competencies that develop during palliative care training programs are communication skills, spiritual, symptom and quality-of-life assessment, and family-centered care among others [141]. The benefits of PC implementation in the care of patients with advanced cancer have been demonstrated in diverse clinical trials. In ENABLE II study, for example, a cohort of 322 patients diagnosed with gastrointestinal, lung, genitourinary, or breast cancer were randomized to palliative care or standard oncologic care. It was reported significantly higher quality of life, reduced depression, and lower intensity of symptoms compared with standard care group.

Furthermore, on a cohort of 151 patients with metastatic non-small-cell lung cancer who underwent randomization it was observed a better quality of life in early palliative care group compared with patients assigned to standard care. In addition, patients in palliative care group presented significantly lower depressive symptoms and higher median survival [142]. Prior studies demonstrated that early integration of PC reduced ICU admissions in the end-of-life and was associated with improved patients' outcomes [143]. It has been discussed if patients with knowledge of their terminal condition and assisted by palliative care die sooner [144]. However, there is published data demonstrating that being assigned to a palliative care or ICU did not impact patients' survival [145].

In the literature, there are only a few studies addressing the effects of palliative care use for patients with cancer admitted to the ICU. According to studies disponible in the literature, palliative care contributes for pain reduction and improvement in mental health and life quality [140, 146]. The impact of PC on symptoms distress and outcomes in the ICU was characterized in a cohort of 88 admitted in the ICU with advanced disease (76% diagnosed with metastatic disease and 24% had locally recurrent and relapsed hematologic disease). The comorbidities identified among those patients include pulmonary disease, congestive heart failure, thromboembolic disease, diabetes mellitus, and anxiety/depression. The majority of patients presented more than one comorbidity listed [140]. The main interventions by PC team were made in management and pain control using opioids in the majority of patients (99%) and steroids (70% of patients). It was provided family counseling and spiritual support, besides symptom management and psychosocial support for all patients and their families. It was observed an improvement in several symptoms as pain, nausea, dyspnea and anxiety [141, 147].

Palliative care is a support offered at any point along the disease trajectory, independently of prognosis. It is recommended as an important and necessary standard part of cancer care and other serious illness. It is estimated that if the proportion of people needing palliative care remains the same, the number of patients needing PC will increase. According to those projections of future palliative care need, it would be beneficial a massive increase in training of specialist nurses, physicians, and other PC professionals and health services improvement to support the growing number of patients who will need this service [147].

## References

1. Markham MJ, Wachter K, Agarwal N, et al. Clinical cancer advances 2020: annual report on progress against cancer from the American Society of Clinical oncology. J Clin Oncol. 2020;38:1081–101.
2. Puxty K, McLoone P, Quasim T, Sloan B, Kinsella J, Morrison DS. Risk of critical illness among patients with solid cancers: a population-based observational study. JAMA Oncol. 2015;1:1078–85.

3. Sauer CM, Dong J, Celi LA, Ramazzotti D. Improved survival of cancer patients admitted to the intensive care unit between 2002 and 2011 at a U.S. Teaching Hospital. Cancer Res Treat. 2019;51:973–81.
4. Bos MMEM, De Keizer NF, Meynaar IA, Bakhshi-Raiez F, De Jonge E. Outcomes of cancer patients after unplanned admission to general intensive care units. Acta Oncol (Madr). 2012;51:897–905.
5. Tan AC, Jacques SK, Oatley M, Guminski AD. Characteristics and outcomes of oncology unit patients requiring admission to an Australian intensive care unit. Intern Med J. 2019;49:734–9.
6. Lee DS, Suh GY, Ryu JA, Chung CR, Yang JH, Park CM, Jeon K. Effect of early intervention on long-term outcomes of critically ill cancer patients admitted to ICUs. Crit Care Med. 2015;43:1439–48.
7. Mokart D, Lambert J, Schnell D, et al. Delayed intensive care unit admission is associated with increased mortality in patients with cancer with acute respiratory failure. Leuk Lymphoma. 2013;54:1724–9.
8. Mokart D, Darmon M, Resche-Rigon M, et al. Prognosis of neutropenic patients admitted to the intensive care unit. Intensive Care Med. 2015;41:296–303.
9. Brenner H, Hakulinen T. Long-term cancer patient survival achieved by the end of the 20th century: Most up-to-date estimates from the nationwide Finnish cancer registry. Br J Cancer. 2001;85:367–71.
10. Maringe C, Belot A, Rachet B. Prediction of cancer survival for cohorts of patients most recently diagnosed using multi-model inference. Stat Methods Med Res. 2020;29:3605–22.
11. Esposito M, Ganesan S, Kang Y. Emerging strategies for treating metastasis. Nat Cancer. 2021;2:258–70.
12. Bassford C. Decisions regarding admission to the ICU and international initiatives to improve the decision-making process. Crit Care. 2017;21:1–3.
13. Dao L, Ragoonanan D, Yi S, Swinford R, Petropoulos D, Mahadeo KM, Li S. The organ trail: a review of biomarkers of organ failure. Front Oncol. 2020;10:1–10.
14. Feliu J, Heredia-Soto V, Gironés R, Jiménez-Munarriz B, Saldaña J, Guillén-Ponce C, Molina-Garrido MJ. Can we avoid the toxicity of chemotherapy in elderly cancer patients? Crit Rev Oncol Hematol. 2018;131:1–26.
15. Liu J, Pandya P, Afshar S. Therapeutic advances in oncology. Int J Mol Sci. 2021;22:1–39.
16. Silbermann M, Pitsillides B, Al-Alfi N, et al. Multidisciplinary care team for cancer patients and its implementation in several middle Eastern countries. Ann Oncol. 2013;23:1–7.
17. Robert R, Reignier J, Tournoux-Facon C, Boulain T, Lesieur O, Gissot V, Souday V, Hamrouni M, Chapon C, Gouello JP. Refusal of intensive care unit admission due to a full unit: impact on mortality. Am J Respir Crit Care Med. 2012;185:1081–7.

18. Murthy S, Leligdowicz A, Adhikari NKJ. Intensive care unit capacity in low-income countries: a systematic review. PLoS One. 2015;10:1–12.
19. Cardoso LTQ, Grion CMC, Matsuo T, Anami EHT, Kauss IAM, Seko L, Bonametti AM. Impact of delayed admission to intensive care units on mortality of critically ill patients: a cohort study. Crit Care. 2011;15:1–8.
20. Azoulay E, Mokart D, Kouatchet A, Demoule A, Lemiale V. Acute respiratory failure in immunocompromised adults. Lancet Respir Med. 2019;7:173–86.
21. Chi AK, Soubani AO, White AC, Miller KB. An update on pulmonary complications of hematopoietic stem cell transplantation. Recent Adv Chest Med. 2013;144:1913–22.
22. Soares M, Depuydt PO, Salluh JIF. Mechanical ventilation in cancer patients: clinical characteristics and outcomes. Crit Care Clin. 2010;26:41–58.
23. César BN, de Souza DM. Acute kidney injury in cancer patients. Rev Assoc Med Bras. 2020;66:25–30.
24. Salahudeen AK, Doshi SM, Pawar T, Nowshad G, Lahoti A, Shah P. Incidence rate, clinical correlates, and outcomes of AKI in patients admitted to a comprehensive cancer center. Clin J Am Soc Nephrol. 2013;8:347–54.
25. Pitello N, Treon M, Jones K, Kiel P. Approaches for administering chemotherapy in the intensive care unit. Curr Drug Saf. 2010;5:22–32.
26. Pearce A, Haas M, Viney R, Pearson S, Haywood P, Brown C, Ward R. Incidence and severity of self-reported chemotherapy side effects in routine care: a prospective cohort study. PLoS One. 2017;12:1–12.
27. Akhlaghi E, Lehto RH, Torabikhah M, Sharif Nia H, Taheri A, Zaboli E, Yaghoobzadeh A. Chemotherapy use and quality of life in cancer patients at the end of life: an integrative review. Health Qual Life Outcomes. 2020;18:1–9.
28. Gudiol C, Albasanz-Puig A, Cuervo G, Carratalà J. Understanding and managing sepsis in patients with cancer in the era of antimicrobial resistance. Front Med. 2021;8:1–15.
29. Rosolem MM, Rabello LSCF, Lisboa T, Caruso P, Costa RT, Leal JVR, Salluh JIF, Soares M. Critically ill patients with cancer and sepsis: clinical course and prognostic factors. J Crit Care. 2012;27:301–7.
30. Taberna M, Gil Moncayo F, Jané-Salas E, Antonio M, Arribas L, Vilajosana E, Peralvez Torres E, Mesía R. The multidisciplinary team (MDT) approach and quality of care. Front Oncol. 2020;10:1–16.
31. Soares M, Bozza FA, Azevedo LCP, et al. Effects of organizational characteristics on outcomes and resource use in patients with cancer admitted to intensive care units. J Clin Oncol. 2016;34:3315–24.
32. Wang Y, Dai Y, Lau AH, Yang J, Chen W, Li G. Oncology clinical pharmacy services in Chinese hospitals. J Am Coll Clin Pharm. 2020;3:988–96.

33. Coutsouvelis J, Adams J, Bortz H, et al. Standard of practice in oncology and haematology for pharmacy services. J Pharm Pract Res. 2020;50:528–45.
34. Holle LM, Segal EM, Jeffers KD. The expanding role of the oncology pharmacist. Pharmacy. 2020;8:1–5.
35. Moukafih B, Abahssain H, Mrabti H, Errihani H, Rahali Y, Taoufik J, Chaibi A. Impact of clinical pharmacy services in a hematology/oncology ward in Morocco. J Oncol Pharm Pract. 2020;27:305–11.
36. Delpeuch A, Leveque D, Gourieux B, Herbrecht R. Impact of clinical pharmacy services in a hematology/oncology inpatient setting. Anticancer Res. 2015;35:457–60.
37. Lin G, Huang R, Zhang J, Li G, Chen L, Xi X. Clinical and economic outcomes of hospital pharmaceutical care: a systematic review and meta-analysis. BMC Health Serv Res. 2020;20:1–14.
38. World Health Organization. Action Programme on Essential Drugs and Vaccines. Good pharmacy practice (GPP) in community and hospital settings, vol. 1. Geneva: World Health Organization; 1996. p. 1–11.
39. Aguiar K, Santos J, Cambrussi MC, Picolotto S, Carneiro MB. Patient safety and the value of pharmaceutical intervention in a cancer hospital. Einstein (São Paulo, Brazil). 2018;16:1–7.
40. Brilli RJ, Spevetz A, Branson RD, et al. Critical care delivery in the intensive care unit: defining clinical roles and the best practice model. Crit Care Med. 2007;29:2007–19.
41. Haupt MT, Bekes CE, Brilli RJ, Carl LC, et al. Guidelines on critical care services and personnel: recommendations based on a system of categorization of three levels of care. Crit Care Med. 2003;31:2677–83.
42. Keely JL. American College of Physicians-American Society of internal medicine. Pharmacist scope of practice. Ann Intern Med. 2002;136:79–85.
43. Maclaren R, Devlin JW, Martin SJ, Dasta JF, Rudis MI, Bond CA. Critical care pharmacy services in United States hospitals. Ann Pharmacother. 2006;40:612–8.
44. Preslaski CR, Lat I, MacLaren R, Poston J. Pharmacist contributions as members of the multidisciplinary ICU team. Chest. 2013;144:1687–95.
45. Valle TD, Garcia PC. Oncology patient admission criteria in intensive care units of general care hospitals. Rev Ciênc Med. 2018;27:73–84.
46. Jairam V, Lee V, Park HS, et al. Treatment-related complications of systemic therapy and radiotherapy. JAMA Oncol. 2019;5:1028–35.
47. Bos MMEM, Verburg IWM, Dumaij I, Stouthard J, Nortier JWR, Richel D, et al. Intensive care admission of cancer patients: a comparative analysis. Cancer Med. 2015;4:966–76.
48. Taconne FS, Artigas AA, Spring CL, Moreno R, Sakr Y, Vincent JR. Characteristics and outcomes of câncer patients in European ICUS. Crit Care. 2009;13:1–10.

49. Parack S, Piggin A, Neeman T, Mitchell I, Crispin P, Davis A. Outcomes of haematology/oncology patients admitted to intensive care unit at the Camberra Hospital. Intern Med J. 2014;44:1087–94.
50. Charles LS, et al. Consensus statement on the triage of critically ill patients. Society of Critical Care Medicine Ethics Committee. JAMA. 1994;271:1200–3.
51. Lecuyer L, Chevret S, Thiery G, Darmon M, Schlemmer B, Azoulay E. The ICU trial: a new admission policy for cancer patients requiring mechanical ventilation. Crit Care Med. 2007;35:808–14.
52. Sung H, Ferlay J, Siegel RL, Laversanne M, Soerjomataram I, Jemal A, Bray F. Global cancer statistics 2020: GLOBOCAN estimates of incidence and mortality worldwide for 36 cancers in 185 countries. CA Cancer J Clin. 2021;71:209–49.
53. Silva LCA, et al. Contributions of pharmaceutical care to patients on oncological treatment. Rev Investig Bioméd. 2017;9:216–22.
54. Richter A, Bates I, Thacker M, et al. Impact of the introduction of a specialist critical care pharmacist on the level of pharmaceutical care provided to the critical care unit. Int J Pharm Pract. 2016;24:253–61.
55. Mabasa VH, Malyuk DL, Weatherby EM, Chan A. A standardized, structured approach to identifying drug-related problems in the intensive care unit: FASTHUG-MAIDENS. Can J Hosp Pharm. 2011;64:366–9.
56. Flannery AH, Pandya K, Laine ME, et al. Managing the rising costs and high drug expenditures in critical care pharmacy practice. Pharmacotherapy. 2016;37:54–64.
57. Neufeld NJ, Elnahal SM, Alvarez RH. Cancer pain: a review of epidemiology, clinical quality and value impact. Future Oncol. 2017;13:833–41.
58. DAS-Taskforce 2015, Baron R, Binder A, Biniek R, et al. Evidence and consensus based guideline for the management of delirium, analgesia, and sedation in intensive care medicine. Revision 2015 (DAS-guideline 2015) – short version. Ger Med Sci. 2015;13:1–42.
59. Jacobi J, Fraser GL, Coursin DB, et al. Task Force of the American College of Critical Care Medicine (ACCM) of the Society of Critical Care Medicine (SCCM), American Society of Health-System Pharmacists (ASHP), American College of Chest Physicians. Clinical practice guidelines for the sustained use of sedatives and analgesics in the critically ill adult. Crit Care Med. 2002;30:119–41.
60. Argelia LS, Marisol AO, Amparito de los ABP. American guidelines for cancer pain management. Pain Manag. 2017;7:287–98.
61. Kress JP, Pohlman AS, O'Connor MF, Hall JB. Daily interruption of sedative infusions in critically ill patients undergoing mechanical ventilation. N Engl J Med. 2000;342:1471–7.
62. Geerts WH, Bergqvist D, Pineo GF, et al. Prevention of venous thromboembolism: American College of Chest Physicians Evidence-Based Clinical Practice Guidelines (8th edition). Chest. 2008;133:381–453.

63. Lima IM, Vidigal SB, Lima NM, et al. Application of FASTHUG-MAIDENS mnemonic and evaluation of its impact in pharmaceutical intervention in an adult intensive care unit. Rev Bras Farm Hosp Serv Saude. 2021;12:1–8.
64. Ely EW, Inouye SK, Bernard GR, et al. Delirium in mechanically ventilated patients: validity and reliability of the confusion assessment method for the intensive care unit (CAM-ICU). JAMA. 2001;286:2703–10.
65. Bergeron N, Dubois MJ, Dumont M, Dial S, Skrobik Y. Intensive care delirium screening checklist: evaluation of a new screening tool. Intensive Care Med. 2001;27:859–64.
66. Siddiqui F, Ahmed M, Abbasi S, et al. Gastrointestinal bleeding in patients with acute respiratory distress syndrome: a National Database Analysis. J Clin Med Res. 2018;11:42–8.
67. Krag M, Perner A, Wetterslev J, Wise MP, et al. Prevalence and outcome of gastrointestinal bleeding and use of acid suppressants in acutely ill adult intensive care patients. Intensive Care Med. 2015;41:833–45.
68. Hapani S, Chu D, Wu S. Risk of gastrointestinal perforation in patients with cancer treated with bevacizumab: a meta-analysis. Lancet Oncol. 2009;10:559–68.
69. Plummer MP, Blaser AR, Deane AM. Stress ulceration: prevalence, pathology and association with adverse outcomes. Crit Care. 2014;18:1–7.
70. Daley RJ, Rebuck JA, Welage LS, Rogers FB. Prevention of stress ulceration: current trends in critical care. Crit Care Med. 2004;32:2008–13.
71. Hershey DS, Hession S. Chemotherapy and glycemic control in patients with type 2 diabetes and cancer: a comparative case analysis. Asia Pac J Oncol Nurs. 2017;4:224–32.
72. Bell CM, Brener SS, Gunraj N, et al. Association of ICU or hospital admission with unintentional discontinuation of medications for chronic diseases. JAMA. 2011;306:840–7.
73. Bosma LBE, Hunfeld NGM, Quax RAM, et al. The effect of a medication reconciliation program in two intensive care units in the Netherlands: a prospective intervention study with a before and after design. Ann Intensive Care. 2018;8:1–19.
74. Manias E, Williams A, Liew D. Interventions to reduce medication errors in adult intensive care: a systematic review. Br J Clin Pharmacol. 2012;74:411–23.
75. Santos JP, Azevedo RMHS, Araújo PL, et al. Pharmaceutical care in oncology UTI. Braz J Hea. 2020;3:5697–704.
76. Lin Q, Wang G, Ma G, et al. The role of pharmaceutical care in the oncology department. Eur J Hosp Pharm. 2015;22:128–31.
77. Chagastelles PC, Nardi NB. Biology of stem cells: an overview. Kidney Int Suppl. 2011;1:63–7.
78. Hawley RG, Ramezani A, Hawley TS. Hematopoietic stem cells. In: Methods Enzymol Academic Press Inc. 2006;365:149–79.

79. Henig I, Zuckerman T. Hematopoietic stem cell transplantation – 50 years of evolution and future perspectives. Rambam Maimonides Med J. 2014;5:1–15.
80. Park M, Seo JJ. Role of HLA in hematopoietic stem cell transplantation. Bone Marrow Res. 2012;20:1–7.
81. Lennard AL, Jackson GH. Topic in review: stem cell transplantation. West J Med. 2001;175:42–6.
82. Balassa K, Danby R, Rocha V. Haematopoietic stem cell transplants: principles and indications. Br J Hosp Med. 2019;80:33–9.
83. Choo SY. The HLA system: genetics, immunology, clinical testing, and clinical implications. Yonsei Med J. 2007;48:11–23.
84. Gahrton G, Svensson H, Björkstrand B, et al. Syngeneic transplantation in multiple myeloma - a case-matched comparison with autologous and allogeneic transplantation. Bone Marrow Transplant. 1999;24:741–5.
85. Bayraktar UD, Nates JL. Intensive care outcomes in adult hematopoietic stem cell transplantation patients. World J Clin Oncol. 2016;7:98–105.
86. Randolph BV, Ciurea SO. What the intensivist needs to know about hematopoietic stem cell transplantation? Oncol Crit Care Springer International Publishing. 2019;1:1531–46.
87. Jantunen E, Itälä M, Lehtinen T, et al. Early treatment-related mortality in adult autologous stem cell transplant recipients: a nation-wide survey of 1482 transplanted patients. Eur J Haematol. 2006;76:245–50.
88. Bulley SR, Strahm B, Doyle J, Dupuis LL. Defibrotide for the treatment of hepatic veno-occlusive disease in children. Pediatr Blood Cancer. 2007;48:700–4.
89. Bayraktar UD, Shpall EJ, Liu P, Ciurea SO, Rondon G, De Lima M, Cardenas-Turanzas M, Price KJ, Champlin RE, Nates JL. Hematopoietic cell transplantation-specific comorbidity index predicts inpatient mortality and survival in patients who received allogeneic transplantation admitted to the intensive care unit. J Clin Oncol. 2013;31:4207–14.
90. Sorror ML, Maris MB, Storb R, Baron F, Sandmaier BM, Maloney DG, Storer B. Hematopoietic cell transplantation (HCT)-specific comorbidity index: a new tool for risk assessment before allogeneic HCT. Blood. 2005;106:2912–9.
91. Saillard C, Blaise D, Mokart D. Critically ill allogeneic hematopoietic stem cell transplantation patients in the intensive care unit: reappraisal of actual prognosis. Bone Marrow Transplant. 2016;51:1050–61.
92. Justiz AA, Vaillant RV, Zito PM. Immediate hypersensitivity reactions. Immunotoxicol Risk Assess. 2006;1:155–71.
93. Kanji S, Chant C. Allergic and hypersensitivity reactions in the intensive care unit. Crit Care Med. 2010;38:162–8.
94. Marwa K, Kondamudi NP. Type IV hypersensitivity reaction. StatPearls Publishing. 2020;2:1–8.
95. Justiz Vaillant AA, Zito PM. Immediate hypersensitivity reactions. StatPearls Publishing. 2018;1:1–10.

96. Ericson-Neilsen W, Kaye AD. Steroids: pharmacology, complications, and practice delivery issues. Ochsner J. 2014;14:203–7.
97. Liu D, Ahmet A, Ward L, Krishnamoorthy P, Mandelcorn ED, Leigh R, Brown JP, Cohen A, Kim H. A practical guide to the monitoring and management of the complications of systemic corticosteroid therapy. Allergy Asthma Clin Immunol. 2013;9:1–25.
98. Buchman AL. Side effects of corticosteroid therapy. J Clin Gastroenterol. 2001;33:289–94.
99. Schäcke H, Döcke WD, Asadullah K. Mechanisms involved in the side effects of glucocorticoids. Pharmacol Ther. 2002;96:23–43.
100. Vatti RR, Ali F, Teuber S, Chang C, Gershwin ME. Hypersensitivity reactions to corticosteroids. Clin Rev Allergy Immunol. 2014;47:26–37.
101. Patel A, Bahna SL. Immediate hypersensitivity reactions to corticosteroids. Ann Allergy Asthma Immunol. 2015;115:178–82.
102. Watkins T, Surowiecka MK, McCullough J. Transfusion indications for patients with cancer. Cancer Control. 2015;22:38–46.
103. Bayer WL, Bodensteiner DC, Tilzer LL, Adams ME. Use of platelets and other transfusion products in patients with malignancy. Semin Thromb Hemost. 1992;18:380–91.
104. Montenegro H. World Health Organisation: global status report on blood safety and availability. Licence: CC BYNC-SA 3.0 IGO. Geneva. 2016.
105. Iqbal N, Haider K, Sundaram V, Radosevic J, Burnouf T, Seghatchian J, Goubran H. Red blood cell transfusion and outcome in cancer. Transfus Apher Sci. 2017;56:287–90.
106. Hogshire L, Carson JL. Red blood cell transfusion: what is the evidence when to transfuse? Curr Opin Hematol. 2013;20:546–51.
107. Sapiano MRP, Savinkina AA, Ellingson KD, Haass KA, Baker ML, Henry RA, Berger JJ, Kuehnert MJ, Basavaraju SV. Supplemental findings from the National Blood Collection and Utilization Surveys, 2013 and 2015. Transfusion. 2017;57:1599–624.
108. Velásquez JF, Cata JP. Transfusions of blood products and cancer outcomes. Rev Esp Anestesiol Reanim. 2015;62:461–7.
109. Vincent JL, Jaschinski U, Wittebole X, Lefrant JY, Jakob SM, Almekhlafi GA, Pellis T, Tripathy S, Rubatto Birri PN, Sakr Y. Worldwide audit of blood transfusion practice in critically ill patients. Crit Care. 2018;22:1–9.
110. Vlaar AP, Oczkowski S, de Bruin S, et al. Transfusion strategies in non-bleeding critically ill adults: a clinical practice guideline from the European Society of Intensive Care Medicine. Intensive Care Med. 2020;46:673–96.
111. Hendrickson JE, Tormey CA. Red blood cell antibodies in hematology/oncology patients: interpretation of immunohematologic tests and clinical significance of detected antibodies. Hematol Oncol Clin North Am. 2016;30:635–51.

112. Tas F, Eralp Y, Basaran M, Sakar B, Alici S, Argon A, Bulutlar G, Camlica H, Aydiner A, Topuz E. Anemia in oncology practice: relation to diseases and their therapies. Am J Clin Oncol Cancer Clin Trials. 2002;25:371–9.
113. Abdel-Razeq H, Saadeh SS, Malhis R, Yasser S, Abdulelah H, Eljaber R, Kleib A, Ismael R. Treatment of anemia in cancer patients undergoing chemotherapy with intravenous ferric carboxymaltose without erythropoiesis-stimulating agents. Ther Adv Med Oncol. 2020;12:1–9.
114. Chantepie SP, Mear JB, Parienti JJ, et al. Blood transfusion in hematologic intensive care unit. Transfusion. 2017;57:296–302.
115. Leal-Noval SR, Muñoz-Gómez M, Jiménez-Sánchez M, Cayuela A, Leal-Romero M, Puppo-Moreno A, Enamorado J, Arellano-Orden V. Red blood cell transfusion in non-bleeding critically ill patients with moderate anemia: is there a benefit? Intensive Care Med. 2013;39:445–53.
116. Hébert PC, Wells G, Blajchman MA, Marshall J, Martin C, Pagliarello G, Tweeddale M, Schweitzer I, Yetisir E. A multicenter, randomized, controlled clinical trial of transfusion requirements in critical care. N Engl J Med. 1999;340:409–17.
117. Webert KE, Cook RJ, Couban S, Carruthers J, Lee K-A, Blajchman MA, Lipton JH, Brandwein JM, Heddle NM. A multicenter pilot-randomized controlled trial of the feasibility of an augmented red blood cell transfusion strategy for patients treated with induction chemotherapy for acute leukemia or stem cell transplantation. Transfusion. 2008;48:81–91.
118. Carson JL, Stanworth SJ, Roubinian N, Fergusson DA, Triulzi D, Doree C, Hebert PC. Transfusion thresholds and other strategies for guiding allogeneic red blood cell transfusion. Cochrane Database Syst Rev. 2016;10:1–118.
119. Carson JL, Carless PA, Hébert PC. Outcomes using lower vs higher hemoglobin thresholds for red blood cell transfusion. JAMA. 2013;309:83–4.
120. Carson JL, Brooks MM, Abbott JD, et al. Coronary artery disease liberal versus restrictive transfusion thresholds for patients with symptomatic coronary artery disease. Am Heart J. 2013;165:964–71.
121. Fleming A. On the antibacterial action of cultures of a penicillium, with special reference to their use in the isolation of B. Bull World Health Organ. 1929;79:780–90.
122. Tverdek FP, Rolston KV, Chemaly RF. Antimicrobial stewardship in patients with cancer. Pharmacotherapy. 2012;32:722–34.
123. Başaran NÇ, Karaağaoğlu E, Hasçelik G, Tanrıöver MD, Akova M. Prospective evaluation of infection episodes in cancer patients in a tertiary care academic center: microbiological features and risk factors for mortality. Turkish J Hematol. 2016;33:311–9.

124. Srinivasan A, Wang C, Srivastava DK, Burnette K, Shenep JL, Leung W, Hayden RT. Timeline, epidemiology, and risk factors for bacterial, fungal, and viral infections in children and adolescents after allogeneic hematopoietic stem cell transplantation. Biol Blood Marrow Transplant. 2013;19:94–101.
125. Rolston KVI. Infections in cancer patients with solid tumors: a review. Infect Dis Ther. 2017;6:69–83.
126. Blennow O, Ljungman P. Infections in hematology patients. In: Concise guide to hematology. Cham: Springer International Publishing; 2019. p. 503–18.
127. Zembower TR. Epidemiology of infections in cancer patients. Cancer Treat Res. 2014;161:43–89.
128. Napolitano LM, Edmiston CE Jr. Clostridium difficile disease: Diagnosis, pathogenesis, and treatment update. Surgery. 2017;162: 325–48.
129. Chopra T, Alangaden GJ, Chandrasekar P. Clostridium difficile infection in cancer patients and hematopoietic stem cell transplant recipients. Expert Rev Anti-Infect Ther. 2010;8:1113–9.
130. Abughanimeh O, Qasrawi A, Kaddourah O, Al Momani L, Abu Ghanimeh M. Clostridium difficile infection in oncology patients: epidemiology, pathophysiology, risk factors, diagnosis, and treatment. Hosp Pract. 2018;46:266–77.
131. Sipsas NV, Kontoyiannis DP. Invasive fungal infections in patients with cancer in the intensive care unit. Int J Antimicrob Agents NIH Public Access. 2012;39:464–71.
132. Rello J, Sarda C, Mokart D, Arvaniti K, Akova M, Tabah A, Azoulay E. Antimicrobial stewardship in hematological patients at the intensive care unit: a global cross-sectional survey from the nine-i investigators network. Eur J Clin Microbiol Infect Dis. 2020;39:385–92.
133. Montassier E, Batard E, Gastinne T, Potel G, De La Cochetière MF. Recent changes in bacteremia in patients with cancer: a systematic review of epidemiology and antibiotic resistance. Eur J Clin Microbiol Infect Dis. 2013;32:841–50.
134. Leekha S, Terrell CL, Edson RS. General principles of antimicrobial therapy. Mayo Clin Proc Elsevier. 2011;15:156–67.
135. Ibrahim EH, Sherman G, Ward S, Fraser VJ, Kollef MH. The influence of inadequate antimicrobial treatment of bloodstream infections on patient outcomes in the ICU setting. Chest. 2000;118:146–55.
136. Dellit TH, Owens RC, McGowan JE, et al. Infectious Diseases Society of America and the Society for Healthcare Epidemiology of America guidelines for developing an institutional program to enhance antimicrobial stewardship. Clin Infect Dis. 2007;44:159–77.
137. Radbruch L, De Lima L, Knaul F, et al. Redefining palliative care-a new consensus-based definition. J Pain Symptom Manag. 2020;60:754–64.

138. Etkind SN, Bone AE, Gomes B, Lovell N, Evans CJ, Higginson IJ, Murtagh FEM. How many people will need palliative care in 2040? Past trends, future projections and implications for services. BMC Med. 2017;15:1–10.
139. Rietjens JAC, Sudore RL, Connolly M, et al. Definition and recommendations for advance care planning: an international consensus supported by the European Association for Palliative Care. Lancet Oncol. 2017;18:543–51.
140. McCaughan D, Roman E, Smith AG, Garry AC, Johnson MJ, Patmore RD, Howard MR, Howell DA. Palliative care specialists' perceptions concerning referral of haematology patients to their services: findings from a qualitative study. BMC Palliat Care. 2018;17:1–11.
141. Delgado-Guay MO, Parsons HA, Li Z, Palmer LJ, Bruera E. Symptom distress, interventions, and outcomes of intensive care unit cancer patients referred to a palliative care consult team. Cancer. 2009;115:437–45.
142. LeBlanc TW, El-Jawahri A. When and why should patients with hematologic malignancies see a palliative care specialist? Hematol (United States). 2015;2015:471–8.
143. Temel JS, Greer JA, Muzikansky A, et al. Early palliative care for patients with metastatic non–small-cell lung cancer. N Engl J Med. 2010;363:733–42.
144. Romano AM, Gade KE, Nielsen G, Havard R, Harrison JH, Barclay J, Stukenborg GJ, Read PW, Blackhall LJ, Dillon PM. Early palliative care reduces end-of-life intensive care unit (ICU) use but not ICU course in patients with advanced cancer. Oncologist. 2017;22:318–23.
145. Connor SR, Pyenson B, Fitch K, Spence C, Iwasaki K. Comparing hospice and nonhospice patient survival among patients who die within a three-year window. J Pain Symptom Manag. 2007;33:238–46.
146. Yun YH, Lee MK, Kim SY, et al. Impact of awareness of terminal illness and use of palliative care or intensive care unit on the survival of terminally ill patients with cancer: prospective cohort study. J Clin Oncol. 2011;29:2474–80.
147. Smith TJ, Temin S, Alesi ER, et al. American Society of Clinical Oncology provisional clinical opinion: the integration of palliative care into standard oncology care. J Clin Oncol. 2012;30:880–7.

# Chemotherapy for the Surgery Center

# 15

Alessandro Menegon

## 15.1 Introduction

The operating room has been an ally in cancer treatment since the beginning of the discovery of the disease. Even several lines of curative cancer treatment include tumor removal. That is why it is important for surgeons to have extensive knowledge of the use and mechanism of action of chemotherapy drugs, which can be used before, after, and during the surgical procedure.

According to a report by the World Health Organization, 80% of approximately 15.2 million new cases of cancer that occurred in 2015 must have required a surgical procedure at some point in the evolution of the disease. Another point to note is that some authors state that, despite advances in radiotherapy and chemotherapy, surgery remains the basis of support for cancer-related care, from curative treatment to treatment support measures [1].

Within this entire context, we have the importance of chemotherapy within the operating room itself. Some chemotherapy treatments are performed inside an operating room, as a result of the route that will be used to administer the drug, e.g., chemo-embolization, intrathecal chemotherapy, either through the

A. Menegon (✉)
Clinical Pharmacist of Pharmaceutical Assistance Department, July 9th Hospital, São Paulo, São Paulo, Brazil





C. W. P. Schmidt, K. M. Otoni (eds.), *The Golden Guide to Oncologic Pharmacy*, https://doi.org/10.1007/978-3-030-98596-7_15

Ommaya catheter or lumbar puncture with sedation, hyperthermic intraperitoneal chemotherapy (HIPEC), aerosolized, and pressurized intraperitoneal chemotherapy (PIPAC), among other therapies.

In this chapter, we will address the main chemotherapy treatments that are performed within the operating room itself, the care to be taken by the entire multidisciplinary team that will have contact with the antineoplastic drug, and how a chemotherapy agent can make the procedure more dangerous with its possible clinical repercussions and interactions.

## 15.2 Hyperthermic Intraperitoneal Chemotherapy (HIPEC)

### 15.2.1 Overview

This therapy is associated with cytoreductive surgery (CRS); after this procedure, this technique is used to complete the treatment. CRS, together with HIPEC, appeared as a treatment option for peritoneal surface neoplasms, especially those that remain confined in the abdominal–pelvic cavity with minimal invasion of underlying organs and without extra-abdominal dissemination, and it has been evolving more and more (Table 15.1) [2].

These two combined procedures have become a treatment with a curative proposal for a certain group of patients, being the standard for peritoneal pseudomyxoma (PMP) and diffuse malignant peritoneal mesothelioma (MPMD), as well as an alternative for several other oncological diseases, such as peritoneal carcinomatosis due to tumors colorectal, appendicular, gastric and ovarian, gastrointestinal tumors perforated or invading adjacent organs, rare tumors complicated by isolated peritoneal diffusion, in addition to prophylaxis for peritoneal metastatic disease in patients at high risk of peritoneal metastases and palliative care for malignant ascites [2, 3].

After CRS, where the tumor foci are completely resected, it is time for the heated chemotherapy to take effect. In addition to the cytotoxic action of the antineoplastic drug, heat causes a synergism

**Table 15.1** Chronology of development of cytoreductive surgery (CRS) and hyperthermic intraperitoneal chemotherapy (HIPEC) [3]

| Period | Development |
|---|---|
| 30s | Description of debulking of solid ovarian tumors and adjuvant chemotherapy or radiation |
| 60s | Improved survival of patients with stage IV ovarian cancer associated with aggressive CRS |
| 1969 | Success reports of aggressive regional therapy in a patient with pseudomyxoma peritonei |
| 1977 | Infusion and filtration systems made for hyperthermic intracavitary perfusion; reports of tumor burden reduction with systemic thermotherapy |
| 1979 | First case of pseudomyxoma peritonei treated with hyperthermic thiotepa |
| 80s | Technique tested in various gastrointestinal malignancies; development of targeted chemotherapy; first trials of intraperitoneal chemotherapy vs. intravenous |
| 90s | Peritoneal cancer index development; formal description of peritonectomy |
| 00s | Description of the debulking score calculation used to measure the degree of CRS performed |

that increases the cytotoxic effect and potentiates the chemotherapeutic, even improving its penetration into the tumoral tissues of the peritoneal and pelvic cavity [4].

HIPEC allows drug perfusion in the cavity and causes poorly vascularized tumor tissue to be exposed to high doses of cytotoxic agents before the formation of adhesions that limit the circulation of peritoneal fluid. The barrier that forms between blood and peritoneal fluid prevents the passage of high doses of chemotherapy into the plasma, reducing its systemic effects and consequently its toxicity [2].

Some studies also report that, in addition to the cytotoxic effect of heat, it potentiates the effect of some antimitotic agents (such as mitomycin, cisplatin, and oxaliplatin) and increases tissue penetration, reduces resistance mechanisms to certain antineoplastic drugs, and induces an anticancer immune response efficiently [2].

When we talk about HIPEC, we have several variables that can determine one technique or another. Temperature, dose and choice of chemotherapy agents, time of abdominal closure, and the circuit used for perfusion and its time are determining factors among the techniques used. However, neither technique has managed to show considerable superiority over the other [4].

Comparing the data we found about everything related to HIPEC, these are quite heterogeneous, especially in relation to technical particularities. However, CRS/HIPEC therapy has shown reasonable morbidity and mortality and survival over some more conventional treatments in several centers around the world, such as in Brazil, where the Brazilian Society of Oncology Surgery (SBCO) reinforces this idea, even though there is no standardization of the technique in the country [2].

A point to be highlighted in relation to HIPEC is that a few years ago, the so-called bidirectional HIPEC began to be used, in which, in addition to the drug administered intraperitoneally, neoplastic agents are concomitantly administered intravenously, which proved beneficial in some cases [5].

### 15.2.2 Pharmacokinetics

After intraperitoneal administration, cytotoxic drugs can reach highs in the region, without increasing their systemic levels. This difference in concentration is partly due to the slow rate of drug movement between the cavity and the plasma, due to the aforementioned plasma–peritoneum barrier. Another situation that seems to favor the technique is that the drainage of blood present in the cavity occurs through the portal vein, favoring first-pass metabolism and increasing its exposure to liver micrometastases that can occur there. Antineoplastic drugs are transported by lymphatic vessels, generating a greater concentration of the drug in the lymph than in the plasma itself. In relation to tissue penetration, this seems to be a disadvantage of the technique, as studies show a maximum value between 3 and 5 mm, hence the importance of an adequate CRS.

The area under the curve (AUC) of the concentration/time ratio of the drugs between the intraperitoneal cavity and the blood demonstrates the advantage of this procedure. Transferring its lipophilicity, molecular weight, first-pass metabolism, and hepatic clearance, the AUC ratio of the drug administered intraperitoneally in relation to the intravenous route may be greater than 1000 (as in the case of paclitaxel) [5].

### 15.2.3 Temperature Effects

According to several studies, the temperature range between 41 and 43 °C is ideal for killing cancer cells. Even though the interruption of mitosis and the inhibition of RNA synthesis are reversible and non-selective of hyperthermia, the increase in the amount of lysosomes and their enzymatic action are selective effects on malignant cells. Heat makes these structures more unstable, increasing their destructive capacity. Another direct action of hyperthermia on tumor cells is the decrease in blood flow in the microcirculation.

Hyperthermia causes a reduction or complete inhibition of oxidative metabolism in malignant cells, leading to an increase in lactic acid and a lower pH in the cellular environment, which is an extremely selective effect. Increased acidity also increases the action of lysosomes, resulting in increased cell death.

As already mentioned, the combination of cytotoxic drugs and temperature increase causes a good synergistic effect, which ranges from increased cell membrane permeability, which improves absorption, as well as changes in drug pharmacokinetics and cell metabolism. In fact, several drugs had their therapeutic index and efficacy apparently increased, both in vitro and in experimental studies in vivo, as is the case of alkylating agents [5].

### 15.2.4 Drug Choice

When thinking about using chemotherapy in the intraperitoneal cavity, we must consider certain aspects, such as which drug to use and its dosage. It is extremely important that the drug used does not have direct toxicity at the administered site, as well as that this drug has known and well-established activity against the target cancer. One point to consider is that drugs that need to be metabolized before they can actually start working should be disregarded. In the HIPEC procedure, it is necessary to use direct cytotoxic chemotherapy.

As systemic exposure occurs and this is variable, it is very important to think about the possible toxicity subsequent to this exposure and the relation between the volume of the carrier solution and the body surface. In patients over 60 years of age, dose adjustment is also recommended [5].

One thing to consider is the carrier solution to be used. Each one has a chemical property that can make a difference, but in general, the most used is the peritoneal dialysis solution with 1.5% glucose. However, other crystalloid solutions or even high molecular weight starch can be used [5]. Table 15.2 lists the HIPEC regimens commonly used around the world.

### 15.2.5 Techniques

The CRS/HIPEC procedure is performed in 3 steps:

- Exploration: It consists of an exploratory laparoscopy or direct a complete laparotomy followed by cancer assessment.
- Cyto-reduction: It is also called debulking; it is at this stage that the surgeon removes visible tumors.
- Chemoperfusion: This is when the abdominal cavity is washed with the warm chemotherapy solution [3].

It is in the last stage where differences can occur between one or another CRS/HIPEC technique, and in general, there are two types: open (also known as coliseum technique) or closed.

In the open abdomen technique, a Tenckhoff catheter is used and four closed suction drains are placed in the abdominal wall. Temperature probes are also placed for control. From there, the skin edges of the abdominal incision are lifted, creating an open space.

**Table 15.2** Commonly used HIPEC regimens around the world [2, 5]

| Drugs and doses | Duration (min) | Indication |
|---|---|---|
| Mitomycin C 15 $mg/m^2$ Doxorubicin 15 $mg/m^2$ | 90 | Appendiceal and colorectal carcinomatosis |
| Cisplatin 50 $mg/m^2$ Doxorubicin 15 $mg/m^2$ | 90 | Gastric cancer, peritoneal mesothelioma, ovarian cancer |
| Oxaliplatin 130 $mg/m^2$ | 60 | Appendiceal and colorectal carcinomatosis |
| Melphalan 50–70 $mg/m^2$ | 60 | Carcinomatosis with incomplete cytoreduction |
| Oxaliplatin 460 $mg/m^2$ | 30 | Colorectal carcinomatosis |
| Mitomycin C 35 $mg/m^2$ | 90 | Appendiceal and colorectal carcinomatosis |
| Cisplatin 43 mg/L Doxorubicin 15.25 mg/L | 90 | Peritoneal mesothelioma and advanced ovarian cancer |
| Mitomycin C 3.3 $mg/m^2/L$ Cisplatin 25 $mg/m^2/L$ | 90 | Appendiceal, colorectal carcinomatosis, advanced ovarian cancer, and peritoneal mesothelioma |
| Mitomycin 0.5 mg/kg Cisplatin 0,7 mg/kg | 90 | Peritoneal mesothelioma |
| Cisplatin 20 $mg/m^2/L$ | 90 | Recurrent and chemoresistant stage III ovarian cancer |
| Cisplatin 250 $mg/m^2$ | 90 | Peritoneal mesothelioma |
| Oxaliplatin 360 $mg/m^2$ | 30 | Pseudomyxoma peritonei and peritoneal mesothelioma |
| Cisplatin 100 $mg/m^2$ + Doxorubicin 15mg/$m^2$ | 60 | Pseudomyxoma peritonei |
| Carboplatin 800 $mg/m^2$ | 60 | Peritoneal mesothelioma |

The solution is infused for approximately 90 minutes, and all anatomical structures in the peritoneal cavity are evenly exposed to heat and cytotoxic agents by continuous manipulation of the perfusate. The solution is perfused through a Tenckhoff catheter through a pump and removed from the cavity through drains at a rate of around 1 L/min. At this first moment, only the carrier solution is infused, without chemotherapy. There is also a heat exchanger that keeps the infused solution between 43 and 45 °C, causing the intraperitoneal fluid to remain between 41 and 43 °C. After adjusting all these steps, the chemotherapy is added and the infusion time is started. It is important to note that a plastic protection is placed over the system to protect and prevent possible leakage.

During the open technique, the heated chemotherapy is properly distributed throughout the cavity and there is no accumulation of temperature or chemotherapy, having a better distribution of fluids when compared to the closed technique. The fact that the cavity remains open during the procedure favors its main disadvantages. During this technique, there is greater heat dissipation, making temperature control difficult, in addition to the exposure of professionals involved by direct contact with the drug or aerosols formed by heating the fluid.

The closed technique uses the same catheter and the same probes as the open technique, but the edges are sutured in order to perfuse in a closed system. After starting the infusion of fluids, the patient's abdominal wall must be manually agitated at all times to obtain an even distribution of heat. Therefore, a larger volume of perfusate is usually needed. Because the system is closed, greater pressure is achieved, which may eventually facilitate the penetration of cytotoxic agents into tissues. After finishing the perfusion, the abdomen is opened again and all the contents are removed.

As the system is closed, the ideal temperature is more easily reached and maintained when we camp with the open technique. Another advantage is the minimal exposure of professionals to cytotoxic drugs, either in fluid form or in aerosols. On the other hand, there is an uneven distribution of chemotherapy and heat, which can cause injuries due to high temperatures and undertreated areas [5].

### 15.2.6 Safety

Because this entire process involves chemotherapy, the pharmacist has an essential role, from preparation to administration, even though this last step takes place in the operating room without the supervision of a pharmacist. The orientation process must be very well done and strictly followed by professionals.

First of all, the professional who is carrying the bag prepared with the chemotherapy or even the professionals who will be present in the room must be properly dressed with a waterproof disposable apron, gloves, cap, glasses, mask, among others, in addition to paying attention to any leak in the bag or precipitation.

The operating room itself must also be prepared and organized with disposable and waterproof materials, especially sheets, properly identified disposal containers, in addition to the materials needed in case of extravasation or even spillage. The room must be identified, indicating that HIPEC will take place there, and after CRS to start the perfusion, circulation must be restricted. If the technique to be used is open, a smoke evacuator is used to minimize contamination by aerosols [5].

If chemotherapy spills, room cleaning should be started immediately, and all contaminated clothing should be discarded in the proper location. If the cytotoxic agent comes into contact with the skin, it must be washed with water and mild soap. If the affected area is the eyes, they should be washed with water or saline solution [5], remembering that the parts of the body that have had contact with chemotherapy can be considered contaminated for 48 hours [3].

The patient must always be aware of the risks and adverse effects arising from the use of chemotherapy, so the pharmacist must always guide the patient and family.

## 15.3 Aerosolized and Pressurized Intraperitoneal Chemotherapy (PIPAC)

### 15.3.1 Overview

In an attempt to improve the techniques used to administer intraperitoneal chemotherapy and avoid the difficulties found in peritoneal hyperthermic chemotherapy, the PIPAC model was designed. However, it should not be considered an alternative to CRS/HIPEC in all cases. This new technique has certain advantages compared to techniques that use drugs in liquid form, such as reduced morbidity, better tissue penetration, an efficient distribution of the chemotherapeutic drug, and fewer adverse effects. Because this technique forms aerosols, a disadvantage is the safety of the professionals involved due to the difficult control of the gases formed [6].

In this technique, chemotherapy is nebulized with carbon dioxide ($CO_2$) to create an aerosol, a pharmaceutical form that has two phases: liquid (droplets) and gas. The aerosol is applied directly into the pressurized peritoneal cavity, causing a pressure difference between the intraperitoneal and extraperitoneal means; consequently, the diffusion of substances in the peritoneum is increased [7].

One of the main differences between PIPAC and other techniques, in addition to the pharmaceutical form of the chemotherapy, is the preparation of the operating room. Before starting the procedure, we must pay attention to the presence of three resources present at the site: unidirectional airflow, port with hermetic seal, and negative pressure. Another important point is patient monitoring. The professional must be able to monitor the patient remotely, so he needs the proper equipment such as a remote monitor [8].

As PIPAC is a relatively new technique, there are little data on the drugs used. However, the most used are cisplatin 7.5 mg/m$^2$ in nebulization for around 3 to 6 minutes, followed by doxorubicin 1.5 mg/m$^2$ [7].

### 15.3.2 Technique

When preparing the patient and the room for the PIPAC, the position he will be in must be taken into account, as he needs to be observed from outside the room. To apply the aerosol, a longitudinal incision is made in the abdomen and the device that will administer the drug into the cavity is introduced. After that, a pneumoperitoneum is provoked. From there, we can aspirate the ascetic fluid, if necessary, or proceed to the aerosolization of intraperitoneal chemotherapy.

When the patient, operating room and materials are ready and protected, the team supplies the chemotherapy in the injector and leaves the room, which must be sealed. Only after all these steps begins the administration of the chemotherapy drug. After the aerosolization procedure, the pressure is maintained to remain with the therapeutic pneumoperitoneum. After this time, professionals return to the operating room dressed, the insufflator is turned off, and the drug is aspirated. The medical professional checks the intraperitoneal cavity and then closes the patient's abdomen [8].

### 15.3.3 Safety

In general, care related to chemotherapy is the same as in CRS/HIPEC, where attention must be paid during the transport and administration of the chemotherapy agent and any suspicion of spillage. Pharmaceutical guidance and room preparation continue to be extremely important.

Due to the fact that it generates a lot of aerosols, in theory, this technique offers much more risk to the professionals involved. However, several studies point to the safety of the procedure if the room is properly prepared and professionals properly dressed. Even so, toxicological analysis must be considered.

If there is a spillage of chemotherapy or any aerosol leakage due to failure to prepare the room, cleaning must be started immediately and all the steps mentioned above in relation to HIPEC must be followed: All contaminated clothing must be discarded in the proper place. If the cytotoxic agent comes into contact with the skin, it must be washed with water and mild soap. If the affected area is the eyes, they should be washed with water or saline solution [5], remembering that the parts of the body that have had contact with chemotherapy can be considered contaminated for 48 hours [6–8].

As with HIPEC, the patient must always be aware of the risks and adverse effects arising from the use of chemotherapy, and the pharmaceutical professional is also essential at this time.

## 15.4 Chemoembolization

### 15.4.1 Overview

Another therapy performed in a surgical environment, but which this time is not related to major surgeries or administration routes different from the usual one, is chemoembolization. This procedure is an interventional technique and widely used mainly for the treatment of hepatocellular carcinomas, which is nothing more than the intra-arterial infusion of chemotherapeutic agents with embolic particles, thus causing microinfarctions associated with the local action of chemotherapy.

Hepatocellular carcinomas originate from the malignant transformation of the hepatocyte, possibly associated with chronic liver complications, cirrhosis being the main one. It is also one of the cancers that cause the most deaths worldwide. The main treatment is liver transplantation, given the extensive liver dysfunction caused by the lesions. However, the discovery of this type of cancer may be late, which requires an urgency that cannot always wait for a transplant. This is why chemoembolization is so important in this context.

Chemoembolization is a therapeutic method aimed mainly at slowing down the evolution of hepatocarcinoma and keeping the patient in a position to reach liver transplantation. It can be performed several times with certain time intervals to be defined by the medical team. However, there is no consensus in the literature on how to proceed with chemoembolization in the best way due to several factors that vary according to the institution, such as waiting time.

As there is no consensus, each center uses the chemotherapy drug and the embolic particles they prefer. Mitomycin C, doxorubicin, and cisplatin are the most used neoplastic agents, the former being less toxic, but apparently less effective than the others. The same goes for embolic agents, with lipiodol apparently being less toxic and less effective when compared to gelatin sponge and polyvinyl alcohol. The choice of these agents varies from the severity and stage of the disease to the state of liver function at the time of the procedure.

The infusion of the chemotherapy–embolic agent mixture can be done through several arteries. The main ones are proper hepatic artery, right hepatic artery, and left hepatic artery via femoral artery puncture. Occasionally, access may be via the radial, brachial, or axillary arteries [9].

### 15.4.2 Safety

As a less complex procedure and an exclusively injectable route, chemoembolization offers less risk to the professionals involved. Even so, you need to be very careful during the transport and administration of the drug. The professional's proper attire must also be guided by the pharmacist, as well as the team that will be with the patient after the surgical procedure. It is a consensus and precaution with the patient's excreta for at least 48 hours after administration. Patient and family must also be oriented about the richness and effects of drugs [9].

## 15.5 Intrathecal Chemotherapy

### 15.5.1 Overview

Although the administration of drugs via the intrathecal route is not exclusive to the surgical environment, it can be done via lumbar puncture at the bedside, but there are cases of patients who are taken to the operating room to benefit from this technique, such as those who need sedation or even use the Ommaya catheter.

The prevention of neoplastic infiltration or even the treatment of central nervous system (CNS) neoplasms is done through the intrathecal route, showing considerable efficacy. Even to prevent the relapse of acute lymphoblastic leukemia (ALL), chemotherapy drugs are used in this way.

Due to the existence of the blood–brain barrier (BBB), it is difficult to reach adequate concentrations of several drugs in the CNS. This barrier is a structure formed by endothelial cells from the central nervous system's capillary network, preventing the free passage of molecules and ions. We must also highlight the presence and importance of the cerebrospinal fluid (CSF), which regulates the environment in the central nervous system, and is through it that we are able to diagnose various diseases.

The drugs to be used, volume and diluents, and the administration technique and the professional's preparation are factors that totally influence the effectiveness and appearance of adverse effects [10].

## 15.5.2 Techniques

Basically, intrathecal administration is nothing more than the direct infusion of the drug in the CNS and can be done through two methods: lumbar puncture (LP) or in the lateral ventricle through an Ommaya catheter [10].

### 15.5.2.1 Lumbar Puncture

The aim of this technique is to reach the subarachnoid space with a diagnostic objective, when a certain volume is collected for investigation, or therapeutic, where the drug is infused. One of the determining factors for the technique is the position in which the patient will be during the procedure: preferably in lateral decubitus for adults and sitting for children.

This procedure can be quite painful depending on the professional's experience, the gauge of the needle, and even the patient's pain threshold, which is why local anesthetics are commonly used. Children almost always undergo the procedure with pharmacological sedation before the procedure, and occasionally some adults do too.

In diagnostic lumbar puncture, a small amount of CSF is removed, being 2–3 mL in newborns, 5–8 mL in children and adolescents, and 6–8 mL in adults. The therapeutic objective LP is a continuation of the diagnostic technique, where after removing a certain volume of CSF, the drug is slowly administered between 3 and 5 minutes, in order to avoid headaches. In general, there is no consensus in the literature on drug dilution, but usually a volume of CSF similar to that of the diluted drug is extracted in order to avoid increased intracranial pressure and several other adverse effects.

After intrathecal administration, the patient should be in a position that facilitates the drug penetration or reduces side effects such as post-puncture headache. But this guidance is at the discretion of the medical professional and may vary from 1 hour in the prone position to 12 hours in the supine position.

The most common adverse effects and complications related to the LP technique are post-puncture headache, low back pain, hemorrhages, and even infections [10].

#### 15.5.2.2 Ommaya Catheter

Ommaya reservoir or catheter is an intraventricular device inserted into the lateral ventricles of the brain via the subcutaneous tissue of the scalp. Its main indication is for patients who need frequent and prolonged treatment in the CNS. The placement of this reservoir increases the risk of bleeding and infections, in addition to complications associated with misuse and functioning.

One of the advantages of this technique in relation to LP is the homogeneous distribution of the chemotherapy drug in the subarachnoid space. When we compare the concentrations of drugs in the CSF soon after administration in the two techniques, we observe that the infusion through the catheter reaches a concentration much higher and faster than that of the lumbar puncture. In addition, the patient's position after LP is proven to be very important to reach the desired concentrations, and if the patient does not follow the guidelines, it can affect the treatment.

In intrathecal administration via an Ommaya catheter, the drug is injected into the ventricular reservoir. First, a certain amount of CSF is removed, ranging from 12 to 20 mL, and after that, the chemotherapy is infused at a rate of approximately 1 mL/minute. After the infusion, approximately 10 mL of previously extracted CSF will be reinfused, both to clean the needle and the catheter [10].

### 15.5.3 Drug Choice

Because CSF is a specific medium (Table 15.3), some precautions during drug preparation should be considered, such as pH, osmolarity, and ionization level, as well as diluent characteristics, such as sterility, apyrogenicity, and no preservatives.

It is at this stage of drug preparation that the pharmacist is again present and plays an important role, to guarantee a product with these qualities. Solutions with pH and osmolarity very different from those of CSF can reduce tolerability, the presence of preservatives can cause the most diverse adverse effects, and drug contamination can cause even worse adverse effects.

The main chemotherapy drugs used in practice are methotrexate (MTX), cytarabine (Ara-C), and glucocorticoids. Recent studies have also shown the effectiveness of two monoclonal antibodies: rituximab and trastuzumab.

Methotrexate is not metabolized in the CSF, so its pharmacokinetics are different when administered intravenously. Its elimination depends on CSF flow and usually reaches very low doses considered subtherapeutic after 4 days of intrathecal administration.

**Table 15.3** Physical–chemical properties of CSF [10]

| Parameter | Normal LCR |
|---|---|
| Aspect | Crystalline |
| Cells | 0–5/mm$^3$ (lymphocytes) |
| Proteins | 15–45 mg/dL |
| Glucose | 50–80 mg/dL |
| Chlorides | 116–122 mEq/L |
| Sodium | 117–137 mEq/L |
| Potassium | 2.3–4.6 mEq/L |
| Osmolarity | 292–297 mOsm/L |
| Density | 1.0005–1.0007 g/mL |
| pH | 7.31 |

The dose should not be calculated either by weight or by body surface, as children may have the same volume of CSF as adults. Therefore, to calculate the dose, age is used. The older the age, the higher the dose, which may vary from 6–8 mg in patients under 2 years old, up to 15 mg in adult patients over 18 years old.

Intrathecal administration of MTX can cause both acute and long-term neurotoxicity. Usually after drug infusion, symptoms such as headache, nausea, and neck stiffness may appear, the main adverse effect reported being aseptic meningitis or chemical arachnoiditis. Occasionally, dizziness, seizures, and subacute encephalopathy may occur. To try to minimize the effects, the concomitant administration of corticosteroids is indicated.

Cytarabine has basically the same pharmacokinetic characteristics as MTX, its metabolization in the CSF is practically insignificant, and drug elimination depends on the flow of the cerebrospinal fluid.

Intrathecal ARA-C doses should also be calculated by age not body surface area or weight, ranging from 20 mg mainly for children under 1 year to 100 mg for adults. As undesirable effects of cytarabine, we can point out aseptic meningitis, seizures, encephalopathy, and transverse myelopathy. There is also the alternative of liposomal cytarabine, which is nothing more than a controlled release formulation of aqueous cytarabine encapsulated in spherical and multivesicular particles. Basically, this presentation has as main feature the longer elimination half-life in the LCR. On the other hand, its toxicity is higher and may cause seizures and encephalopathy more frequently, in addition to cauda equina syndrome and pseudotumor cerebri. In general, there is a consensus that the dose to be used is always 50 mg in adults.

Although glucocorticoids are not chemotherapeutic agents, they will be mentioned here because of their importance in the technique of intrathecal administration of antineoplastic agents. Although they are quickly cleared from the CSF, when combined with ARA-C and MTX, they have two main effects: increasing effectiveness and decreasing the incidence of meningeal irritation.

In general, they are drugs with few adverse effects, being related to cases of headache, nausea, and confusion, in addition to isolated cases of depressive syndromes and psychosis. The main drugs of this class used in practice are dexamethasone and prednisolone, but hydrocortisone and methylprednisolone can be used. The doses to be used vary widely from center and which corticosteroid will be used.

Speaking of monoclonal antibodies, trastuzumab is indicated for the treatment of HER2-positive breast cancer and rituximab for B-cell lymphoma. The first one can be administered intrathecally alone or with MTX, in a regimen of up to 25 mg, showing good results. The second can also be administered alone or in combination with liposomal cytarabine, in doses that can reach 50 mg, with good results. Expected effects after infusion of these drugs are headache, nausea, and vomiting.

Finally, intrathecal triple therapy consisting of the administration of MTX, ARA-C, and glucocorticoids, in the same syringe, has shown several promising results, without increasing adverse effects. This mixture has a synergistic effect for both prophylaxis and treatment of neoplastic meningitis [10].

### 15.5.4 Safety

As much as this technique uses low volumes, the drugs used are quite aggressive. Therefore, all the precautions already mentioned above, such as proper attire of all professionals who will participate in the procedure and care with handling, must be considered. In addition to orienting the multidisciplinary team regarding these risks, patient and family guidance is also extremely important.

## 15.6 Clinical Repercussions of Chemotherapy

So far, we have covered several ways in which we can use chemotherapy within the operating room. However, this is not the only point to be considered when relating these two variables. It is extremely important that not only the surgeon has extensive knowledge of drugs, but also the anesthesiologist.

We have seen that in the various techniques presented, patients are sedated; therefore, chemotherapeutic agents will not be the only drugs that will be circulating in the patient's bloodstream. Even patients who will undergo a surgical procedure, other than those already mentioned, such as other oncological surgeries or catheter insertion, may be using curative chemotherapy, neoadjuvants, and adjuvants that may have a clinical repercussion if they interact with other drugs. Today, there are several pharmacological classes of chemotherapeutics (Table 15.4), each with its specificity, action, and adverse effects. As examples, we can mention that the alkylating agents that cause the disruption of the purine ring and blocking mitosis are the largest group of cytotoxic drugs and have nausea, vomiting, and myelosuppression as adverse effects; antimetabolites that have structures similar to several structures in our body, acting on enzymes and blocking the normal cell cycle that mainly causes inflammation and ulcerations; "vinca" alkaloids that break down microtubules present in mitosis are potent neurotoxic and cause hyperuricemia; and anthracyclines that form stable complexes with DNA inhibiting its synthesis, among others.

Citing just a few classes, we can already see how important it is to have knowledge of all the mechanisms of chemotherapy to measure their clinical repercussions (Table 15.5) and possible interactions.

**Table 15.4** Classification of the main chemotherapy drugs [11]

| Classification | Examples |
|---|---|
| Alkylants | Cyclophosphamide, melphalan, thiotepa, busulfan, and carmustine |
| Antimetabolites | Methotrexate, cytarabine, 5-fluoracil, azathioprine, mercaptopurine |
| Antitumor antibiotics | Daunorubicin, doxorubicin, bleomycin |
| Enzymes | Asparaginase |
| Vinca alkaloids | Vincristine, vinblastine, paclitaxel |
| Platinum analogs | Cisplatin, carboplatin |
| Hormones | Tamoxifen, estrogens |
| Drugs that alter the immune response | Cytotoxic immunosuppressants, corticosteroids, immunostimulants |
| Others | Hydroxyurea, procarbazine |

**Table 15.5** Main side effects of some of the most used drugs in clinical practice [11]

| | Cardiovascular | Pulmonary | Renal | Hepatic | Neurological | Immunosuppression |
|---|---|---|---|---|---|---|
| Cyclophosphamide | | | x | x | | xxxx |
| Busulfan | | xx | xx | | | x |
| Melphalan | | x | | x | x | x |
| Carmustine | | x | x | | | |
| Methotrexate | | x | xx | x | | xxx |
| 5-Fluoracil | | | | | x | xxxx |
| Cytarabine | | x | | x | | xxx |
| Azathioprine | | | | xx | | xxxx |
| Vincristine | | | | x | | xx |
| Vinblastine | | | | | x | xx |
| Paclitaxel | x | | | | | xx |
| Daunorubicin | xxx | | | | | x |
| Doxorubicin | xxx | | | x | | |
| Bleomycin | xxx | xxx | | | | |
| Mitomycin | x | x | | | x | |
| Asparaginase | | | x | xx | x | xx |
| Cisplatin | x | | xxxx | | xx | x |

Captions: x= minimum, xx = low, xxx = moderate, xxxx = severe

When we analyze each system in the body, we see how much of the effects chemotherapy drugs can have the following:

- Cardiovascular: cardiomyopathy, myocardial fibrosis, myocardial ischemia.
- Pulmonary: pneumonitis, pulmonary edema, pleural effusion.
- Gastrointestinal: nausea and vomiting, electrolyte disturbances, mucositis.
- Hematopoietic: myelosuppression.
- Liver: liver dysfunction.
- Renal: renal dysfunction, nephropathy.
- Immunological: anaphylactic reactions.
- Neurological: autonomous and peripheral neuropathies, seizures.
- Metabolic: inadequate suppression of hormones.

Patients exposed to these chemotherapeutic agents must have their anamnesis well done and their history well explored. A major surgery with a lot of volume infusion can be fatal for a patient who is already experiencing some chemotherapy-related cardiotoxicity [11].

## 15.7 Drug Interactions of Chemotherapy Agents

Drug interactions, on the other hand, can be considered a little more predictable and can be avoided or even monitored. Table 15.6 shows us some of the main interactions that can occur.

In addition to the interactions shown in the table, several others can be cited and entered the radar of professionals responsible for the patient, such as physicians and pharmacists, for example:

- Vincristine or vinblastine: It can cause peripheral neuropathy, which added to the effect of vasodilators can cause hypotension in the preoperative period.
- Methotrexate: It may increase the sedative effect of barbiturate and opioid drugs.

**Table 15.6** Main interactions between chemotherapy and drugs used in anesthesia [11]

| Chemotherapeutic agent | Anesthetic agent | Interaction effect |
|---|---|---|
| Cyclophosphamide | Succinylcholine | Increased effect of succinylcholine |
| Azathioprine | Neuromuscular blockers | "Resistance" |
| Procarbazine | CNS depressants | Increased effects of sympathomimetics |
| Bleomycin | Oxygen | Pulmonary fibrosis |
| Thiotepa | Succinylcholine | Increased effect of succinylcholine |
| Methotrexate | Nitrous oxide | Increased cytotoxic effect and toxicity of methotrexate |

- Estrogens and androgens: They can lead to hypercalcemia, which requires strict monitoring of calcium and renal output.
- Azathioprine: It may reduce the metabolism of ester-type anesthetics.

Due to this fact, the guidelines are given by the pharmacists to the entire team that will participate in the procedure and the good relationship of these with surgeons and anesthetists facilitates the exchange of knowledge about interactions and increases the chance to avoid them.

## 15.8 Conclusion

Since the surgical treatment of several cancers is increasing, knowledge about the entire process of using chemotherapeutics in operating rooms or even preoperatively becomes extremely important. Knowing how a given anticancer drug works and how to manage it is one of the great challenges.

The pharmacist has an outstanding role in this entire process, as he is the professional who will prepare the chemotherapy, and at the same time, he is the professional who guides the entire team regarding the risks inherent in the use of chemotherapy in the various techniques already mentioned.

Analyzing the techniques presented in the chapter, we see room for improvement in all of them, whether in the study of new drugs, evolution of the techniques themselves, and awareness of all the professionals involved.

Knowing how to manage the clinical repercussions of a chemotherapy drug is still for few and that makes a difference, as it can save lives. Likewise, managing an interaction between chemotherapy and any other drug used in the procedure is still very important.

## References


1. Silva, Luiz Antonio Santini Rodrigues Da. Oncologic surgery: a great challenge. Revista do ColégioBrasileiro de Cirurgiões [online]. 2016; 43(03):139–140. Accessed 18 Aug 2021. Available in: https://doi.org/10.1590/0100-69912016003012. ISSN 1809-4546.
2. Batista, Thales Paulo et al. A proposal of Brazilian Society of Surgical Oncology (BSSO/SBCO) for standardizing cytoreductive surgery (CRS) plus hyperthermic intraperitoneal chemotherapy (HIPEC) procedures in Brazil: pseudomixoma peritonei, appendiceal tumors and malignant peritoneal mesothelioma. Revista do Colégio Brasileiro de Cirurgiões [online]. 2017, 44, n. 05. 530–544. Accessed 18 Aug 2021. Available in: https://doi.org/10.1590/0100-69912017005016. ISSN 1809-4546. https://doi.org/10.1590/0100-69912017005016.
3. Kearsley Rosemarie, Egan Sinead, Mc McCaul Conan. Anesthesia for cytoreductive surgery (CRS) with hyperthermic intraperitoneal chemotherapy (HIPEC). ATOTW 379. 2018. Accessed 18 Aug 2021. Available in: https://resources.wfsahq.org/wp-content/uploads/379_english.pdf.
4. Batista, Thales Paulo, Badiglian, Levon, Leão, Cristiano Souza. Exploring flow rate selection in HIPEC procedures. Revista do Colégio Brasileiro de Cirurgiões [online]. 2016, 43, 6. 476–479. Accessed 18 Aug 2021. Available in: ISSN 1809-4546. https://doi.org/10.1590/0100-69912016006014.
5. González-Moreno S, González-Bayón LA, Ortega-Pérez G. Hyperthermic intraperitoneal chemotherapy: Rationale and technique. World J Gastrointest Oncol. 2010; 2(2): 68–75. Accessed 18 Aug 2021. Available in: https://www.ncbi.nlm.nih.gov/pmc/articles/PMC2999165/. 10.4251/wjgo.v2.i2.68. PMID: 21160924; PMCID: PMC2999165.

6. Willaert W, Sessink P, Ceelen W. Occupational safety of pressurized intraperitoneal aerosol chemotherapy (PIPAC). Pleura Peritoneum. 2017; 2(3): 121–128. Accessed 18 Aug 2021. Available in: https://www.ncbi.nlm.nih.gov/pmc/articles/PMC6328076/. 10.1515/pp-2017-0018. Epub 12 de agosto de 2017. PMID: 30911641; PMCID: PMC6328076.
7. Solass W, Giger-Pabst U, Zieren J, Reymond MA. Pressurized intraperitoneal aerosol chemotherapy (PIPAC): occupational health and safety aspects. Ann Surg Oncol. 2013;20(11):3504–3511. Accessed 18 Aug 2021. Available in: https://pubmed.ncbi.nlm.nih.gov/23765417. 10.1245/s10434-013-3039-x. Epub 2013 Jun 14. PMID: 23765417; PMCID: PMC3764316.
8. Seitenfus, Rafael et al. Aerosolized and Pressurized Intraperitoneal Chemotherapy (PIPAC) via single port: alternative application in the control of peritoneal metastases. Revista do ColégioBrasileiro de Cirurgiões [online]. 2018, 45, 4:e1909. Accessed August 18, 2021. Available in: https://doi.org/10.1590/0100-6991e-20181909. Epub 20 Ago 2018. ISSN 1809–4546.
9. Langer, Luís Francisco et al. Contribution of chemoembolization of hepatocarcinomas in cirrhotic patients awaiting liver transplantation. Radiologia Brasileira [online]. 2005, 38, 1 1-6. Accessed 18 Aug 2021. Available in: https://doi.org/10.1590/S0100-39842005000100003. Epub 23 Mar 2005. ISSN 1678–7099.
10. Olmos-Jiménez Raquel, Espuny-Miró Alberto, Cárceles-Rodríguez Carlos, Díaz-Carrasco María Sacramento. Practical aspects of the use of intrathecal chemotherapy. Farm Hosp. [Internet]. 2017. 41(1): 105–129. Accessed 18 Aug 2021; Available in: http://scielo.isciii.es/scielo.php?script=sci_arttext&pid=S1130-63432017000100105&lng=es. https://doi.org/10.7399/fh.2017.41.1.10616.
11. Lacerda, Márcio Augusto. Chemotherapy and anesthesia. Revista Brasileira de Anestesiologia [online]. 2001, 51, 3. 250-270. Accessed 18 Aug 2021. Available in: https://doi.org/10.1590/S0034-70942001000300009. Epub 10 Fev 2011. ISSN 1806-907X. https://doi.org/10.1590/S0034-70942001000300009.

**Alessandro Menegon** Clinical Pharmacist at the Onco-Hematology and Adult and Pediatric Bone Marrow Transplant Unit of Hospital 9 de Julho. Graduated in Pharmacy from the ABC Medical School (FMABC). Postgraduation degree in Clinical Pharmacy with emphasis in pharmaceutical prescription by the Institute of Research and Education in Health of São Paulo (IPESSP).

# Chemotherapy for Rheumatology

# 16

Celina de Jesus Guimarães,
Pedro Mikael da Silva Costa,
José de Brito Vieira Neto,
and Anderson Cavalcante Guimarães

C. de Jesus Guimarães (✉)
Postgraduate Program in Pharmacology, Department of Physiology and Pharmacology, Faculty of Medicine, Federal University of Ceará, Laboratory of Experimental Oncology, Center for Research and Development of Medicines (NPDM), Fortaleza, CE, Brazil

Hospital Pharmacy, Fundação Centro de Controle de Oncologia do Estado do Amazonas (FCECON-AM), Manaus, AM, Brazil

P. M. da Silva Costa
Postgraduation Program in Biotecnology – RENORBIO, Laboratório de Oncologia Experimental, Núcleo de Pesquisa e Desenvolvimento de Medicamentos (NPDM), Fortaleza, CE, Brazil

J. de Brito Vieira Neto
Postgraduate Program in Pharmacology, Department of Physiology and Pharmacology, Faculty of Medicine, Federal University of Ceará, Laboratory of Experimental Oncology, Center for Research and Development of Medicines (NPDM), Fortaleza, CE, Brazil

A. C. Guimarães
Chemistry Department, Exact Science Instituit, Universidade Federal do Amazonas, Manaus, AM, Brazil



C. W. P. Schmidt, K. M. Otoni (eds.), *The Golden Guide to Oncologic Pharmacy*, https://doi.org/10.1007/978-3-030-98596-7_16

## 16.1 Introduction

Rheumatology is a branch of medicine related to the different conditions that affect any structure that makes up the musculoskeletal system, such as joints, bones, cartilage, tendons, ligament, and muscles [1]. Rheumatic diseases, also called arthritis or musculoskeletal diseases, include a common symptoms like joint pain, loss of motion in a joint or joints, and inflammatory processes. There exists a complex relationship between malignancies diseases and the development of autoimmune and rheumatic diseases, as a function of the cancer progress or the use of cancer chemotherapeutic agents, which can also lead to manifestations of rheumatologic diseases and other kinds of adverse effects, as anomalies of the immune system, which augment risks of infections or a frail immunity [2, 3].

Chemotherapy refers to treatment with drugs that are used often to kill or slow the reproduction of rapidly growing cancer cells. But there are also other uses for chemotherapy. Rheumatology is designed to alter the abnormal behavior of cells. In many cases, inflammation results from autoimmunity, a malfunction of the immune system in which a person's own tissues or organs are mistakenly attacked by the body's immune system.

Consequently, rheumatic and malignant diseases sometimes occur in the same patient, either as consequence or simultaneously. It is important to clarify that there are records that establish an increased risk of developing malignant diseases due to systemic inflammatory diseases, such as rheumatoid arthritis (RA), Sjögren's syndrome, or systemic lupus erythematosus. This condition requires that the decision regarding treatment is made by the oncologist in association with the rheumatologist, and once the management is decided, these patients need intensive monitoring.

It is possible to establish a causal relationship between the two conditions. In principle, it is plausible that a healthy person could develop a malignant disease and, over time, develop a rheumatologic disease, with no apparent cause connected with each other. However, the treatment of malignant disease can induce a rheumatic condition (such as osteoporosis), and in some cases, anticancer treatment itself can be used to treat some rheumatic complications, such as rituximab and can be used to treat lymphoma and RA [4]. On the other hand, if the initial situation starts with a rheumatic disease, it is important to note that some supportive drugs used in rheumatology have the potential to induce or promote a malignant disease or can also be used in the treatment of malignant diseases [4]. Considering these aspects, it is possible to observe that there is a close complex relationship between oncological and rheumatological complications.

In this chapter, it is intended to gather information on some rheumatic diseases, relate their pathophysiology, epidemiology, and their respective treatments, including the treatments that are common between rheumatic and oncological diseases, such as antimetabolites and monoclonal antibodies, and, additionally, list some reports of case of occurrence of malignant disease simultaneously or because of rheumatic disease. The indication for the use of NSAIDs and corticosteroids will not be addressed, despite being the first line of treatment in many rheumatologic diseases.

## 16.2 Systemic Lupus Erythematosus

Systemic lupus erythematosus (SLE) is a chronic autoimmune disease with a wide range of clinical manifestations and multisystem involvement. Etiology of SLE is complex because disease initiation and progression involve environmental, immunological, genetic, and hormonal factors. SLE immunopathogenesis includes dysregulation of the innate and adaptive immune systems, presence of autoantibodies and immunocomplexes, activation of the complement system, production of several cytokines including type I interferons, and disturbance on the elimination of nucleic acids after cell death [5, 6].

More than 80 risk loci for SLE susceptibility have been identified, and many genes were related to adaptive and innate immunity like HLA, BLK, IRF5, ITGAM-ITGAX, and PXK, but several genetics risk associations such JAZF1, XKR6, UHRF1BP1, or WDFY4 still remain unexplained. Environmental triggers related to lupus are ultraviolet light, drugs/supplements (sulfa-drugs), smoking, infection by Epstein–Barr Virus, vitamin D deficiency, and silica [7, 8].

Female gender and hormonal influence are expressive risk factors for SLE. While androgens are considered protective, prolactin and estrogens stimulate autoimmunity, lymphocyte activation, and higher levels of B-cell activation factor [5].

Both innate and adaptive immune systems participate in the pathogenesis of SLE. Apoptotic cells (like UV-light exposed keratinocytes) release DAMPs activating Toll-like receptors 2, 4, and 6 (TLRs) leading to activation of transcription factors for the expression of proinflammatory mediators, for example, IFN-b (interferon B). TLRs 7 and 9 are recognized single-stranded RNA and demethylated DNA causing increase in the production of interferon-alpha and RNA-binding autoantibodies such as Ro, La, Sm, and RNP. Additionally, RNA sensors (RIG-1, MDA-5) and DNA sensors (IFI16, DAI) placed in cytoplasm promote activation of transcription factors IRF3 and NF-κB in an TLR-independent pathway. Damaged cell-derived antigens can be presented to T cells by antigen-presenting cells. T-cell gene expression is dysregulated in SLE, and these T cells express cytokines related to altered regulatory T-cell production (IL2) and increase in mononuclear cell production (IL-6, IL-10, IL-12, and IL-23). High expression of interferon-γ results in defective T-cell production. Autoreactive B cells are activated by CD40L and cytokine produced by T cells. Autoantibodies produced by activated B cells are pathogenic and can induce tissue and organ damage by immune complex deposition, complement and neutrophil activation, and disrupting cell function resulting in apoptosis [5, 7, 9].

Around the world, women are more affected by SLE than men. Black, Hispanic, and Asian populations have higher incidence and prevalence rates than white populations. Mortality among patients with SLE is two to three times higher than that of the general population, and the main causes of death include are infections and cardiovascular disease [7, 8].

SLE treatment seeks to ensure low degree of activity by immunomodulators and immunosuppression, preventing organ damage and reducing exposition to known triggers. Immunomodulators are important in the immune system regulation reducing the risk of infection or malignancy, and in this approach, drugs are used like hydroxychloroquine, which is the drug of choice for most dermatologic manifestations, vitamin D, and dehydroepiandrosterone (DHEA), which is a precursor for androgens and is related to regulation of several proinflammatory cytokines. Corticosteroid administration in high doses or "pulsed" is important to reduce the autoimmune response preventing damage in cases of nephritis, vasculitis, central nervous system lupus, myocarditis, or alveolitis [7, 9].

SLE treatment can also include cytotoxic and immunosuppressants as cyclophosphamide, which is a drug that causes depletion of T and B cells and suppression of antibody production. Cyclophosphamide therapy is associated with premature ovarian failure, hemorrhagic cystitis, increased risk of bladder and other malignancies, and leukopenia along with an increased risk of infections [7]. A nasal type of an extranodal NK/T-cell lymphoma has been diagnosed in a 68-year-old woman with SLE treated with various immunosuppressive agents including steroids, cyclophosphamide, and tacrolimus [10]. In other studies, two women with SLE had developed bladder cancer after prolonged treatment with cyclophosphamide [11]. In non-Hodgkin's lymphoma, cyclophosphamide therapy had also strong relation to bladder cancer. Administration of cumulative doses of 50 g or more increases the risk to approximately seven excess bladder cancers per 100 NHL patients [12]. Due to its toxicity, cyclophosphamide had been replaced by less toxic immunosuppressive medications such as mycophenolate, calcineurin inhibitors, and azathioprine for nephritis and rituximab for severe central nervous system lupus treatment [7].

Mycophenolate mofetil treatment in lupus patients has been associated with the development of several central nervous system lymphoma [13, 14], including diffuse large B-cell lymphoma [15, 16]. Methotrexate had induced Hodgkin's disease in a 48-year-old man with a history of systemic lupus erythematosus (SLE), and its discontinuation facilitated Hodgkin's disease reversal [17]. A 24-year-old woman with SLE methotrexate-associated

Hodgkin's lymphoma had tumoral mass reduced 3 weeks after withdrawing the methotrexate treatment [18]. Additionally, bone marrow metastasis of Merkel cell carcinoma had been described for a 73-year-old woman with SLE and Sjögren's syndrome, who had been treated with prednisolone and methotrexate for 10 years [19]. A patient with SLE and family history of immunological aberrations and malignancies was diagnosed with immunoblastic lymphoma. This patient had done 3 years of treatment with azathioprine and prednisone [18].

It was described that SLE is also a risk factor for developing cervical neoplasia, especially pre-malignant cervical lesions. The risk is higher when SLE patients are treated with immunosuppressants than when they are treated with antimalarials [20]. It was also observed that patients with SLE are at higher risk of developing hematological malignancies than the general population. Hematological malignancies diagnosed before or concurrent with SLE had a better prognostic than the ones diagnosed after SLE, and diffuse large B-cell lymphoma was the most common type of lymphoma in these patients [21].

Therapeutic antibodies had become an option to treat SLE patients, which had developed resistance to conventional treatments or that are non-responders to therapy with steroids and immunosuppressants [21]. Complete remission of mucosa-associated lymphoid tissue lymphoma of the lacrimal glands was observed in a SLE patient after treatment with four once-weekly doses of rituximab 375 mg/m$^2$ every 6 months for 2 years [22].

New promising treatments for SLE are being developed, many of them based on a specific target or pathway. These new approaches must consider a precise characterization of disease phenotypes based on molecular and clinical features to allow more effective and less toxic regimens in the future [7].

## 16.3 Sjögren's Syndrome

Sjögren's syndrome (SS) is a relatively common autoimmune rheumatic disease, which is most common in women in the fifth decade of life, being nine times more common among women than among men, with peak onset during menopause [23, 24]. SS is a slowly progressive chronic disease, characterized by a lymphocytic infiltrate that affects the epithelium of exocrine (mainly salivary and tear) glands, leading to a decreased production of tears and saliva [23–25], and can occur in association with other autoimmune diseases such as systemic lupus erythematosus (SLE) and rheumatoid arthritis (RA) [24, 25]. The latter is manifested by hyper-gammaglobulinemia and the presence of serum autoantibodies, including antinuclear antibodies, rheumatoid factor, cryoprecipitable immunoglobulins, and antibodies against two ribonucleoprotein complexes named Ro/SSA and La/SSB; these antibodies are considered hallmarks of the disease [23, 25]. Although SS is classically considered to be localized disease of the exocrine glands, mainly manifested with oral and ocular dryness, and connective tissue disease [23], this is a systemic disease with high risk of transformation to lymphoma, with a small number of cases that can be complicated by the development of non-Hodgkin lymphoma [24]. It also has a wide range of systemic clinical manifestations that affect essentially any organ system. SS can be "primary" if it occurs alone (pSS) or "secondary" (sSS) when it is associated with another autoimmune disease [26]. Primary Sjögren's syndrome affects the joints, lungs, central nervous system (CNS), peripheral nervous system (PNS), and kidneys in approximately 50% of patients [24, 25]. The secondary Sjögren's syndrome is associated with an established connective tissue disease [23].

SS is considered a multifactorial process originating from the interaction between genetic factors and exogenous and endogenous agents that are able to trigger an abnormal autoimmune response mediated by T and B lymphocytes. Some recurrent events are usually associated with SS, including trigger phase factors induced by environmental factors, specific epigenetic changes, genetic predisposition or hormonal regulation; followed by dysregulation of the function of the epithelial cells of the salivary and lacrimal glands; and consequently, chronic inflammation with lymphocytic infiltrates (especially B lymphocytes) and autoantibody production [26].

Targeted therapy for Sjögren's syndrome is focused on relieving symptoms of oral (xerostomia) and ocular dryness, in addition to preventing complications such as tooth decay, dysphagia, and oral candidiasis. In most patients, the main aim of therapy is to improve quality of life by treating the ocular and oral dryness and fatigue symptoms [25]. The use of artificial saliva containing mucin or mucin with xanthan or guar gum [27], and eye lubricants containing either sodium hyaluronate or hydroxypropyl methylcellulose has been shown to improve subjective symptoms of oral and ocular dryness, respectively. Other kinds of care means mouth hygiene, thorough dental follow-up, stimulation of salivary flow (sugar-free gum or citrus juice), and muscarinic agonists, such as pilocarpine and cevimeline, for the treatment of oral dryness and, to a lesser extent, ocular dryness in patients with primary SS [23, 28]. Furthermore, alcohol, smoking, and medications such as diuretics, antidepressants (except for selective serotonin reuptake inhibitors, especially escitalopram and fluoxetine), and antihistamines should be avoided because they exacerbate mucosal dryness, just like air conditioning should also be avoided [23].

However, when it comes to a patient with systemic complications related to the syndrome, the recommended approach includes other therapeutic agents common to the practice of cancer therapy and should be adapted to organs affected and their severity [24]. In such cases, in patients with inflammatory arthritis, methotrexate (MTX) can usually be recommended [23, 24]. For cases of persistent arthritis, rituximab has been shown to significantly improve the tender and swollen joint count [23]. It is effective in improving many manifestations in SS, such as glandular involvement, fatigue, disease activity, immunological parameters, glandular lymphocytic infiltration, systemic manifestations, and quality of life [24]. Cytotoxic drugs, such as cyclophosphamide, are reserved for severe extraglandular manifestations, including cutaneous vasculitis and glomerulonephritis [23]. Abatacept and belimumab are promising drugs to improve disease activity, immunological profile, and quality of life. These drugs can be considered in the treatment of SS in refractory cases and with high systemic disease activity [24, 26].

Malignant non-Hodgkin lymphoma (NHL) of B-cell lineage occurs in about 5% of patients with SS, who are at a significantly increased risk of developing NHL compared with the general population [25, 27]. These lymphomas are mostly B-cell non-Hodgkin's lymphomas, with a predominance of the low-grade, marginal-zone histologic type [28]. These patients belong to a high-risk group and require monitoring at closer intervals and, if necessary, additional diagnostic investigations, such as chest radiography and abdominal ultrasound [25]. In these cases, the conduct must follow the established NHL treatment protocols.

On the other hand, there are already registers about cases of the cancer treatment that induces SS. Ghosn and coworkers, in 2018, made the first case report of a patient who developed a complication of severe neuro-Sjögren's syndrome induced by pembrolizumab treatment. In this case, a melanoma patient treated for 8 months with pembrolizumab developed a right trigeminal neuropathy, with a salivary gland biopsy showing inflammatory changes suggestive of Sjögren's syndrome. The treatment initially began by intravenous frontline methylprednisone that changed for rituximab, which led to a quick clinical improvement [29]. Other register includes the use of other immune checkpoint inhibitor, nivolumab, for the treatment of gastric cancer. In this case, xerostomia developed after two cycles and the use of prednisone and pilocarpine did not improve either the subjective symptoms or the salivary flow rates, maybe because the treatment with nivolumab was not discontinued until the tumor cessation [30].

## 16.4 Psoriatic Arthritis

Psoriatic arthritis (PsA) is a chronic inflammatory musculoskeletal and skin disease. The musculoskeletal is associated with psoriasis, manifesting most commonly with peripheral arthritis, dactylitis, enthesitis, and spondylitis [31, 32] and presents its similar impact on quality of life and functional ability as in rheumatoid arthritis [33]. The skin complications are associated with psoriasis and nail disease [31]. The incidence of PsA is approximately 6 for each 100,000 per year, and the prevalence is around

1–2 per 1000 in the general population and can affect both men and women in the same proportion [32, 34].

The physiopathology involving psoriasis and psoriatic arthritis is associated with class I MHC alleles. Genome-wide association scans have shown that certain polymorphisms in the gene encoding interleukin-23 receptor (IL23R), along with variants in nuclear factor κB (NF-κB) gene expression (TNIP1) and signaling (TNFAIP3), and TNF expression are associated with psoriatic arthritis. Association studies have identified additional risk alleles in patients with psoriasis and in those with psoriatic arthritis, including interleukin-12A (IL-12A), interleukin-12B (IL-12B), IL-23R, and genes that regulate NF-κB. In addition, it has been shown that T cells are important in psoriasis and psoriatic arthritis. A central role for CD8+ T cells in disease pathogenesis is supported by the association with HLA class I alleles, oligoclonal CD8+ T-cell expansion, and the association of psoriatic arthritis with human immunodeficiency virus disease [34].

Beyond the musculoskeletal and skin features, patients with PsA experience fatigue, physical function limitations, sleep disturbance, and diminished work capacity and social participation. In addition to the association with extra-articular manifestations such as uveitis and inflammatory bowel disease (IBD), PsA is also associated with several comorbidities including obesity and metabolic disease (diabetes, hypertension, hyperlipidemia, fatty liver disease, cardiovascular outcomes), depression, and anxiety [31].

To choose the appropriate conduct, it is necessary to differentiate psoriatic arthritis from rheumatoid arthritis, osteoarthritis, gout, pseudogout, systemic lupus erythematosus, and other forms of spondyloarthritis. Psoriatic arthritis tends to be oligoarticular and less symmetric than rheumatoid arthritis, although with time, psoriatic arthritis may become polyarticular and symmetric. The affected joints are less tender in psoriatic arthritis than in rheumatoid arthritis and may have a purplish discoloration [33, 34].

Treatment for PsA includes traditional or conventional disease-modifying antirheumatic drugs (MTX, sulfasalazine, cyclosporine, leflunomide, apremilast), biologic therapies such as TNF inhibitors (TNFi) (etanercept, infliximab, adalimumab, golimumab, certolizumab pegol), IL-17 inhibitors (IL-17i) (secukinumab, ixekizumab), IL-12/23 inhibitor (IL-12/23i) (ustekinumab), and new targeted oral agents including a phosphodiesterase-4 inhibitor and a Janus kinase (JAK)/signal transducer and activator of transcription (STAT) inhibitor (tofacitinib) and anti-CTLA-4 (abatacept) [31–34]. In reference to psoriasis, therapies are possible to include IL-17R blockers, such as brodalumab and IL-23 inhibitors, such as guselkumab, tildrakizumab, and risankizumab [31].

Skin cancer, particularly nonmelanoma skin cancer (NMSC), is among the most reported cancers in patients with PsA. Studies in psoriasis report up to a sevenfold increase in the risk of skin cancer and risk of squamous cell carcinoma (but not basal cell carcinoma), in patients treated with phototherapy, including high-dose psoralen plus ultraviolet (PUVA), methotrexate, and both combined [35]. Law-Ping-Man and coworkers in 2016 registered a case of psoriasis and psoriatic arthritis induced by nivolumab, an immune checkpoint inhibitor, in a patient with advanced lung cancer. It was identified in a patient with no personal or family history of psoriasis who developed psoriatic skin lesions associated with peripheral inflammatory arthritis after the eighth infusion of nivolumab, during therapy for metastatic lung cancer. The occurrence of nivolumab-induced psoriasis temporally coincided with regression of the lung cancer lesions. The management of this adverse reaction was conducted with the withdrawal of nivolumab for 4 weeks, and then, a therapy with oral MTX at a dose of 10 mg/week in combination with a low dose of oral prednisone (15 mg/day) and topical corticosteroids was introduced. After 1 month of therapy, both psoriatic skin lesions and joint symptoms gradually resolved, allowing gradual tapering of MTX and prednisone. Thereafter, nivolumab was restarted with continued response and without recurrence of the psoriasis [36]. Another case reported by Ruiz-Banobre and colleagues, in 2017, describes a patient treated by nivolumab for therapy for metastatic non-small cell lung cancer, and after the eleventh cycle of nivolumab, the patient complained of joint pain again and with the clinical suspicion of inflammatory arthritis. In this last case, the nivolumab therapy was not discontinued and the use of sulfasalazine was introduced, with no positive response and changed for methotrexate

10 mg associated with folate 5 mg per week (to minimize toxicity), with a great improvement in the patient quality of life [37].

## 16.5 Takayasu's Arteritis

Takayasu arteritis (TA) is an idiopathic, granulomatous, large-vessel arteritis that predominantly involves the aorta, its major branch arteries, and (less frequently) the pulmonary arteries, with variable presentation in different ethnicities and countries [38–41]. It is more common in younger women [38, 41]. The clinical manifestations include constitutional symptoms, elevated levels of inflammation markers, and arterial stenosis and/or aneurysms resulting in limb claudication and absent pulses [38]. Its overall incidence has been estimated to be 2/1000,000 per year and occurs more frequently in women, representing 90% of cases in adults, while series on childhood TA have shown different female/male ratios, depending on location. For example, in the Japanese population where TA was originally described, the majority (80–90%) of the patient consists of females, contrary to what was observed in Indian, Thai, and Israeli with a proportion of male patients around 31–38% [40].

As for the age group, some registers have found a double peak incidence: one at age 10–15 years and a second one at age 20–24 years. Female patients seem to have a major incidence peak between age 15 and 19 years representing the leading cause of stenotic aorto-arteriopathy and one of the most prevalent causes of vascular hypertension in childhood [39].

TA has been described as the infiltration of inflammatory cells into the adventitia and media resulting in a cell-mediated immune response, involving NK T cells and CD4 T cells, which form characteristic granulomas and giant cells [40], with three possible theories for its pathology: the genetic hypothesis, associated with the HLA complex (human leukocyte antigen); the infection hypothesis involving case reports of HIV patients, post-vaccination patients against hepatitis B and tuberculosis, with evidence of expression of circulating antibodies against aortic endothelial cells induced by the expression of adhesion molecules and secretion of pro-inflammatory cytokines by endothelial cells of the aortic arteries, which suggests a potential pathogenic role of these autoantibodies [39, 41]; and finally the immunological hypothesis that suggests the both circulating anti-endothelial cell antibodies and autoantibody-producing B-cell infiltrates in inflamed vessels point to a role of humoral immunity [41].

The treatment of TA is aimed at controlling vascular inflammation and preventing irreversible organ damage and is dependent on the stage and presentation of the disease [39, 40]. After the use of glucocorticoids [42], the second line of treatment indicated is the MTX. Methotrexate is often used as the initial immunosuppressive agent, but other therapies such as tumor necrosis factor inhibitors and azathioprine can be considered as well [38, 39, 42]. Other therapies have been indicated such as mycophenolate mofetil (MMF), leflunomide [39, 42], and cyclophosphamide (CYC) [39]. Considering pediatric patients, TNF inhibitors, such as etanercept, and anti-TNF-α monoclonal antibodies, such as adalimumab, and infliximab [39, 40], furthermore the IL-6 inhibitor, tocilizumab (TCZ), and B-cell-directed strategies such as the monoclonal anti-CD20 antibody, such as rituximab, have been increasingly used in the treatment of TA in children [39].

A retrospective cohort study, developed by Park and colleagues, in 2013, estimates the incidence of cancer in Takayasu arteritis patients and compares it with the incidence in general population. They conclude that overall cancer incidence is not increased compared with the general population, but that the incidence of myelodysplastic syndrome (MDS) might be increased, probably due to the patients exposed to cyclophosphamide years before, considering that an alkylating agent can increase the risk of [43].

## 16.6 Rheumatoid Arthritis

Rheumatoid arthritis (RA) is an autoimmune disease characterized by its chronic inflammation state that mainly causes impairment and damage to the joints, therefore leading to disability, early death, and social economics health issues [44, 45]. The prevalence of RA worldwide is about 2%, and Australia is the country with the highest indices [46].

The etiology of RA is not well understood; however, different studies show that environmental factors and genetics play an important role in RA development [44, 47]. Environmental factors like infection, smoking, alcohol, red meat, and location of birth seem to be relevant aspects related to RA [47, 48]. Despite that, heritability and genetics are associated with risk factors for developing RA. Studies show that a family history of RA rises the chance of developing this disease by five times [44, 49]. In addition, the human leukocyte antigen (HLA) is a complex of genes with high indices of polymorphism, which is responsible for different mechanisms on the immune system, for example, presentation of intracellular antigens and relation with antigen-specific immune response [50]. Moreover, some HLA alleles are related to increased risk of developing autoimmune diseases, such as RA [50].

The pathogenesis of RA is mainly linked to the process of citrullination, that is a post-translational modification of protein amino acids from arginine to citrulline by the action of peptidyl-arginine) deiminase enzymes (PADs) [51]. These citrullinated proteins are recognized by an abnormal response of anti-citrullinated protein antibodies (ACPAs) that may be related to the expression of two genes, HLA-DR1 and HLA-DR4 [45].

As mentioned above, RA is complex disease, where there is no cure. However, there is a range of pharmacologic therapies based on early treatment or support. The main treatment is based on the use of conventional disease-modifying antirheumatic drugs (cDMARDs), which can be classified as a group of immunosuppressive and immunomodulatory drugs [52]. Among cDMARDs, the most used one is methotrexate that can have different mechanisms for its clinical benefits in RA, such as increasing adenosine signaling that promotes an anti-inflammatory response, induction of T-cell death, and interfering with the methyl donation cascade [53]. Another important DMARDs is the cyclophosphamide that has proven benefit in treating patients with RA. In addition, cyclophosphamide is an alkylating agent that binds to DNA, therefore impairing DNA replication in immune-competent cells [54].

Leflunomide is a newer cDMARD that acts by suppressing the production of pyrimidines through inhibition of dihydroorotate dehydrogenase [54]. Besides the cDMARDs, there are the biologic DMARDs that present a more specific mechanism of action, such as hindering cytokine activity and impairing signaling for T-cell activation [52]. Adalimumab is monoclonal antibody that specifically targets the tumor necrosis factor (TNF), an important cytokine that promotes inflammation and damage to the joints in RA [55]. In addition, rituximab is also used to treat RA, because of its ability to bind to CD20, therefore inducing reduction in different B cells culminating in a decrease in cytokine, autoantibody production, and B-cell antigen presentation ability [56].

Interestingly, some of the drugs cited above were first developed for the treatment of cancer. However, there is a risk of patients with RA under the use of antineoplastic drugs of developing cancer. A study conducted by Buchbinder and colleagues (2008) in Australia showed that patients with RA treated with methotrexate have a higher risk of developing different types of cancer, such as melanoma, non-Hodgkin's lymphoma, and lung cancer when compared to general population. Moreover, different studies present that the use of cyclophosphamide increases the chances of developing some cancer, for example, hematologic and bladder cancer [57–59]. However, a meta-analysis study showed that there is no increased risk of developing cancer for RA patients treated with biologic DMARDs [60].

Besides that, chemotherapy for the treatment of cancer can induce a range of adverse effects, such as RA in a discrete way [3]. Moreover, different reports suggest that gefitinib and sunitinib, both tyrosine kinase inhibitors, were able to induce RA in cancer patient [61–63]. In addition, another report described that a cancer patient treated with irinotecan developed RA [64].

## 16.7 Spondyloarthritis

Spondyloarthritis (SpA), also known as spondyloarthropathy, is a group of inflammatory diseases of the joints and spine with various clinical manifestations. Clinically, the SpA was divided into subtypes: ankylosing spondylitis (AS), reactive arthritis (ReA), psoriatic arthritis (PsA) (previously discussed), arthritis associated with inflammatory bowel disease (SpA-IBD), and undifferentiated spondyloarthritis (uSpA) [65, 66]. And about the skeleton lesion, SpA can be classified as axial SpA (ax-SpA) and peripheral SpA if the involvement is of the spine or axial skeleton [67].

The physiopathology of spondyloarthritis development remains unclear until these data, however some theories relate it to genetic susceptibility, environmental factors, and gut disease, with an important role related to infection by microorganisms [65]. There is an important relationship with the major histocompatibility complex (HMC) class I antigen, with predominant allele of HLA-B*27 [65, 67], a highly polymorphic molecule of which provides advantage to the immune system against the diversity of microorganisms and their antigens. However, if exacerbated, it can induce the development of autoimmune diseases such as SpA [65]. There are no specific diagnostic tests for SpA; it is necessary to observe the clinical symptoms and radiographic changes in sacroiliac joints [67], such as joint pain in fingers or toes; chronic back pain, enthesitis, dactylitis, psoriasis (including psoriatic nail symptoms); and some factors risk factors like recent genitourinary infection, family history of spondyloarthritis, and family history of psoriasis [68].

The treatments recommended for SpA in adults, in addition to treatment with NSAIDs (first line), are strongly recommended treatment with TNFi, such as adalimumab, infliximab, etanercept, golimumab, and certolizumab pegol [66, 69]. Treatment with sulfasalazine and MTX is recommended primarily for patients with prominent peripheral arthritis and few or no axial symptoms [66, 69]. Secukinumab or ixekizumab, both IL-17 inhibitors, can help reduce or slow inflammation, but it is recommended only in cases of TNFi unavailability access [69].

People with ankylosing spondylitis (AS) have an increased risk of developing cancer due to the higher levels of chronic inflammation, and in addition, just like other rheumatological diseases, some medications (like biologics) used to treat AS may increase the risk of certain cancers [70]. Among various kinds of cancer, AS seems to be involved in someone such as colon cancer, esophageal cancer, liver cancer, and cancer of the stomach or small intestine, multiple myeloma (a type of blood cancer), lymphoma, and prostate cancer [70]. Nam and coworkers, in 2019, made the comparison of a general male population group, and the overall incidence of cancer was increased in male patients with AS. The authors concluded that for male AS patients were at increased risk of cancer, especially for male reproductive system and pancreatic cancer [71].

## 16.8 Scleroderma

Scleroderma is a disease characterized by fibrosis (hardening) of the skin and internal organs, involvement of small blood vessels, and formation of antibodies against the body's own structures (autoantibodies). It can be classified into two types: a) the systemic form—systemic sclerosis, and the localized form—localized scleroderma. Three primary mechanisms contribute to the development of the scleroderma: vascular anomalies, excess fibrosis, and autoimmune phenomenon.

Systemic sclerosis is a chronic autoimmune disease characterized by excess collagen synthesis, leading to fibrosis of the skin and organs, which can promote high morbidity and mortality [72]. It is widely more frequent in females than in males, affecting mainly the fourth decade of life [72–73]. Systemic sclerosis is classified into 3 subtypes, according to the extent and pattern of cutaneous involvement: limited cutaneous, diffuse cutaneous, and sine scleroderma. These subtypes are associated with clinical and laboratory manifestations and distinct natural histories [73, 74]. The events that underlie susceptibility to systemic sclerosis probably include both genetic and environmental factors, which result in microvascular dysfunction and autoimmune phenomena [75].

The management of systemic sclerosis (SSc) will be determined considering the presence and severity of any organ-based complications, since it is possible to generate various damages, such as digital vasculopathy, gastrointestinal complications, lung fibrosis, pulmonary hypertension, cardiac fibrosis, scleroderma renal crisis, digital contractures, calcinosis, and acro-osteolysis

[75]. For the treatment of scleroderma renal crisis, the angiotensin-converting enzyme inhibitors (ACEi) can be indicated, followed by adding calcium channel blockers (CCb) or the alternative use of angiotensin receptor blockers (ARb) [76, 77]. For pulmonary arterial hypertension (PAH), the endothelin receptor antagonists (ERAs) are an important part of the treatment [76, 78]. Other therapies include eculizumab associated with ACEi in refractory cases [78, 79]. For Raynaud's phenomenon (RP) treatment, can include CCb, followed by, or in addition to, prostaglandins and endothelin-1 receptor antagonists [76, 80]. For interstitial lung disease, the induction therapy can be mycophenolate mofetil (MMF), intravenous cyclophosphamide, and rituximab, respectively [76].

Considering the risk of development of cancer, registers show a number of studies indicating possible associations between SSc and breast, gastrointestinal, urogenital, lung, and hematologic malignancies [81]. Morrisroe and colleagues quantified the burden of cancer in systemic sclerosis and conclude that the patients had increased risk of developing cancer, particularly lung cancer associated with Interstitial lung disease (ILD), breast cancer, and melanoma, and observed an association of some of these phenomena with anti-RNA polymerase III antibodies [82].

The localized form of scleroderma (LoS) affects a restricted area of the skin, sparing the internal organs, being more common in children. It generally evolves in three consecutive phases: edematous, indurated, sclerotic, and then atrophic [83]. Depending on the localized scleroderma, it can be classified as morphea or linear scleroderma [84].

In terms of LoS treatment, the first line of systemic treatment is methotrexate, with mycophenolate used as a second-line treatment in cases of methotrexate nonresponse. Further studies in patients with localized scleroderma using rituximab and abatacept have been reported [85]. Fage and coworkers determined if abatacept may have a positive effect on disease activity in LoS and concluded that the abatacept may be an appropriate treatment option for treatment-resistant LoS disease of different subtypes [86]. As to the study carried out by Foeldvari and colleges, in a small cohort of LoS young patients, tocilizumab seems to be a promising rescue medication [85].

### 16.8.1 Behçet's Disease

Behçet's disease (BD) is an immune-mediated multisystem vasculitis affecting any type and size of blood vessels. The disease has been regarded as the outcome of an autoimmune process that is triggered by the same factors such as infectious process and environmental factors and genetically predisposed [87].

The BD incidence varies according to the geographical location, with the highest prevalence in Turkey, followed by Iran, Japan, northern China, and Korea. In pediatric patients, BD was defined if the disease was fully manifested and diagnosed up to the age of 16 years [88].

Considering the clinical manifestations, recurrent oral ulceration occurred in almost all patients, and the painful ulcers may appear on the lips, tongue, and palate. Eye lesions can occur, and it is common in pediatric population with BD, and vascular disease can affect all types and sizes of vessels with a predominance of venous involvement, as in adults as in pediatric BD population. Other clinical manifestation includes central nervous system disease, with development of chronic headaches; gastrointestinal involvement, with presentation of various symptoms, such as nausea, diarrhea, abdominal pain, ulceration of the ileum, cecum, and colon, melena, or hematochezia; and some symptoms of arthritis/arthralgia, with predominant effect in knees, ankles, elbows, and wrists [88].

For the treatment of the population with BD, it is recommended that the long-term use of corticosteroids is avoided and that a combination of different disease-modifying antirheumatic drugs (DMARDs), such as azathioprine, cyclophosphamide, or cyclosporine A, can be used, with the prospect of positive benefits [88], in both adult and pediatric population. Other registers demonstrated that tocilizumab was effective and can serve as an alternative treatment for refractory disease with ocular, neuro, and vascular clinical manifestation in BD, but was not recommended for patients with mucocutaneous and articular involvement [89]. Other therapeutic choices have been suggested for BD, including the interleukin (IL)-1 inhibitors (anakinra and canakinumab), TNF-α inhibitors, such as infliximab, followed by antibody anti-TNF-α, adalimumab, used as monotherapy and after the primary or secondary failure to other anti-TNF agents. Similarly, etanercept has proved to be effective in controlling almost all BD manifestations with a good safety profile. Few reports have demonstrated benefits with the use of golimumab, with better clinical results when associated with DMARDs [89, 90]. Lymphocyte-targeted therapies, such as rituximab, alemtuzumab, and daclizumab, seem to show efficacy, principally in case of BD with ocular involvement [90].

Just like other types of rheumatic disease, chronic uncontrolled inflammation and chronic infections are among the main causes of cancer development. So, Behçet's disease is also reported to be related to an increased risk of malignancy in multiple studies [87]. In a study reported by Lin and colleagues, in 2014, identified the clinical characteristics of BD associated with malignancies. In this study, about 41 of 651 patients with BD were diagnosed with some type of malignancies, between hematological and solid malignancies. The research concludes that myelodysplastic syndrome (MDS) and colorectal cancer were the most common hematologic malignancy and malignant solid neoplasm associated with BD, respectively, and the possibility of increased risk of developing malignancies in BD patients should not be neglected [91].

## 16.9 Gout

Gout is a common inflammatory arthritis associated with high serum uric acid levels of 6.8 mg/dL (404 μmol/L) [92, 93]. It is characterized by the precipitation of monosodium urate crystals in the synovial fluid of the joints, as well as in other tissues [93, 94]. The most common symptom is sudden and severe pain in the joint along with swelling redness and loss of function, with the first metatarsophalangeal, ankle, knee, and joint of the big toe being the most frequently affected [94, 95].

This disease has been addressed in four phases that include: asymptomatic hyperuricemia, ie, high serum urate levels, but no clinical symptoms; deposition of urate crystals in joints or periarticular tissues, triggered by hyperuricemia, resulting in an acute flare-up of inflammatory arthritis (acute gouty arthritis); patients with untreated gout remain hyperuricemia which can increase tissue crystal deposition (intercritical gout); and after long-term joint inflammation occurs complications such presence of tophi, bone/joint damage, and pain, associated with joint pain at rest and/or on movement (chronic tophaceous gout) [96, 97].

The management of gout has been based on nonpharmacological and pharmacological therapy. Nonpharmacological therapy includes patient education, dietary recommendations, and resting of the joint. One approach to gout treatment is patient education. Lifestyle modification is very important, so gout patients should avoid overweight, soft drinks and drinks containing fructose, reduce alcohol consumption, and decrease the intake of high purine food contents such as meat, ofal, crustaceans, and yeast. Hyperuricemia is more common with current lifestyle trends. Gout patient should introduce physical activity since they are at increased risk of cardiovascular disease and diabetes mellitus [95, 97].

Pharmacological therapy is aimed at anti-inflammatory therapy as the first-line treatment option, using nonsteroidal anti-inflammatory drugs (NSAIDs), glucocorticoids, and colchicine. The decision of which of the 3 substance groups to use depends on the patient's comorbidities. Engel et al. (2017) described an overview of treatment options. In addition, according to a Cochrane review, interleukin-1 antagonists (canakinumab SC) can be considered as an alternative option if all 3 standard treatment options are contraindicated or not tolerated [97]. According to the 2017 guidelines of the British Society of Rheumatology and British Health Professional in Rheumatology, allopurinol, which is a xanthine oxidase inhibitor, should be prescribed for all patients without waiting for any complications or recurrent gout attacks [95].

Gout flares are driven by uptake of deposited monosodium urate crystals by macrophages and subsequent release of inflammatory mediators such as interleukin-1, cytokines, prostaglandins, and chemokines, which lead to infiltration of neutrophils and monocytes and subsequent amplification of joint inflammation. A prompt interruption of this auto-inflammatory process is needed to achieve control of symptoms, which is the main goal in the management of gout flares [98].

Gout is associated with an excess of mortality, mainly due to cardiovascular causes, but also by renal disease, diseases of the digestive system, and infections, with a lower probability of dementia [99].

To date, studies in the available literature have reported conflicting data regarding the association between gout and cancer. Here, we list some research about that association.

Veljkovi'c et al. (2020) reported the relation in xanthine oxidase/dehydrogenase activity as a source of oxidative stress in prostate cancer tissue [99]. Huang and colleagues (2020) related high levels of serum uric acid (SUA) can be a risk factor for pancreatic cancer in women and gallbladder cancer in men [100]. Uric acid may be an important risk factor for cancer when humans develop a high concentration of high uric acid serum level. Hyperuricemia may also contribute to the metastasis of some cancers [101]. Oh al (2021) investigated the association between gout and cancer risk in a retrospective cohort study using the Korean National Health Insurance Service Database related to a significantly high risk of cancer [102]. Their findings indicated that esophageal, stomach, colon, liver, pancreatic, lung, ovarian, renal, and bladder cancers were higher in Korean gout patients.

Oxidative stress, which is a hallmark of cancer, seems to be involved in a relationship with hyperuricemia. All papers point to antioxidant and pro-oxidant activities of uric acid. These dual papers can be beneficial as protective against neurodegenerative diseases, such as Parkinson's disease, Alzheimer's disease, and amyotrophic lateral sclerosis. In contrast, acid uric can contribute to the free radical formation, resulting in oxidative cell damage, low-grade inflammation, insulin resistance, and negative cardiovascular effects. Although the high uric acid is associated with a high incidence of cancer, more research is needed to confirm their findings.

## References


1. Khan WA. Introductory chapter: introduction to rheumatology. In: Newest updates in rheumatology. London: InTech; 2018.
2. Almoallim H, Abdulaziz S, Fallatah E, Alhazmi H, Meraiani N, Bazuhair T, et al. Clinical characteristics and outcomes of cancer patients with post-chemotherapy arthritis: a retrospective case series report. Open Access Rheumatol Res Rev. 2017;9:111–6.
3. Jayashree S, Nirekshana K, Guha G, Bhakta-Guha D. Cancer chemotherapeutics in rheumatoid arthritis: a convoluted connection. Biomed Pharmacother. Elsevier Masson SASs. 2018;102:894–911.
4. Elandt K, Aletaha D. Treating rheumatic patients with a malignancy. Arthritis Res Ther [Internet]. 2011;13(3):223. Available from: http://arthritis-research.biomedcentral.com/articles/10.1186/ar3352
5. Vaillant AAJ, Goyal A, Bansal P, Varacallo M. Systemic lupus erythematosus. In: StatPearls [Internet]. Treasure Island (FL): StatPearls Publishing [Internet]; 2021. [cited 2021 Aug 25]. Available from: https://pubmed.ncbi.nlm.nih.gov/30571026/.
6. Pan L, Lu MP, Wang JH, Xu M, Yang SR. Immunological pathogenesis and treatment of systemic lupus erythematosus. Vol. 16. World J Pediatr. 2020;16:19–30. Institute of Pediatrics of Zhejiang University.
7. Fava A, Petri M. Systemic lupus erythematosus: diagnosis and clinical management. J Autoimmunity. 2019. 96 p. 1–13. Academic Press
8. Barber MRW, Drenkard C, Falasinnu T, Hoi A, Mak A, Kow NY, et al. Global epidemiology of systemic lupus erythematosus. Nat Rev Rheumatol [Internet]. 2021;17(9):515–32. Available from: https://www.nature.com/articles/s41584-021-00668-1
9. Fanouriakis A, Tziolos N, Bertsias G, Boumpas DT. Update in the diagnosis and management of systemic lupus erythematosus. Ann Rheum Dis. BMJ Publishing Group. 2021;80:14–25.
10. Ichikawa S, Fukuhara N, Shirai T, Ishii T, Ichinohasama R, Harigae H. Extranasal extranodal NK/T-cell lymphoma associated with systemic lupus erythematosus. Int J Hematol. 2020;112(4):592–6.
11. Elliott RW, Essenhigh DM, Morley AR. Cyclophosphamide treatment of systemic lupus erythematosus: risk of bladder cancer exceeds benefit. BMJ. 1982;284(6323):1160.

12. Travis LB, He He R, Curtis E, Glimelius B, Holowaty EJ, Van Leeuwen FE, et al. Bladder and kidney cancer following cyclophosphamide therapy for non-hodgkin's lymphoma [Internet]. Available from: http://jnci.oxfordjournals.org/.
13. Dasgupta N, Gelber AC, Racke F, Fine DM. Central nervous system lymphoma associated with mycophenolate mofetil in lupus nephritis. Lupus. 2005;14(11):910–3.
14. Balci MA, Pamuk GE, Unlu E, Usta U, Pamuk ON. Development of primary central nervous system lymphoma in a systemic lupus erythematosus patient after treatment with mycophenolate mofetil and review of the literature. Lupus. 2017;26(11):1224–7.
15. Tsang H, Trendell-Smith N, Wu A, Mok M. Diffuse large B-cell lymphoma of the central nervous system in mycophenolate mofetil-treated patients with systemic lupus erythematosus. Lupus. 2010;19(3):330.
16. Svobodova B, Hruskova Z, Rysava R, Tesar V. Brain diffuse large B-cell lymphoma in a systemic lupus erythematosus patient treated with immunosuppressive agents including mycophenolate mofetil. Lupus. 2011;20:1452–4.
17. Sliesoraitis S, Khan R, Rothman J. Methotrexate-induced Hodgkin disease in a patient with systemic lupus erythematosus. J Osteopath Med. 2009;109(6):325–8.
18. Berliner S, Shoenfeld Y, Sidi Y, Santo M, Weinberger A, Luria D, et al. Systemic lupus erythematosus and lymphoma a family study. Scand J Rheumatology. 1983;12:310–4.
19. Nemoto I, Sato-Matsumura KC, Fujita Y, Natsuga K, Ujiie H, Tomita Y, et al. Leukaemic dissemination of Merkel cell carcinoma in a patient with systemic lupus erythematosus. Clin Exp Dermatol. 2008;33(3):270–2.
20. Wadström H, Arkema EV, Sjöwall C, Askling J, Simard JF. Cervical neoplasia in systemic lupus erythematosus: a nationwide study. Rheumatol (United Kingdom). 2017;56(4):613–9.
21. Knight JS, Blayney DW, Somers EC. Patients with systemic lupus erythematosus and haematological malignancy at a tertiary care centre: timing, histopathology and therapy. Lupus Sci Med [Internet]. 2014;1:51. Available from: http://lupus.bmj.com/
22. Yang B, Zhao M, Wu H, Lu Q. A comprehensive review of biological agents for lupus: beyond single target. Front Immunol. 11: 539797. 2020. Frontiers Media S.A.
23. Mavragani CP, Moutsopoulos HM. Sjögren syndrome. CMAJ. 2014;186:E579–86. Canadian Medical Association
24. Valim V, Trevisani VFM, Pasoto SG, Serrano EV, Euzébio Ribeiro SL, de Alencar Fidelix TS, et al. Recommendations for the treatment of Sjögren's syndrome. Revista Brasileira de Reumatologia. 2015;55:446–57. Elsevier Editora Ltda.

25. Stefanski AL, Tomiak C, Pleyer U, Dietrich T, Burmester GR, Dörner T. The diagnosis and treatment of Sjögren's syndrome. Dtsch Arztebl Int. 2017;114(20):354.
26. Parisis D, Chivasso C, Perret J, Soyfoo MS, Delporte C. Current state of knowledge on primary Sjögren's syndrome, an autoimmune exocrinopathy. J Clin Med. 2020;9(7):2299.
27. Łysik D, Niemirowicz-Laskowska K, Bucki R, Tokajuk G, Mystkowska J. Artificial saliva: challenges and future perspectives for the treatment of xerostomia. Int J Mol Sci MDPI AG. 2019;20:3199.
28. Mariette X, Criswell LA. Primary sjögren's syndrome. Solomon CG, editor. N Engl J Med [Internet]. 2018;378(10):931–9. Available from: http://www.nejm.org/doi/10.1056/NEJMcp1702514.
29. Ghosn J, Vicino A, Michielin O, Coukos G, Kuntzer T, Obeid M. A severe case of neuro-Sjögren's syndrome induced by pembrolizumab. J Immunother Cancer. 2018;6(1):110.
30. Higashi T, Miyamoto H, Yoshida R, Furuta Y, Nagaoka K, Naoe H, et al. Sjögren's syndrome as an immune-related adverse event of nivolumab treatment for gastric cancer. Intern Med. 2020;59(20):2499–504.
31. Ogdie A, Coates LC, Gladman DD. Treatment guidelines in psoriatic arthritis. Rheumatol. 2021;59:I37–46.
32. Singh JA, Guyatt G, Ogdie A, Gladman DD, Deal C, Deodhar A, et al. Special article: 2018 American College of Rheumatology/National Psoriasis Foundation Guideline for the Treatment of Psoriatic Arthritis. Arthritis Rheumatol. 2019;71(1):5–32.
33. Coates LC, Helliwell PS. CMJv17n1-CME_Helliwell.indd [Internet]. Clin Med. 2017;17. Available from: www.bad.org.
34. Ritchlin CT, Colbert RA, Gladman DD. Psoriatic arthritis. Longo DL, editor. N Engl J Med [Internet]. 2017;376(10):957–70. Available from: http://www.nejm.org/doi/10.1056/NEJMra1505557.
35. Karmacharya P, Shahukhal R, Ogdie A. Risk of malignancy in spondyloarthritis: a systematic review. Rheum Dis Clin N Am. 2020;46:463–511. W.B. Saunders.
36. Law-Ping-Man S, Martin A, Briens E, Tisseau L, Safa G. Psoriasis and psoriatic arthritis induced by nivolumab in a patient with advanced lung cancer. Rheumatol. 2016;55(11):2087–9.
37. Ruiz-Bañobre J, Pérez-Pampín E, García-González J, Gómez-Caamaño A, Barón-Duarte FJ, López-López R, et al. Development of psoriatic arthritis during nivolumab therapy for metastatic non-small cell lung cancer, clinical outcome analysis and review of the literature. Lung Cancer. 2017;108:217–21.
38. Maz M, Chung SA, Abril A, Langford CA, Gorelik M, Guyatt G, et al. 2021 American College of Rheumatology/Vasculitis Foundation Guideline for the management of giant cell arteritis and takayasu arteritis. Arthritis Care Res. 2021;73(8):1071–87.

39. Russo RAG, Katsicas MM. Takayasu arteritis. Vol. 6, Frontiers in pediatrics. Lausanne: Frontiers Media S.A.; 2018.
40. Lim RW, Yann M, Khung KS, Narendra YK, et al. Takayasu's arteritis: a review of the literature and the role of endovascular treatment. Asia Intervention. 2018;4:117–25.
41. Hrisrova D, Marchev S. Takayasu arteritis - a systematic review. Acta Medica Bulgarica. 2019;46:56–64.
42. Agueda AF, Monti S, Luqmani RA, Buttgereit F, Cid M, Dasgupta B, et al. Management of Takayasu arteritis: a systematic literature review informing the 2018 update of the EULAR recommendation for the management of large vessel vasculitis. RMD Open. 2019;5(2):e001020.
43. Park JK, Choi IA, Lee EY, Song YW, Lee EB. Incidence of malignancy in Takayasu arteritis in Korea. Rheumatol Int. 2014;34(4):517–21.
44. Karami J, Aslani S, Jamshidi A, Garshasbi M, Mahmoudi M. Genetic implications in the pathogenesis of rheumatoid arthritis; an updated review. Gene. 2019;702:8–16.
45. Guo Q, Wang Y, Xu D, Nossent J, Pavlos NJ, Xu J. Rheumatoid arthritis: pathological mechanisms and modern pharmacologic therapies. Bone Res. 2018;6:15.
46. Almutairi K, Nossent J, Preen D, Keen H, Inderjeeth C. The global prevalence of rheumatoid arthritis: a meta-analysis based on a systematic review. Rheumatol Int. 2021;41(5):863–77.
47. Silman Alan J, Pearson JE. Epidemiology and genetics of rheumatoid arthritis. Arthritis Res. 2002;4 Suppl 3:S265.
48. Liao KP, Alfredsson L, Karlson EW. Environmental influences on risk for rheumatoid arthritis. Curr Opinion Rheumatol. 2009;21:279–83.
49. Stahl EA, Raychaudhuri S, Remmers EF, Xie G, Eyre S, Thomson BP, et al. Genome-wide association study meta-analysis identifies seven new rheumatoid arthritis risk loci. Nat Genet. 2010;42(6):508–14.
50. Van Drongelen V, Holoshitz J. A reciprocal HLA-disease association in rheumatoid arthritis and pemphigus vulgaris. 2018.
51. Gazitt T, Lood C, Elkon KB. Citrullination in rheumatoid arthritis—a process promoted by neutrophil lysis? Rambam Maimonides Med J. 2016;7(4):e0027.
52. Benjamin O, Bansal P, Goyal A, Lappin SL. Disease modifying anti-rheumatic drugs (DMARD). In 2018 [cited 2021 Aug 24]. Available from: https://europepmc.org/article/NBK/nbk507863#free-full-text.
53. Brown PM, Pratt AG, Isaacs JD. Mechanism of action of methotrexate in rheumatoid arthritis, and the search for biomarkers. Nat Rev Rheumatol. 2016;12(12):731.
54. Brummaier T, Pohanka E, Studnicka-Benke A, Pieringer H. Using cyclophosphamide in inflammatory rheumatic diseases. Eur J Intern Med. 2013;24(7):590.

55. Mease PJ. Adalimumab in the treatment of arthritis. Thera Clin Risk Manag. 2007;3:133–48.
56. Cohen MD, Keystone E. Rituximab for rheumatoid arthritis. Rheumatol Ther. 2015;2(2):99–111.
57. Wilton KM, Matteson EL. Malignancy incidence, management, and prevention in patients with rheumatoid arthritis. Rheumatol Ther. 2017;4(2):333–47.
58. Bernatsky S, Clarke AE, Suissa S. Hematologic malignant neoplasms after drug exposure in rheumatoid arthritis [Internet]. 2008. Available from: http://archinte.jamanetwork.com/.
59. Asten P, Barrett J, Symmons D. Risk of developing certain malignancies is related to duration of immunosuppressive drug exposure in patients with rheumatic diseases. J Rheumatol [Internet]. 1999;26(8):1705–14. Available from: https://pubmed.ncbi.nlm.nih.gov/10451066/.
60. Maneiro JR, Souto A, Gomez-Reino JJ. Risks of malignancies related to tofacitinib and biological drugs in rheumatoid arthritis: systematic review, meta-analysis, and network meta-analysis. Semin Arthritis Rheum. 2017;47(2):149–56.
61. Kitazaki T, Oka M, Nakamura Y, Tsurutani J, Doi S, Yasunaga M, et al. Gefitinib, an EGFR tyrosine kinase inhibitor, directly inhibits the function of P-glycoprotein in multidrug resistant cancer cells. Lung Cancer. 2005;49(3):337–43.
62. Ohara G, Satoh H, Kohno M, Goto D, Sumida T, Hizawa N. Development of rheumatoid arthritis during the course of gefitinib therapy. Sao Paulo Med J. 2009;127:177–8.
63. Ohtsuka T. Sunitinib-induced hand-foot syndrome in a renal cell carcinoma: a sclerodermatous and rheumatoid arthritis-like case. J Dermatol. 2012;39:943–4.
64. Yau TC, Chu KW, Mok MY, Liang RH, Epstein RJ. Acute presentation of rheumatoid arthritis following cancer chemotherapy using the topoisomerase I inhibitor irinotecan [3]. Acta Oncologica. 2005;44:771–2.
65. Sharip A, Kunz J. Understanding the pathogenesis of spondyloarthritis. Biomolecules. 2020;10:1–20.
66. Sieper J, Poddubnyy D. Axial spondyloarthritis. The Lancet. 2017;390:73–84.
67. Ramdin D, Moorthy A, Rennie WJ. Classification terminology and definitions in reporting of MRI in axial spondyloarthritis. J Belgian Soc Radiol. 2017;101:11.
68. Van Tubergen A, Weber U. Diagnosis and classification in spondyloarthritis: Identifying a chameleon. Nat Rev Rheumatol. 2012;8:253–61.
69. Ward MM, Deodhar A, Gensler LS, Dubreuil M, Yu D, Khan MA, et al. 2019 update of the American College of Rheumatology/Spondylitis Association of America/Spondyloarthritis Research and Treatment

Network recommendations for the treatment of ankylosing spondylitis and nonradiographic axial spondyloarthritis. Arthritis Rheumatol. 2019;71(10):1599–613.
70. Chang C-C, Chang C-W, Nguyen P-AA, Chang T-H, Shih Y-L, Chang W-Y, et al. Ankylosing spondylitis and the risk of cancer. Oncol Lett. 2017;14(2):1315.
71. Nam B, Kim H, Jang EJ, Cho SK, Sung YK, Kim TH. Malignancy risk in Korean male patients with ankylosing spondylitis. Rheumatol Int. 2019;39(10):1741–8.
72. da Silva AM, Roque LCSC, Gonçalves RSG, Duarte ALBP, da Tenório A, S, Dantas AT. Evaluation of quality of life, functionality and disability in patients with systemic sclerosis in a University Hospital. ABCS Heal Sci. 2020;45:e020025.
73. Sticherling M. Systemic sclerosis - dermatological aspects. Part 1: pathogenesis, epidemiology, clinical findings. JDDG J Ger Soc Dermatol. 2012;10(10):705–16.
74. Varga J, Abraham D. Systemic sclerosis: a prototypic multisystem fibrotic disorder. J Clin Investigation. 2007;117:557–67.
75. Denton CP, Khanna D. Systemic sclerosis. The Lancet. 2017;390:1685–99.
76. Fernández-Codina A, Walker KM, Pope JE. Treatment algorithms for systemic sclerosis according to experts. Arthritis Rheumatol. 2018;70(11):1820–8.
77. Bütikofer L, Varisco PA, Distler O, Kowal-Bielecka O, Allanore Y, Riemekasten G, et al. ACE inhibitors in SSc patients display a risk factor for scleroderma renal crisis - A EUSTAR analysis. Arthritis Res Ther. 2020;22(1):59.
78. Nagaraja V. Management of scleroderma renal crisis. Curr Opinion Rheumatol. 2019;31:223–30.
79. Devresse A, Aydin S, Le Quintrec M, Demoulin N, Stordeur P, Lambert C, et al. Complement activation and effect of eculizumab in scleroderma renal crisis. Medicine. 2016;95(30):e4459.
80. Belch J, Carlizza A, Carpentier PH, Constans J, Khan F, Wautrecht JC, et al. ESVM guidelines – the diagnosis and management of Raynaud's phenomenon. Vasa Eur J Vasc Med. 2017;46:413–23.
81. Abu-Shakra M, Guillemin F, Lee P. Cancer In systemic sclerosis.
82. Morrisroe K, Hansen D, Huq M, Stevens W, Sahhar J, Ngian GS, et al. Incidence, risk factors, and outcomes of cancer in systemic sclerosis. Arthritis Care Res. 2020;72(11):1625–35.
83. Careta MF, Romiti R. Localized scleroderma: clinical spectrum and therapeutic update. An Bras Dermatol. 2015;90(1):62–73.
84. Venturi M, Pinna AL, Pilloni L, Atzori L, Ferreli C, Rongioletti F. Bullous morphoea: a retrospective study. Clin Exp Dermatol. 2017;42(5):532–5.

85. Foeldvari I, Anton J, Friswell M, Bica B, de Inocencio J, Aquilani A, et al. Tocilizumab is a promising treatment option for therapy resistant juvenile localized scleroderma patients. J Scleroderma Relat Disord. 2017;2(3):203.
86. Fage S, Arvesen K, Olesen A. Abatacept improves skin-score and reduces lesions in patients with localized scleroderma: a case series. Acta Derm Venereol. 2018;98(4):465.
87. Guven DC, Bolek EC, Altintop SE, Celikten B, Aktas BY, Kiraz S, et al. Cancer incidence in Behçet's disease. Ir J Med Sci. 1971;189(4):1209.
88. Hu Y-C, Chiang B-L, Yang Y-H. Clinical manifestations and management of pediatric behçet's disease. Clin Rev Allergy Immunol. 2021;61(2):171.
89. Akiyama M, Kaneko Y, Takeuchi T. Effectiveness of tocilizumab in Behcet's disease: a systematic literature review. Semin Arthritis Rheum. 2020;50(4):797.
90. Bulur I, Onder M. Behçet disease: new aspects. Clin Dermatol. 2017;35(5):421.
91. Lin Y, Li G, Zheng W, Tian X, Zhang F. Behcet's disease associated with malignancy: a report of 41 Chinese cases [Internet]. 2013. Available from: http://www.behcet.ws/pdf/BehcetsDiseaseActivi-.
92. Vora B, Brackman DJ, Zou L, Garcia-Cremades M, Sirota M, Savic RM, et al. Oxypurinol pharmacokinetics and pharmacodynamics in healthy volunteers: influence of BCRP Q141K polymorphism and patient characteristics. Clin Transl Sci. 2021;14(4):1431.
93. Gaviria JL, Ortega VG, Gaona J, Motta A, Medina Barragán OJ. Unusual dermatological manifestations of gout. Plast Reconstr Surg Glob Open. 2015;3(7):e445.
94. Shiozawa A, Szabo SM, Bolzani A, Cheung A, Choi HK. Serum uric acid and the risk of incident and recurrent gout: a systematic review. J Rheumatol. 2017;44(3):388.
95. Alghamdi AA, Mutlaqah MA, Labani AMH, Alahmadi LMA, Alahmari AF, Albalawi RA, et al. Gout management in primary care approach; literature review. Int J Pharm Res Allied Sci. 2021;10(1):19–23.
96. Dalbeth N, Stamp L. Hyperuricaemia and gout: time for a new staging system? Ann Rheum Dis. 2014;73(9):1598.
97. Engel B, Just J, Bleckwenn M, Weckbecker K. Treatment Options for Gout. Dtsch Aerzteblatt Online. 2017 Mar 31.
98. Paré G, Vitry J, Marceau F, Vaillancourt M, Winter P, Bachelard H, et al. The development of a targeted and more potent, anti-inflammatory derivative of colchicine: implications for gout. Biochem Pharmacol. 2020;180:114125.
99. Punzi L, Scanu A, Galozzi P, Luisetto R, Spinella P, Scirè CA, et al. One year in review 2020: gout. Clin Exp Rheumatol. 2020;38(5):807–21.

100. Huang C-F, Huang J-J, Mi N-N, Lin Y-Y, He Q-S, Lu Y-W, et al. Associations between serum uric acid and hepatobiliary-pancreatic cancer: a cohort study. World J Gastroenterol. 2020;26(44):7061.
101. Mi S, Gong L, Sui Z. Friend or Foe? an unrecognized role of uric acid in cancer development and the potential anticancer effects of uric acid-lowering drugs. J Cancer. 2020;11(17):5236–44.
102. Oh Y-J, Lee YJ, Lee E, Park B, Kwon J-W, Heo J, et al. Cancer risk in Korean patients with gout. Korean J Intern Med. 2020.

# Index






C. W. P. Schmidt, K. M. Otoni (eds.), *The Golden Guide to Oncologic Pharmacy*, https://doi.org/10.1007/978-3-030-98596-7

GPSR Compliance

*The European Union's (EU) General Product Safety Regulation (GPSR) is a set of rules that requires consumer products to be safe and our obligations to ensure this.*

*If you have any concerns about our products, you can contact us on ProductSafety@springernature.com*

In case Publisher is established outside the EU, the EU authorized representative is:

Springer Nature Customer Service Center GmbH
Europaplatz 3
69115 Heidelberg, Germany

**Batch number: 10732632**

Printed by Printforce, the Netherlands